Clinical Pharmacology in Dentistry

Clinical Pharmacology in Dentistry

R. A. Cawson
MD (Lond.), BDS, FDS RCPS Glasg., FRC Path.

Emeritus Professor of Oral Medicine and Pathology in the University of London,
Guy's Campus, United Medical Schools, London, UK;
Visiting Professor, Baylor University Medical Center and Dental College,
Dallas, Texas, USA

R. G. Spector
MD, PhD, FRCP, FRC Path.

Professor of Applied Pharmacology,
Guy's Campus, United Medical Schools, London, UK

FIFTH EDITION

CHURCHILL LIVINGSTONE
EDINBURGH LONDON MELBOURNE AND NEW YORK 1989

CHURCHILL LIVINGSTONE
Medical Division of Longman Group UK Limited

Distributed in the United States of America by Churchill
Livingstone Inc., 1560 Broadway, New York, N.Y. 10036, and
by associated companies, branches and representatives
throughout the world.

First edition 1975
Second edition 1978
Third edition 1982
Fourth edition 1985
    Reprinted 1987
Fifth edition 1989
    Reprinted 1990

ISBN 0-443-04043-5

British Library Cataloguing in Publication Data
    Cawson, R.A. (Roderick Anthony)
    Clinical pharmacology in dentistry. — 5th ed.
    1. Pharmacology, — For dentistry
    I. Title II. Spector, R.G. (Roy Geoffrey)
    615'.1'0246176

Library of Congress Cataloguing in Publication Data
    Cawson, R.A.
    Clinical pharmacology in dentistry/R.A. Cawson, R.G.
Spector. — 5th ed.
    p.   cm.
    Includes bibliographies and index.
    ISBN 0-443-04043-5
    1. Dental pharmacology. 2. Pharmacology.
    I. Spector, R. G. (Roy Geoffrey) II. Title.
    [DNLM: 1. Dentistry. 2. Pharmacology, Clinical. QV 50
C383c]
    RK701.C33 1989
    615'.1'0246176--dc19
    DNLM/DLC
    for Library of Congress
    89-571 CIP

Produced by Longman Singapore Publishers (Pte) Ltd
Printed in Singapore

Preface

The teaching of pharmacology and therapeutics to dental students is a subject which provokes strong feelings among those who have anything to do with it, and even more among those who do not.

It is true that the subject arouses among many – often those who should be most concerned – a violent upsurge of apathy. But it would be fair to suggest of the remainder that there are those at one extreme who regard pharmacology as hardly more relevant to dentistry than, and at least as pretentious as (say), Middle Period Etruscan Studies. At the other extreme there seems to be the belief that the dental student should have a detailed knowledge of the intricacies of actions and interactions of a remarkable number of drugs. It is even possible that there are extremists who believe that the level of knowledge of pharmacology might be at least comparable to that of dental materials. This comparison is perhaps not so bizarre when it is remembered that 'Materials Science' also deals with substances which are used on patients but, unlike drugs, these materials have, or should have, little effect on his health or life.

Some mischief-makers have even suggested that pharmacology and therapeutics are unpopular with students (and some teachers) because, unlike most of the rest of the clinical dental curriculum, they are mildly intellectually demanding. This is a frightening thought. Nevertheless, the dental student has had a broadly based scientific education at least until the start of his clinical years. It seems a pity if this has to go entirely to waste in the all too successful conversion of the dental student into a high-grade technician.

It would be rash indeed to suggest that this book could by any stretch of the imagination provide a compromise acceptable to such deeply entrenched and widely separated forces. If, however, there is any academic dentist (or dental academic) who believes that pharmacology is a subject from which his students should be protected, he forgets that he himself practises the niceties of his craft in an unusually sheltered environment. He shuts his mind to the fact that when anything goes wrong – if, for instance, the patient is tactless enough to have a heart attack – the experts are called in and the matter is dealt with. The student who happens to see such events does not perhaps appreciate that, once qualified and in practice, he is quite on his own and in a very much more vulnerable position.

The general dental practitioner is giving – not prescribing, but giving – drugs, particularly local or general anaesthetics, on a far greater scale than his medical colleague. As it happens, the pharmacology of these groups of agents is far from simple, and if they are to be used safely and intelligently some understanding of basic pharmacology has somehow to be acquired.

The dental surgeon can also prescribe (even within the confines of the National Health Service) nearly a dozen different groups of drugs in well over a hundred different preparations. Added to all this, a quite remarkably high proportion of his patients are already taking drugs for medical purposes. Either these drugs or the disease for which they are given can, now and then, make some dental procedures distinctly hazardous.

As a consequence dental practitioners have – if the demand for postgraduate courses is any guide – a lively interest in this subject. It is hoped, therefore, that this book may also be of help to those already in practice.

Some attempt has to be made to reconcile the predominantly technical nature of the dentist's training with these medical problems he has to assess and manage.

As far as possible, a clinical approach to the subject has been adopted as being more relevant to dental practice and to relate the subject matter to the medicine and surgery courses.

The writing of this book has had, inevitably, to be based on several assumptions.

First, some basic knowledge of pharmacology is necessary to use the drugs relevant to dentistry to best advantage and to protect the patient.

Second, a somewhat wider (but not detailed) knowledge of drugs is needed to understand both how these drugs act and how some of the reactions or interactions can develop.

Third, a rather more detailed knowledge of a few drugs is needed to deal with the various emergencies – uncommon though they may be – that can happen in the dental surgery.

Fourth, it is, to say the least, useful to have some understanding of the nature of the threats which hover over the dental patient under medical treatment.

Finally, it would be pleasant to think that a few dental students might even become interested in pharmacology and its clinical applications. It is, unlike dentistry, one of the areas of advance which in the past 50 years has made most impact on the physical and, perhaps, the mental welfare of the world. If nothing else is certain, there is little doubt that the dentist and the doctor too – unless quite exceptionally lucky – will sooner or later be a recipient of some of these over-numerous drugs.

Somehow, arbitrary decisions have to be made as to how much of this admittedly vast and sometimes difficult subject can be covered adequately but without suffocating detail. Drugs used in dental practice should presumably be considered more extensively than those which affect dentistry more peripherally, and some sort of balance has to be struck between these different requirements.

Since a brave attempt has been made to keep the text as short as possible, some suggestions have been made as to further reading. This is so rapidly advancing a subject that the choice has been restricted mainly to recent review articles and a few others which seem to be of particular relevance.

No doubt this book will turn out to be both too long *and* too short (according to whoever reads it), so that the treatment of the different types of subject matter is hopelessly unbalanced and that the proposals for additional reading are wildly capricious.

No doubt, too, the title is ill-chosen and some of the facts are wrong. But sad though it may be, this is the best that we can do.

Alas, things do not get easier for the reader, as pharmacology and therapeutics have an unfortunate tendency to advance. New editions of the British National Formulary appear every 6 months and the latest edition at the time of writing had 50 new preparations added. Only a few of these, of course, are major new drugs and, as a result of clinical experience, many other drugs are discarded.

Change is nevertheless forced upon us and there have been more than enough changes in this field to make another edition necessary.

London, 1989   R. A. C.
                                                R. G. S.

Acknowledgements

We would like to express our grateful appreciation to Professor Frank Ashley, Dr Richard Palmer, Professor Crispian Scully and Miss Meg Skelly for their invaluable comments, and to Mr Sidney Luck for his unstinting help with the references.

R. A. C.
R. G. S.

Contents

1. Drugs: administration, absorption and fate

A drug is any substance used for the treatment or diagnosis of disease, or to modify a physiological process. Obviously enough, penicillin given for an infection is a drug, but occasionally the category of some substances is more difficult to decide. A soap used for the usual hygienic or cosmetic reasons is obviously not a drug, but a soap could be a drug if used to treat a skin disease such as acne vulgaris. More difficult still is the status of vitamins: these are foods, present in a normal diet; but in a disease such as pernicious anaemia, vitamin B_{12} has to be administered as a drug since it cannot be absorbed from food.

Originally, all drugs were crude plant, animal or mineral substances, but currently used drugs are highly purified or even entirely synthetic products built up from relatively simple chemical precursors. Aspirin and ephedrine, for example, were originally plant derivatives, but are now synthesized de novo. Nevertheless, many drugs are still extracted from plants, microorganisms or tissues: examples are digoxin, antibiotics and many hormones.

For many patients the term 'drug' conveys unjustifiable overtones of addiction and it is usually better to use the term 'medicine' under such circumstances.

DRUG ACTION

Pharmacokinetics. The way in which drugs are handled in the body is of great clinical importance. The study of the time-course of the absorption, distribution, metabolism and excretion of drugs is the definition of pharmacokinetics. In other words, pharmacokinetics is what the body does to drugs. Although this term may be a discouraging one,

dental surgeons (like Molière's M. Jourdain, who was surprised to learn that he was speaking prose) are unconsciously using their knowledge of pharmacokinetics in the everyday practice of their specialty.

To give a simple example, nitrous oxide is useful for sedation or anaesthesia because, as a gas, it is almost instantaneously absorbed through the lungs into the bloodstream and then acts on receptors in the brain with great rapidity. Since this drug is very little metabolised, it is equally quickly excreted from the lungs and if administration stops, the patient wakes. This is one of the great advantages of nitrous oxide.

By contrast, diazepam, which is also used for sedation, has to be given by injection to get a reliably rapid effect. It affects brain receptors almost as rapidly as nitrous oxide but remains active for very much longer because it has to be metabolised in the liver. Patients require at least an hour to awake but since (among other factors) some of the intermediate metabolites of the drug are also active, take very much longer to recover completely and have to be managed accordingly. Even in a normal person it may be several days before all traces of diazepam metabolites are finally excreted. Further, if the patient has liver disease, recovery may be even more greatly delayed or the dose may have to be reduced.

Local anaesthetics, used many times every day in dental surgery, are an example of the way in which the pharmacokinetics of a drug can be modified. To render lignocaine (the most commonly used local anaesthetic) ionisable and soluble for injection it has to be given as the hydrochloride. To achieve a high tissue concentration the local anaesthetic is injected into close proximity to the nerve, where it

1

penetrates the axonal membrane to block sensory transmission. However, lignocaine is also rapidly absorbed into the blood, carried to the liver and quickly metabolised by amidases. The half-life of lignocaine, once it has entered the circulation, is therefore only a few minutes, although neural transmission recovers rather more slowly. To get a useful duration of analgesia therefore, local is-chaemia is induced by adding a vasoconstrictor (adrenaline) to the solution. Lignocaine is thus held captive in the area and, unaffected by liver en-zymes, maintains its activity often for 2 hours or longer.

Receptor sites

One of the striking features of many drugs is that they can act at remarkably low concentrations and often are so diluted by body fluids that only a few molecules are available to act on each cell. Even so the drug's effect can be profound and widespread. These considerations make it unlikely that the whole cell forms the target of drug action but suggest that there are highly sensitive sites in each cell on which the drug acts. These sites are termed *drug receptors*, and they are specific for different drugs. If the specific receptor is present and a drug binds to it, the receptor becomes changed and stimulates the cell as a whole to produce an observable result. By contrast, cells which lack receptors for a particular drug will not respond to it.

Even minor alterations in the structure of a drug can produce large changes in its effects. Its actions may be enhanced, or abolished or its selectivity changed with the result that its action is enhanced on one organ but diminished on another. An example is the modification of isoprenaline to produce salbutamol.

Isoprenaline relaxes bronchial smooth muscle and also stimulates the rate of heartbeat. Salbuta-mol by contrast relaxes bronchial muscle but has little effect on heart rate. This suggests that iso-prenaline receptors in the bronchi are different from those in the heart – the bronchial receptors can also be stimulated by salbutamol, whilst those in the heart pacemaker are little affected.

The following formulae illustrate the fact that an apparently trivial structural change results in a major difference in effect.

ISOPRENALINE   SALBUTAMOL

Competitive inhibition and receptor blocking drugs

Some drugs can bind to specific receptors but do not necessarily stimulate the cell. Therefore if such a drug and a related agent, which both bind to the same receptor, are given at the same time, they compete for that receptor. The higher the concen-tration of the competitor, the more completely it binds to the receptor and blocks the action of the original drug.

Antihistamines are commonly used drugs, which make use of this principle of *competitive inhibition* to block some of the actions of histamine in allergic diseases. Histamine however stimulates two differ-ent types of receptor, namely H_1 and H_2. Stimu-lation of H_1 receptors causes increased capillary permeability and relaxation of smooth muscle in some organs. An H_1 antihistamine such as chlor-pheniramine blocks these actions of histamine by binding to the receptors on capillary endothelium and smooth muscle and by so doing may lessen the effects of minor allergies.

The H_2 actions of histamine, by contrast, are on receptors on gastric parietal cells to stimulate gastric acid secretion. To prevent this effect a quite different type of antihistamine, an H_2-receptor blocker such as cimetidine, has to be used and is effective in the treatment of peptic ulcer.

Because of this mode of action, antihistamines are *receptor blockers* but other drugs can be used to antagonise the actions of histamine (to continue with the same example) by quite different means as discussed in later chapters.

Species specificity

A final example of some of the many diverse properties of drugs is that of species specificity. Bacterial chemotherapy is an application of this phenomenon. The essential feature of this form of chemotherapy is that some drugs can destroy the cells of bacteria within a patient without harming the patient himself. One mechanism by which this is attained is that the drug can inhibit or destroy a component in the bacterial cell, which is not present in the host's cells. Penicillin and the cephalosporins for example prevent the synthesis of an adequate bacterial cell wall. Animal cells possess no cell wall and are therefore completely un-harmed.

Absorption of drugs

The most important mechanism for drug absorp-tion at cellular level is passive diffusion. This is not dependent on metabolic energy but is determined merely by a concentration gradient and by the ability of the drug to pass through the cell mem-brane. Cell membranes contain a large amount of lipid, and it is generally the lipid-soluble, un-charged forms of the drug which can pass through. Many drugs contain acidic or basic parts in their molecules and these may exist in ionised (charged) or un-ionised (uncharged) forms. It is the un-ionised forms which are more fat soluble and these more readily pass through cell membranes. Thus, basic drugs are best absorbed in an alkaline environ-ment and acidic drugs in an acid environment. Non-polar and lipid substances are usually well absorbed.

Drug administration

The most rapid and certain method of introducing a drug into the body is by injection, but oral administration is simpler, safer, cheaper and less unpleasant. Possible routes of administration are as follows:

1. Oral
2. Parenteral (injections)
   a. subcutaneous and submucosal
   b. intramuscular
   c. intravenous
3. Inhalational
   a. gases and vapours
   b. aerosols and powder inhalers
4. Transcutaneous and transmucosal

Absorption from the alimentary tract

Oral administration, although preferred by patients, is limited by the fact that some drugs, such as benzyl penicillin, are inactivated by gastric acid or destroyed by digestive enzymes. Absorption into the blood stream is also relatively slow and suffi-ciently high plasma levels may not be achieved. In addition, the drug passes via the portal veins to the liver where it may be metabolised to a greater or lesser degree (*first-pass metabolism*). This happens to nitrates used for the treatment of anginal pain. The usual way in which they are given is therefore as a sublingual tablet for transmucosal absorption into veins, avoiding the portal circulation.

A few drugs (such as aspirin and alcohol) are partly absorbed through the stomach wall, but most drugs given by mouth are absorbed in the upper part of the small intestine.

Drugs which are irritant to the stomach can be made tolerable by giving them a coating which only dissolves in the intestine (enteric coating).

Pro-drugs

First-pass metabolism can be a serious limitation on some drugs given by mouth, but, with characteristic ingenuity, pharmaceutical chemists have taken advantage of this phenomenon to produce a variety of pro-drugs. Pro-drugs are drugs which are metab-olised by the liver to release the active component into the systemic circulation. Pivampicillin for example releases the antibiotic, ampicillin; it is more effectively absorbed than the latter and causes less gastric upset. Benorylate releases paracetamol and aspirin and lessens the gastric irritant action of the latter.

Bioavailability

Bioavailability is, in simple terms, the extent to which the drug is taken into the body and can act on the target tissues. The many variables which affect bioavailability include: (1) the drug's physical properties which affect its absorption, (2) gastroin-testinal factors affecting absorption, (3) degree of hepatic metabolism and (4) physical properties of the drug once absorbed. The bioavailability of a drug is measured by the plasma levels achieved by the active component. However, a major factor affecting drugs which are to act on the brain is their ability to penetrate the blood–brain barrier – for this purpose, centrally acting drugs need to be lipid soluble.

The injection of drugs

Subcutaneous injection of a drug is simple but allows only a small volume to be given and absorption is relatively slow. These may however be advantages in the case of a potent drug such as adrenaline.

Submucosal injection is a common route for local anaesthetics as it allows them to act precisely where required.

Intramuscular injection is a common route for giving drugs when a more rapid effect is needed or if, as in the case of penicillin for example, the drug is destroyed in the gastrointestinal tract. Intramuscular injection can however be painful as the muscle fibres are pulled apart, and this may limit the volume of drug that can be administered by this route. Some drugs such as erythromycin are so irritant that they are not given in this way.

Intravenous injection allows a drug to act almost immediately and reach a high plasma concentration; large volumes can also be given but there are disadvantages such as:

a. Skill is required to put the needle into a vein; a haematoma may be produced if the vein wall is torn.

b. Infection may be carried into the blood stream (a major hazard for addicts).

c. The sudden entry of the drug into the blood can cause a toxic reaction (as in the case of adrenaline); other drugs can cause particularly severe allergic reactions when given by this route.

d. Some drugs or their solvents (notably propylene glycol used to dissolve diazepam) are irritant to vessel walls and can cause thrombophlebitis.

Pulmonary absorption

Anaesthetic gases and vapours, liquid aerosols and solid particles are given and absorbed via the lungs. Absorption into the circulation is mainly from the alveoli and alveolar ducts. In the adult human lung the area of these respiratory surfaces is 60 square metres, the area of the deck of a large motor cruiser.

An important advantage of administering bronchodilator aerosols directly into the respiratory tract (such as isoprenaline and salbutamol) by this route is that they are sprayed into the lungs and produce a high local concentration. The blood levels are relatively low and this reduces the danger of systemic toxic effects.

The absorption of anaesthetic gases is governed by their solubility, their rate of entry into the tissues and the rates of pulmonary blood flow and respiration. The longer the time a patient is exposed to an inhaled anaesthetic, the greater the amount of anaesthetic agent that enters the tissues from the plasma. The plasma/tissue difference in concentration therefore falls during exposure to the anaesthetic.

Having entered the body, the main route of excretion of volatile anaesthetics is from the lungs. Some of the drug remains for several hours in adipose tissue and other cells, but this is usually a relatively small proportion.

Liquid aerosols and solid particles can be inhaled as far as the bronchioles if the droplet or particle size is less than 2 μm. Particles of 10 μm reach the small bronchi. Thus the smaller the particle size, the greater the surface area reached for absorption.

Drug absorption through the oral mucosa

Drugs applied to the oral mucosa are mostly used for a purely local effect, but some are absorbed to a significant degree and can have a systemic effect, particularly if they are held under the tongue where there are large superficial veins. Since such drugs are absorbed directly into blood vessels, they avoid the portal circulation and hepatic (first-pass) metabolism.

Drugs which can be given sublingually are nitrates used for angina pectoris (see Ch. 10) and the opiate analgesic, buprenorphine. Morphine can also be given in this way to avoid injections and special adhesive preparations have been made to hold the drug in place in the mouth while it is being absorbed. Injection however remains the most effective route for administration of morphine.

Drug absorption through the skin

Drugs are often applied directly to the skin to treat skin diseases. Apart from the local physical properties of the application – which may in themselves be beneficial – local application gives a high tissue concentration to the affected part, with a much lower concentration elsewhere (assuming there is some diffusion and absorption into the circulation). Even for local effectiveness some of the drug must be absorbed and this takes place through the stratum corneum. Absorption is most rapid where the stratum corneum is thinnest and is further enhanced by warming the skin and increasing its hydration. Plastic occlusive dressings over steroid creams (for instance) greatly enhance and prolong their action, and also increase systemic absorption.

Glyceryl trinitrate, used in the treatment of angina pectoris, can be absorbed following application to the skin in the form of a cream.

Protein binding

Once a drug has been absorbed it travels throughout the body in the plasma. Although some of the drug is simply dissolved in the plasma, some is bound to plasma protein. The protein-bound form is generally inactive, and it is the free form which is pharmacologically active. Many drugs are bound to the albumin component of the plasma proteins. These include the coumarin anticoagulants, indomethacin, aspirin, barbiturates, digitalis and tetracyclines.

One consequence of drugs being protein bound is prolongation of their effect in the body. Drugs which are mainly bound to plasma proteins have a prolonged action because it is only the free, unbound form of the drug which is attacked by drug-metabolising enzymes and later excreted in the urine.

For any particular concentration of a drug in the blood, only a proportion (corresponding to the unbound form) is pharmacologically active. One type of harmful drug interaction can result from this situation. Warfarin, for instance, is a drug used in the prevention of thrombosis because of its anticoagulant action. It is partly protein bound in the plasma. If another drug (such as chloral) is given and displaces warfarin from its binding sites on the albumin molecule, a higher proportion of warfarin is then free to act. The pharmacological effect of the warfarin is therefore increased and this can result in haemorrhage.

Metabolism and fate of drugs in the body (Fig. 1.1)

The effect produced by a drug does not persist indefinitely, but sooner or later ceases. The fall in plasma concentration of the drug often parallels the fall-off in the effect of the drug. The graph of plasma concentration against time generally follows a logarithmic pattern and therefore the rate of descent of the curve can be expressed as a half-life ($t_{1/2}$) in the same way as other processes (such as radioactive decay) which diminish in a logarithmic pattern. This is due partly to metabolic destruction of the drug and partly due to excretion. The relative importance of these two mechanisms varies from drug to drug.

The liver is the principal organ involved in drug metabolism but others, such as kidney and intestine, are also involved to a lesser extent. Within the cell, the most important organelle carrying out metabolic transformations of drugs is the smooth endoplasmic reticulum. This constitutes the so-called microsomal fraction of the cell.

Drugs may be metabolised by two types of mechanism:

1. Conversion.
2. Synthesis.

1. Metabolic conversion. The structure of drugs may be modified in the body by simple chemical reactions. Important examples are oxidation and hydrolysis.

Many drugs are inactivated by oxidation by the microsomal (drug-metabolising) enzymes in the liver. Morphine and most of the barbiturates have their actions terminated in this way. In severe liver disease (such as advanced cirrhosis) or in patients who have been given monoamine oxidase inhibitor drugs (for depression) these oxidising systems do not function adequately. Thus if morphine or a barbiturate is given to such patients, it will cause profound and prolonged sedation with deep depression of respiration.

Suxamethonium is a muscle relaxant drug which acts on the motor end-plate. It has a very short action (usually less than 5 minutes) because it is rapidly hydrolysed by plasma pseudocholinesterase. This drug is therefore used when very short-lived muscular relaxation is wanted. However, about 1 in 4000 of the population lack pseudocholinesterase in their plasma. These people appear perfectly

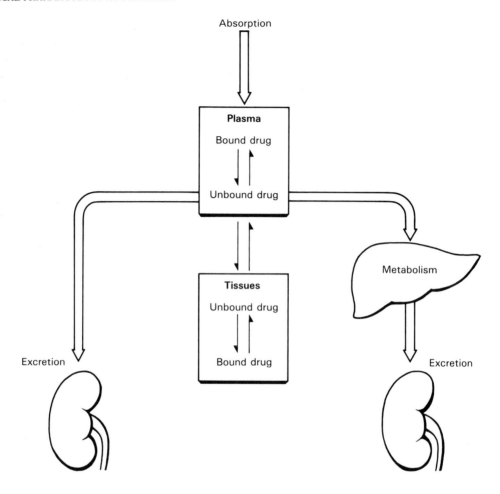

Fig. 1.1   Drug distribution: the essentials of the process of drug handling by the body.

normal until they are given suxamethonium. This produces muscular (including respiratory) paralysis for many hours. During this time, life has to be maintained by applying positive pressure artificial respiration until the effects of the suxamethonium have ceased.

2. Metabolic synthesis. Synthesis in the present context means conjugation of the drug with another chemical grouping or molecule. This may produce an increase in polarity and water solubility, decrease in pharmacological activity and greater ease of excretion.

One form of conjugation of drugs is with glucuronic acid. Glucuronic acid is derived from glucose, and is combined with some drugs in the liver. Such glucuronidation is carried out by the smooth endoplasmic reticulum of the hepatic parenchymal cells. Aspirin and chloramphenicol are examples of two drugs handled in this way. In newborn infants – particularly those born before full term – the drug-conjugating mechanisms may be incompletely developed and fail to function for several days after delivery. If such a child is given chloramphenicol during the early days of life very little of the drug is converted to chloramphenical glucuronide (inactive) and most remains in the nonconjugated active form. Thus unusually high blood levels of the free antibiotic are present and cause toxic effects, in particular circulatory collapse.

Factors which modify drug metabolism

These may be split up into:

1. Genetic
2. Physiological
3. Disease
4. Environmental influences

1. Genetic constitution is a fairly common cause of variation in drug metabolism. Plasma pseudo-cholinesterase for example, which greatly prolongs the action of suxamethonium is inherited as a non sex-linked (i.e. autosomal) recessive trait.

About a third of Europeans have inherited the ability to inactivate some drugs rapidly by acetylation. Thus they quickly inactivate such drugs as the antituberculous agent isoniazid, the antihypertensive hydralazine and the antidepressant nialamid.

Genetic factors may also alter responsiveness to drugs and the ability to develop toxic effects. Thus some patients are resistant to anticoagulants of the coumarin type such as warfarin. Large populations of rats and mice as a result of selection have also developed resistance to warfarin which is a widely used rat poison.

An example of vulnerability to a particular toxic effect is the inherited deficiency of the red cell enzyme glucose-6-phosphate dehydrogenase. Such patients may develop acute haemolytic anaemia when given certain antimalarials (such as primaquine and pamaquine) or antibacterials (such as nitrofurantoin and sulphonamides).

2. Physiological factors. Age is one such variable. In the newborn excessively high levels of drugs such as chloramphenicol may result from immaturity of the microsomal drug-conjugating system. In old age, toxic effects from digoxin (a cardiac glycoside) and streptomycin (an antibiotic) are common, partly due to diminished renal function and impaired excretion.

3. Disease. Malnutrition, if severe, may prolong the action of some drugs (in particular the hypnotics and tranquillisers) due to poor hepatic function. Liver disease – including cirrhosis and obstructive jaundice – may also slow down the removal of drugs which are conjugated and then excreted into the bile.

4. Environmental influences. Previous exposure

to drugs is an example. The barbiturates are powerful inducers of drug-metabolising enzymes. Even a few doses of a barbiturate increase the ability of the liver to metabolise a wide range of drugs. Thus if a patient is taking a barbiturate regularly and at the same time he is given the anticoagulant warfarin the latter has to be given in a higher than usual dose to produce the same anticoagulant effect. This is because the metabolism of warfarin by the liver has been accelerated. A well-recognised danger of this situation is that if the patient suddenly stops taking barbiturates, but continues to take the same dose of warfarin, he may suffer serious haemorrhage. This is because withdrawal of the barbiturate allows the drug-metabolising enzymes in the liver quickly to fall to their previous (non-induced) level of activity. The warfarin is not then broken down so rapidly and attains much higher blood levels. Similarly in women given inducing agents such as the barbiturates, the contraceptive pill may become ineffective unless the dose of the oestrogen component is raised.

By contrast, monoamine oxidase inhibitor drugs (such as nialamid), which are used in the treatment of depression, inhibit oxidising enzymes in the liver. If morphine, which is normally oxidised in the liver, is given at the same time as nialamid, it will have an enhanced effect.

Drug excretion

Drugs may leave the body unchanged or in a metabolically altered form.

The most important organ of excretion is the kidney. Most renal excretion is via the glomerular filtrate. The sequence of events is this: arterial blood flows into the afferent arterioles of the glomeruli of the kidney. Some of the plasma is filtered through the glomerular membrane and enters the lumen of the renal tubules. Some of the solutes in the filtered plasma (which include electrolytes, metabolites and drugs) are to a variable extent reabsorbed via the tubular epithelium into the plasma; the remainder enters the collecting ducts to be excreted in the urine. An important consequence is that the less the tubular reabsorption of drug, the more rapidly will it appear in the urine. To some extent this can be varied with individual drugs, particularly if they are acids or bases. Acids and bases exist in uncharged (undissociated) and charged (ionised) forms.

In acid solutions, acids are mainly undissociated while bases are mainly ionised. In alkaline conditions the situation is reversed: acids are mainly ionised and bases non-ionised.

It is a general rule that drugs can enter cells if they are uncharged and they cannot pass through even the outer cell membrane if they carry a charge. These phenomena are used in the treatment of some forms of drug overdose. Aspirin is a weak acid. When an overdose has been taken, excretion can be greatly accelerated by making the urine alkaline – usually by an infusion of sodium bicarbonate. The alkalinity of the urine encourages dissociation of the aspirin:

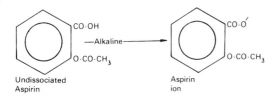

The ion thus formed carries a charge and therefore cannot be reabsorbed by the tubular epithelial cells. The aspirin which has entered the lumen of the renal tubule has then only one way out and this is via the collecting ducts into the urine.

Conversely the base amphetamine can be excreted more rapidly by increasing the acidity of the urine.

Many drugs retain their charge virtually unchanged throughout the entire pH range possible in body fluids. Streptomycin for example remains strongly positively charged at all physiological pH values, and the entire amount of streptomycin is filtered via the glomeruli and is excreted in the urine with almost no renal tubular epithelial reabsorption.

Occasionally renal excretion of a drug exceeds that entering the tubule via the glomerulus. This is due to active secretion of the drug by the renal tubular epithelial cells. These cells take up and concentrate the drug from the plasma and secrete it

directly into the tubular lumen. Penicillin is handled in this way – which explains its extremely high excretion rate. It is possible to block this secretion mechanism with another drug – probenecid. When probenecid is given with penicillin, the blood levels of penicillin are higher and its action more prolonged.

Some drugs, such as the volatile anaesthetics, leave the body partly via the lungs and are exhaled unchanged. This is a great advantage as it allows rapid control of the level of anaesthesia.

Many substances are excreted in the bile. Drugs which appear in the bile are mainly conjugated (e.g. glucuronides or sulphates). These then enter the gut and leave the body in the faeces – although some may be de-conjugated by intestinal organisms and reabsorbed into the circulation.

Some drugs, such as the aminoglycoside antibiotics, many of which are nephrotoxic, may inhibit their own excretion.

Summary

1. Drugs are absorbed through mucous membranes by many mechanisms, but by far the commonest is passive diffusion. As membranes contain a lipid component, mainly uncharged, lipid-soluble drugs are most readily absorbed.

2. Drugs which are eliminated mainly by metabolism are usually inactivated in the liver, although other organs may be involved.

3. The principal organ of drug excretion is the kidney.

SUGGESTED FURTHER READING

Boobis A R, Lewis P (1982) Drugs in pregnancy – altered pharmacokinetics. British Journal of Hospital Medicine 29: 566
Brodie M J 1986 Therapeutic drug monitoring. Practitioner 230: 1003
Feeley J, Brodie M J 1988 Practical clinical pharmacology: drug handling and response. British Medical Journal 296: 1046
Graham G G, Kennedy M (1979) Clinical pharmacokinetics. Medical Journal of Australia I: 383
Lancet 1983 Pharmacokinetics in the elderly. Lancet i: 568
Lindup W E, Orme M C L'E 1981 Plasma protein binding of drugs. British Medical Journal 282: 212
McEinay J C, D'Arcy P F 1983 Protein binding displacement interactions and their clinical importance. Drugs 25: 495

Rawlins M D, James O F W, Williams F M, Wynne H,
Woodhouse K W 1987 Age and the metabolism of drugs.
Quarterly Journal of Medicine, New Series 64: 545
Rylance G 1981 Drugs in children. British Medical Journal
282: 50
Rylance G W 1988 Prescribing for infants and children. British
Medical Journal 296: 984
Scott A K, Hawksworth G M 1981 Drug absorption. British
Medical Journal 282: 462
Vessell E S 1985 Genetic host factors: determinants of drug
response. New England Journal of Medicine 313: 50

2. Prescribing and the Misuse of Drugs Act

The writing of prescriptions usually requires no more than common sense and a formulary for information on such matters as the forms in which the preparation is available and the usual dosage ranges for children and adults.

Pharmacists are not impressed by illegible handwriting and may justifiably regard anyone who sends a formless scrawl as either illiterate or trying to disguise his ignorance.

There is no need to use, or try to remember, obscure Latin abbreviations, but it is acceptable and certainly quicker to put 't.d.s' than to write 'Take three times a day' in full.

The essential information to be put on a prescription is obvious enough, namely:

1. The name and address of the prescriber.
2. The name and address of the patient.
3. The date.
4. The preparation, its form (tablets, mixture or whatever) and the total quantity to be dispensed in metric units.
5. Instructions as to how and when the drug is to be taken, e.g. 'take three times a day before meals'.
6. The prescriber's signature.

Most drugs are available in some easily taken form that ensures adequate absorption and in amounts that form a convenient dose for taking once, twice, three times a day or more often as necessary.

Drugs have a full chemical name but this is almost invariably too complicated for everyday use, and no one but a crank would ask for 6-[(D)-α-aminophenyl acetamido]-penicillanic acid instead of ampicillin which is the official (approved) name. The manufacturers also have their own proprietary or brand name (Ampilar, Penbritin and other proprietary names) which is usually patented. Subsequently other manufacturers often produce the same drug under licence. Chloramphenicol, for example, had no fewer than 45 different proprietary names.

Official (generic) names are incidentally spelt with a small initial letter, e.g. ampicillin. Proprietary names, by contrast, are spelt with an initial capital, e.g. Penbritin.

The prescriber should always use the official name. If a proprietary name is used the pharmacist has to dispense that particular brand, and clearly he cannot keep perhaps 30 proprietary brands of tetracycline for example, in stock. Use of the official name allows the pharmacist to dispense whichever brand is cheapest and available. It has also become apparent that different preparations of the same drug may be absorbed to different degrees. Thus changing brands of the same drug in mid-treatment might swing the response to dangerous under- or overtreatment.

It has to be admitted that it is sometimes much easier to use a proprietary name, and only the most punctilious refer to Librium by its generic name, chlordiazepoxide.

Aspirin is an odd exception in that it was originally the proprietary name for acetysalicylic acid of the first manufacturer (Bayer of Germany) but has since become the official name.

Sources of reference

The Dental Practitioners' Formulary (DPF). The DPF includes all the drugs that can be prescribed under the conditions of the British National Health Service at whatever charge the Government of the day has decided. The charge is the same for all drugs. Thus, at the time of writing, the patient pays £2.60 for a fortnight's course of miconazole tablets, for example, which costs approximately £40. On the other hand, some simple preparations such as aspirin or mouthwashes are cheaper if bought over the counter.

The DPF contains all the preparations that the dental surgeon is likely to prescribe but not preparations such as local anaesthetics which he himself administers.

An attempt is made to ensure that there is reasonable evidence that preparations included in the DPF are effective. Although a few oddments hallowed by tradition still remain, these are being progressively discarded.

There is also information regarding the uses, contraindications and adverse reactions of drugs used in dentistry.

Finally, there are full details of the prescribable drugs and their dosage.

The dentist is not, by the way, limited in his prescribing to the contents of the DPF. He can prescribe anything provided that it does not contravene the Misuse of Drugs Act and that the patient pays the full cost of the prescription of any drugs not included in the DPF.

Currently a combined Dental Practitioners' Formulary and British National Formulary is available to practitioners in the Health Service and (it is planned) there will be a new edition every 2 years.

The British National Formulary (BNF). This (of which the DPF is an offshoot) is a handbook for medical prescribing. It contains a much wider formulary, condensed information about the therapeutic management of almost the whole range of human disease, and much other information. It should be of interest to any dental surgeon who is anxious to widen his knowledge of therapeutics. It is particularly useful, for instance, when the patient's medical history shows that a complicated regimen of treatment is being followed. These drugs have then to be identified and evaluated both in the hope of getting some indication of the patient's physical state and of assessing how it may affect the type of dental treatment proposed.

Like the DPF, the BNF tries to include only drugs of proven effectiveness but also provides basic data on virtually all the different proprietary preparations available. Firm recommendations are made as to the most appropriate drugs to be used in any given circumstance.

The British National Formulary is under constant revision and a new edition is published every 6 months – it is thus more up to date than any textbook of pharmacology.

Basic information about all proprietary preparations available in Britain is also found in the *Monthly Index of Medical Specialties (MIMS).* This gives proprietary and official names for all preparations, formulations and dosage, and also minimal details of side-effects and contraindications. The drugs are grouped according to their main sites and types of action.

Data sheets. Drug companies are now required to publish data sheets for their products. These sheets include a bewildering amount of information, including presentation (tablets, capsules or mixtures as the case may be) and the amounts of the drug in each form, its uses, dosage and administration, contraindications and warnings, effects of overdosage, pharmaceutical precautions, the legal category of the drug, quantities in the manufacturer's packages, further information, which may include information about the pharmacokinetics of the drug, and other facts. Data sheets may sometimes therefore run to two double-sided pages of small print, so that the amount of information provided may unfortunately discourage anyone from reading it.

Misuse of Drugs Regulations 1973

These regulations replace the Dangerous Drugs Act (DDA) but have the same purpose, namely to control the prescribing of drugs of addiction. The dental surgeon can keep in stock, administer or prescribe controlled drugs but only insofar as they are genuinely needed for dental purposes. It would be acceptable for a dental surgeon to keep in stock cocaine for example, for use as a topical analgesic for certain special applications, but it would not be justifiable to prescribe the same drug for its systemic effects as there is no dental condition which can be usefully so treated.

Broadly speaking, the important drugs of dependence (addiction) are:

a. *The opioids* which include both morphine and its derivatives, and synthetic substitutes such as pethidine. These are *depressants* of the CNS.

b. *Stimulants of the CNS*. Cocaine and the amphetamines are the main examples.

Some morphine derivatives such as codeine are also commonly used drugs which rarely lead to dependence. Similarly some medicines (for the control of diarrhoea for instance) contain minute amounts of opium.

Under these regulations controlled drugs are divided into three classes:

Class A drugs are the most addictive and harmful. Morphine, diamorphine (heroin), cocaine and lysergide (LSD) are examples of Class A drugs.

Class B drugs include the oral amphetamines, cannabis, codeine and methylphenidate which, although addictive, are less harmful than Class A drugs.

Class C drugs are related to the amphetamines and include benzphetamine and chlorphentamine.

Among the controlled drugs, only narcotic analgesics might be justifiably prescribed in dentistry for control of severe postoperative pain (for example) or be kept in the dental surgery for use if a patient were to have a myocardial infarction.

Prescribing controlled drugs

Controlled drugs can be dispensed for dental purposes only if certain rules are followed, namely that:

1. The address of the prescriber is within the UK.

2. The pharmacist is familiar with the signature of the prescriber.

3. The drug must not be dispensed before, or later than 13 weeks after, the date of the prescription.

4. The entire prescription must be in the prescriber's own handwriting and in ink (or an indelible equivalent) and must show:

   a. The prescriber's name.

   b. The patient's name and address.

   c. The form of preparation (e.g. capsule or tablet) and its strength (unless only one preparation of the drug is available) must be stated.

   d. The total quantity – in both words *and* figures – of the drug to be supplied must be stated. Alternatively this may be expressed in terms of the number – in both words and figures –of 'dosage units', such as capsules or tablets.

   e. The prescription must be endorsed with the words *For dental treatment only.*

   f. The prescription must be signed with the usual signature of the prescriber and be dated by him and not repeated.

Those then are the rules but it is difficult to imagine any circumstances in dentistry where controlled drugs are worth the effort involved in prescribing them.

Requisition and possession of controlled drugs

To obtain and keep in stock a drug such as cocaine the dental surgeon must:

1. Order the material on a requisition form

   a. signed by him,

   b. stating his name, address and profession, and

   c. specifying the purpose for which the drug is required and the total quantity to be supplied.

2. Keep a register of all such controlled drugs giving precise details both of what has been obtained and what has been administered and the dates of both.

3. Store any controlled drugs in a fixed locked container. The dental surgeon must retain the key. Again, it all seems hardly worth the effort.

SUGGESTED FURTHER READING

Binns, T B 1980 The Committee on Review of Medicines. British Medical Journal, 281: 1614

Bliss, M R 1981 Prescribing for the elderly. British Medical Journal 283: 203

Hartley, B H 1981 Clinical pharmacology. Prescription writing. British Medical Journal 282: 711

Joint Formulary Committee (1986) Dental Practitioners' Formulary, 1986–1988. British Medical Association and The Pharmaceutical Society of Great Britain

Joint Formulary Committee (1988) British National Formulary No. 15. British Medical Association and The Pharmaceutical Society of Great Britain

3. The management of infections

The magic word, antibiotic, inevitably springs to mind whenever an infection has to be dealt with. Nevertheless infection, particularly in dental practice, is generally managed by other means and the role of antibiotics in dentistry, although important, is relatively small. This is partly because severe infections of dental origin are rare while localised infections are usually dealt with more quickly and effectively by surgical means.

Systemic infections are the main realm of use of the antibiotics and many of the severe infections that claimed innumerable lives are now things of the past. The final distressing scenes of *La Traviata* and *La Bohème* were common and true enough in their day but are almost unimaginable now.

Although the antibiotics have conferred enormous benefits it is easy to gain an exaggerated idea of their importance. Overall, many more lives have been saved by preventive measures and improved standards of living.

The water-borne infections, particularly typhoid and cholera, were controlled in large cities even before bacteria were discovered by the apparently simple expedient of keeping excreta out of the drinking water. Where there is no adequate sewage system and water supply, as in underdeveloped countries, these diseases are rampant. Similarly, tuberculosis was declining in Britain long before the introduction of streptomycin, as a result of improved standards of living and (to some degree) by isolation of infected patients. In poorer countries malnutrition and poor standards of living make for greater susceptibility and ease of spread of the infection, for which antibiotics alone are not an effective solution.

Misuse of antibiotics. A different sort of problem has been caused by the *overuse* of antibiotics. In hospitals, cross-infection is common. There are many potential sources of infection and susceptible subjects, particularly those with surgical wounds or those whose resistance is depressed by disease or by drug treatment. Infections are also often due to resistant organisms promoted by the unnecessary use of antibiotics. The hospital staff and other vectors transmit the infection from one patient to another. Rigorous control against overuse of antibiotics combined with strictly applied isolation techniques are needed to deal with this problem.

Viral infections are another very common problem, but there are as yet few effective antiviral drugs.

The lesson is that antibiotics can often provide near-miraculous results, but only if used appropriately and when other circumstances are favourable.

Control of infection in the mouth

The oral cavity is inhabited by enormous numbers of microorganisms which form the normal microflora. Paradoxically perhaps this is a blessing rather than a danger, in that virulent pathogens such as *Staphylococcus aureus* which often cause dangerous infections in other parts of the body rarely cause disease of the mouth or jaws. Giving antibiotics can occasionally, therefore, cause adverse reactions by disturbing the normal microflora. The proliferation of pathogens is thus promoted by the elimination of competitors.

Although organisms of the normal oral microflora are usually harmless it is obviously undesirable to transfer bacteria or viruses from one patient to another on instruments or by hypodermic needles, which can implant organisms deeply.

The control of infection falls into three main

15

categories as follows:

1. Prevention of surgical infections.
   a. Sterilisation of instruments, dressings, work surfaces, etc.
      (i) Physical methods – preferably by autoclaving at 134°C for 3 minutes.
      (ii) Antiseptics (to a small degree only).
   b. Disinfection of the field of operation.
   c. Aseptic operating techniques.
2. Surgical elimination of localised infection, such as extraction of teeth or drainage of pus.
3. Use of antimicrobials when infection cannot otherwise be controlled or surgery is inappropriate.

In addition, special measures are used (with limited success) against dental caries and periodontal disease see (Ch. 4.)

Hepatitis B and the acquired immune deficiency syndrome (AIDS) create special problems which are discussed later.

ANTIBIOTICS AND ANTIBACTERIAL CHEMOTHERAPY

Antimicrobial drugs, in their broadest sense, have a long history. This can be said to have started with the successful use in 1619 of an extract of cinchona bark which proved effective for the treatment of malaria and from which quinine was later derived.

The first synthetic antimicrobials were the organic arsenicals. The first to come into clinical use was Salvarsan, introduced by Ehrlich in 1909 for the treatment of syphilis, which remained in use until superseded by penicillin in the 1940s.

The present era of chemotherapy started with the demonstration in Germany of the antibacterial properties of Prontosil, a dye derivative, by Domagk in 1935. This was the forerunner of many sulphonamides which were spectacularly effective against haemolytic streptococci, pneumococci and a wide range of other bacteria. The sulphonamides were therefore the first antibacterial agents effective against many common infections and remain useful today.

Although the antibacterial effect of a mould had been noticed as early as 1929 by Fleming, the credit for the introduction of penicillin as a practical therapeutic agent belongs to Florey and Chain who, approximately a decade later, started to

develop methods for obtaining this microbial product in usable quantities and ultimately established its effectiveness systemically in experimental infections. The development of large-scale commercial production took several more years so that penicillin did not become widely available until about the mid 1940s. The term *antibiotic* was introduced in 1942 by Waksman (a co-discoverer of streptomycin), although penicillin isolated from the mould *Penicillium notatum* was the first and is still the best-known example.

Chemotherapy does *not* mean treatment with any sort of chemicals (drugs) for any kind of disease. It means only the use of drugs against either microorganisms or cancer cells.

The term 'chemotherapy' alone is probably still most often used to mean antibacterial chemotherapy, but the context usually makes the meaning clear.

Definitions

Antibiotics are substances produced by microorganisms which act in minute concentrations to kill other organisms or prevent them from proliferating.

The overwhelmingly important property of antibiotics is that their action is highly selective, acting specifically against aspects of bacterial metabolism such as their enzyme systems but not against those of tissue cells. There are also wholly synthetic antimicrobials which achieve the same effects.

The main features of antibiotics can be summarised as follows:

1. They are substances produced by microorganisms, but are antagonistic to other microorganisms and either kill them or stop them from proliferating.
2. Antibiotics act in extreme dilution – sometimes less than $0.01 \mu g/ml$ (i.e. a dilution of 1:100 000 000).
3. Antibiotics are highly specific in their action and attack particular metabolic activities or structures of certain bacteria.
4. The specific activity of antibiotics is against microorganisms and not against the host's cells. Antibiotics can be (and usually are) given systemically without ill-effect. Antibiotics can, like any

other drug, have side-effects, but these are relatively uncommon and generally unrelated to the nature of their antibacterial activity.

Although the strict definition of an antibiotic is a substance produced by microorganisms that is antagonistic to the growth or life of others in high dilution, the term tends to be used less precisely. The reason is that many antimicrobials have been produced partially or entirely synthetically, but nevertheless fulfil the functional criteria of antibiotics and are just as specific in their activities.

Antimicrobials include both true antibiotics and synthetic antibacterial drugs.

Chemotherapy, when unqualified, is used as an abbreviation for 'antibacterial chemotherapy' meaning the use of specific antimicrobial drugs for the treatment of infection. In the context of the treatment of cancer the term 'chemotherapy' is used to mean cytotoxic chemotherapy (see Ch. 14), but the context in which these terms are used will make their meanings clear.

In view of the variety of specific antibacterial agents (true antibiotics, semi-synthetic antibiotics and synthetic antimicrobials) these agents will, for the sake of simplicity, be referred to here merely as *antibacterials* or *antibiotics*, whether or not they fulfil the strict, but now somewhat pedantic, definition of the latter.

Antiseptics, in contrast to antibiotics, are crudely toxic substances which have a virtually non-specific action causing as much damage to host cells as to microbes. Antiseptics are therefore useless for systemic infections.

Sources of antibiotics

Streptomycin was the first useful agent to be produced as a result of a deliberate and systematic search for sources of antibiotics. Since then most antibiotics have been discovered as a result of long and painstaking surveys of soil samples from different parts of the world. Soils contain a complex, mixed microflora and analyses of the nature and activity of these organisms has, after immense technical effort, yielded many highly effective antibacterial agents.

Several antibiotics have come from somewhat bizarre sources and many of these agents have a strange history.

It is remarkable enough that the original strain of the mould *Penicillium notatum* should apparently have floated fortuitously through the window of a bacteriology laboratory in St Mary's Hospital, to display its antibacterial properties to someone observant enough to realise its potentialities. Later, a mouldy canteloupe from the market at Peoria (Illinois) yielded the strain of *Penicillium chrysogenum* that is the source of commercially produced penicillin. The cephalosporins came from a sewage outfall in Sardinia, fusidic acid from a Japanese monkey's faeces and framycetin from a damp patch on a wall in Paris. It is not merely that these seem such unlikely sources of potent drugs, but it is hard to imagine why such unpromising materials were chosen and seriously examined.

Many antifungal agents are also derived from microorganisms and are just as specific in their actions as conventional antibacterial antibiotics.

Antiviral agents, which are mostly synthetic, are of recent origin and only a few are available. The lack of synthetic activities by viruses and their intimate interactions with the host cell nucleus for reproduction, make for special difficulties in finding a sufficiently selective line of attack against these organisms.

General aspects and principles of treatment

Antibiotics and synthetic antimicrobials are highly effective drugs for the treatment of infections which might otherwise be fatal. There is obviously a strong temptation to use antibacterials whenever an infection is even faintly suspected. In many other cases an infection is undoubtedly present as in the case of the common cold, for instance, but is caused by a virus and an antibiotic is ineffective. Although it might seem at a superficial level to be better to give an antibiotic whenever an infection seems to be present in the hope that it might help, this is unjustifiable. This approach can cause trouble in the following ways:

1. Antibiotics are all capable of causing side-effects. Fatal reactions have been caused only too often by antibiotics given for trivial conditions.
2. The use of antibiotics has resulted in the emergence of resistant strains of bacteria. This is to some extent unavoidable, but the risk is reduced by

using these drugs only when necessary and in correct dosage.

3. If there is any doubt whether the complaint is an infection, giving an antibiotic may do harm indirectly by causing delay in making an accurate diagnosis.

Indications for antibiotic treatment

An antibiotic should only be given when there is at least reasonable certainty that:

1. An infection is genuinely present.
2. The infection is likely to respond to an antibiotic, e.g. it is not a viral infection.
3. The infection is severe enough to justify treatment.
4. An antibiotic is the best form of treatment, i.e. is more appropriate than surgery.
5. A serious infection (e.g. infective endocarditis) can be prevented.

Infections cannot always be recognised with certainty by their clinical features. A red, tender swelling of the jaw may, for example, be caused by a tumour. An antibiotic would then not merely do no good but could do serious harm by delaying diagnosis.

In most cases, however, the history and physical signs such as fever or rapid onset of symptoms with swelling and tenderness of regional lymph nodes help to make the diagnosis less uncertain. Most infections of the jaws originate from a dead tooth and this should be looked for and dealt with.

It is not possible to lay down hard and fast rules as to how severe an infection should be before an antibiotic is given. Thus, generally speaking, antibiotics are given for infections that are having systemic effects and show no sign of starting to resolve spontaneously. Antibiotics should not, for example, be given for minor attacks of food poisoning (acute diarrhoea and vomiting), but are essential in the treatment of typhoid fever. Another important use of antibiotics is in sites such as the hand or eye where infection could be disabling. Most dental infections are too slight to justify antibiotic therapy and in any case usually respond far more quickly to surgical treatment as mentioned earlier.

It might seem too much to expect to be able to predict whether an infection is likely to respond to an antibiotic, but in many cases it is apparent, for instance, when a viral or fungal infection is present. Most of the acute childhood fevers (chickenpox, measles, rubella, etc.) are caused by viruses, as are the very common respiratory and other infections, such as colds.

Prophlylactic use of antibiotics

Prophylactic use of antibiotics is only justifiable and effective when patients are exposed to and at immediate risk from severe specific infections.

Examples are:

1. Long-term daily penicillin for patients who have had rheumatic fever to prevent recurrences of *Strep. pyogenes* infection.
2. Prevention of infective endocarditis in patients with cardiac valvular disease having dental extractions or some other procedures.
3. Prevention of infection after severe injuries such as maxillofacial fractures, particularly when there is a risk of contamination from the exterior.
4. Susceptible contacts exposed to cases of meningococcal meningitis.
5. Susceptible contacts exposed to tuberculosis.
6. Patients having surgery of the intestine have the gut flora as nearly as possible totally suppressed by means of non-absorbed broad spectrum antibiotics.

More widespread blanket cover may be given to highly susceptible patients such as those having immunosuppressive or cytotoxic therapy, but unless there is exposure to some specific pathogen, protection can at best be only partial.

Classification of antibacterial agents

Antibacterial agents may be divided into two groups according to whether their action is *bactericidal* and therefore kill sensitive organisms or *bacteriostatic* and thus prevent sensitive organisms from proliferating.

The distinction used to be regarded as important in that bacteriostatic drugs depend ultimately on intact humoral and cellular defences to overcome the infection. Further, a few bacteriostatic drugs, particularly tetracycline, may antagonise a bactericidal drug such as penicillin when the two are used in combination. Nevertheless, the distinction is otherwise rarely important clinically.

Broad and narrow spectrum antibiotics

In practice a broad spectrum antibiotic is one which is effective against the Gram-negative bacilli of the intestine or urinary tract as well as Gram-positive cocci. Thus benzyl penicillin, by these criteria, has a narrow spectrum while the closely related drug ampicillin has a broad spectrum.

Choice of antibiotic – preliminary considerations

1. Ideally an antibiotic should only be chosen after the causative organism has been identified and its sensitivity has been tested.

2. Urgent need for treatment of life-threatening infections (such as submaxillary cellulitis) may force a choice on clinical grounds alone; the drug can then, if necessary, be changed when the causative organism has been identified.

3. A few infections, such as acute ulcerative (Vincent's) gingivitis, have such a clear-cut clinical picture and respond so reliably to specific antimicrobials that bacteriological confirmation is rarely sought.

4. Infections in certain sites may give a general indication of the types of antibiotics which may be helpful. Acute infections of dental origin in particular are usually responsive to penicillin. Infections of the gut, by contrast, are caused by organisms (usually Gram-negative bacilli) resistant to penicillin that may respond to ampicillin or other broad spectrum drugs.

ANTIBIOTIC RESISTANCE – ACQUISITION AND MECHANISMS

Bacteria can become resistant to antimicrobial drugs by several mechanisms. Acquired resistance depends, in essence, on genetic material which encodes the information necessary to direct the process. Acquisition of resistance to antibiotics, in turn, is by two main mechanisms, namely:

1. Mutation and therapeutic selection.
2. Transmission of new genetic material from other bacteria.

1. Mutation

In bacterial populations, mutants which are naturally resistant to an antibiotic appear at a rate of less than one per million bacteria for each division. This type of resistance is referred to as *chromosomal resistance* since it depends on changes in the bacterial chromosome.

Once such mutants appear, removal of the dominant antibiotic sensitive strains by administration of an antibiotic allows them to proliferate freely without competition. This phenomenon is well recognised in the case of oral viridans streptococci where a single dose of penicillin produces a resistant population within 24 hours.

2. Transmission of new genetic material

Antibiotic resistance can be transmitted by bacteriophages (bacterial viruses) or by plasmids. The latter consist of extrachromosomal DNA which is transmitted between bacteria during conjugation. Such DNA, known as an r-determinant, directs the production of enzymes which can inactivate one or several antibiotics and is perpetuated by division of the bacterium.

Mechanisms of increased bacterial resistance to antibacterials

The main mechanisms by which bacteria can become resistant is as follows:

1. Alteration of permeability of the bacterial cell for the drug.
2. Changes in the target sites for the drug in the bacterial cell.
3. Bypassing metabolic reactions blocked by the drug.
4. Drug inactivation.

1. Altered permeability for the drug

An antimicrobial has to penetrate the cell membrane to reach target sites in the bacterial cell to exert its action, but the ways in which permeability of the cell can be altered are poorly understood.

2. Changes in target sites in the bacterial cell

Typical mechanisms of action of several antibiotics are by binding to and inactivating bacterial enzymes or nucleic acids. Mutation or episome transfer can, however, change an amino acid or base component of these target substances with the result that the drug can no longer bind to them.

Resistance of staphylococci and streptococci to erythromycin and lincomycin, for example, depends on transfer of plasmid-mediated methylase which interferes with the binding of these antibiotics to ribosomal RNA.

3. Bypassing blocked metabolic reactions

Essential metabolic reactions of bacteria depend on chromosome-coded enzymes which can be blocked by antimicrobials. However, another enzyme, resistant to the drug, may be acquired by plasmid transfer and confer resistance to the antibiotic.

A major example is the blocking of bacterial folic acid production by sulphonamides which inhibit chromosomal-coded dihydrofolate reductase. However, episome-mediated dihydrofolate reductase can be acquired and is not blocked by sulphonamides; such bacteria become sulphonamide resistant as a result.

4. Drug inactivation

This important mechanism is usually mediated by the transmission of r-determinant episomes as described earlier. Inactivation of many of the penicillins by β-lactamases and of chloramphenicol by acetyl transferase are well-known examples.

Broadly speaking, therefore, the mechanisms of bacterial antibiotic resistance are by becoming either:

a. *Antibiotic tolerant.* Reduced permeability to the drug, changes in target substances within bacteria and bypassing blocked metabolic pathways all render bacteria tolerant to an antibiotic.

b. *Antibiotic destructive.* The best-known example of induced enzymic antibiotic destruction

is the production of penicillinases (β-lactamases), but other enzymes can inactivate cephalosporins, aminoglycosides and chloramphenicol.

Cross-resistance. In most cases bacteria resistant to an antibiotic are resistant to variants of the antibiotic which are chemically closely related. Staphylococci resistant to benzyl penicillin, for example, are resistant to most other related penicillins, but are sensitive to the penicillinase-resistant penicillins (cloxacillin and its relatives). Bacteria resistant to penicillins may also show resistance to the cephalosporins which chemically resemble the penicillins. For all practical purposes, bacteria resistant to one tetracycline are resistant to all. The same principle applies to the sulphonamides and other agents where different members of the group have been formed by relatively minor chemical modifications to the basic substance.

Practical aspects of antibiotic resistance. The main points can be summarised as follows:

1. Emergence of antibiotic-resistant strains of bacteria has been an inevitable consequence of the widespread use of antibiotics. This makes a strong case against the use of antibiotics in any circumstances where they are not essential.

2. The organisms which have shown the greatest ingenuity in finding ways of protecting themselves against antibiotics are *Staphylococcus aureus* and the various coliform bacilli. In the mouth penicillin-resistant strains of viridans streptococci rapidly proliferate during penicillin treatment, although in this case penicillin resistance is relative rather than absolute. By contrast, β-haemolytic streptococci appear incapable of developing resistance to penicillin.

3. When an organism is clearly resistant to one antibiotic it is wisest to change to a completely different type of antibiotic preferably as indicated by laboratory tests of sensitivity.

Antibiotic resistance – preventive measures

1. Avoid the use of antibiotics unless they are essential.

The overuse of antibiotics has contributed to the increasing number of antibiotic-resistant infections in hospitals. Even worse, chloramphenicol-resistant *Salmonella typhi* have infected some 100 000 patients in Mexico in recent years and caused more than 14 000 deaths. Resistant strains of *S. typhi* are also widespread in other countries where there is unrestricted public sale of antibiotics, particularly India, Thailand and Vietnam.

2. When an antibiotic has to be given, give it in adequate doses and for long enough to be reasonably certain that the infection has been eliminated. Inadequate treatment can leave sufficient resistant survivors to be troublesome.

3. In the case of dangerous infections, emergence of resistant strains may be prevented by combination therapy. The basis of this procedure is that different antibiotics have different modes of action; if two or more are given the organisms which survive one antibiotic are killed by the other. This measure is mainly used for severe diseases such as tuberculosis or infective endocarditis.

Use of antibiotics in dentistry – general considerations

The usefulness of antibiotics in routine dentistry is limited and these agents are often misused or overused. The abuse of antibiotics is not merely that they may be unnecessary, but side-effects may be more serious than the original complaint. This is especially true of dentistry where infections are rarely serious. Further, if an antibiotic is used 'just in case' there is an infection, serious harm can be done to the patient by delaying the diagnosis.

An antibiotic will not disperse pus once it has formed, although it may limit further spread of infection. Surgical methods are quick, effective and avoid any side-effects that an antibiotic might cause. Acute ulcerative gingivitis, by contrast, responds quickly and reliably to metronidazole and, since this drug seems to have few side-effects, its use is justifiable to prevent rapid destruction of the periodontal tissues.

Infections of the mucous membrane proper are usually caused by viruses such as herpes simplex or fungi, especially *Candida albicans*. Conventional antibiotics are of no direct value and may initiate or worsen fungal infections.

Infections in and around the teeth usually respond far more quickly and reliably to surgical measures (extraction or extirpation of the pulp for example) than to antibiotics which are therefore rarely needed.

The main indications for antibiotics in dentistry are as follows:

1. Prevention of infective endocarditis.
2. Prevention of infection after severe maxillofacial injuries, especially if there is leakage of CSF and a risk of meningitis.
3. Prevention of infections after major oral surgery.
4. Treatment of severe infections such as acute osteomyelitis, cellulitis or actinomycosis (very rarely now).
5. Treatment of acute ulcerative gingivitis.

Antibiotics may also be given for acute pulpitis or periodontitis if surgical treatment has to be delayed, but are of questionable value in such circumstances.

SULPHONAMIDES AND TRIMETHOPRIM

Sulphonamides, the first effective antimicrobials, have been continually developed and improved for over 40 years. Sulphonamides probably reached their peak of application by the Germans during the Second World War, when penicillin was unavailable to them. Their ability to cope with vast numbers of casualties subject to all the infections associated with warfare suggests that sulphonamides are perhaps more useful than many nowadays believe. Nevertheless, so many bacteria have become resistant to the sulphonamides that the latter are mainly used in combination with trimethoprim, particularly as co-trimoxazole.

Mode of action

Sulphonamides act by interfering with bacterial synthesis of folic acid from para-amino benzoic acid (PABA). Folic acid is ultimately needed for production of nucleic acids but bacteria (unlike man) cannot use pre-formed folic acid. Sulphonamides closely resemble PABA chemically and appear to have a stronger affinity for the synthesizing enzyme than the natural substrate; their action illustrates the phenomenon of *competitive inhibition*.

Bacteria can become resistant to sulphonamides by adaptive modifications of their enzyme systems to produce folic acid by other means.

Absorption and excretion

Most sulphonamides are well absorbed from the gut and can also be given by injection. Unlike most antibiotics they cross the blood–brain barrier and readily enter the cerebrospinal fluid.

Sulphonamides are excreted mainly in the urine, both unchanged and in conjugated form. Some sulphonamides or their conjugates are poorly soluble and deposition of crystals and blockage of the renal tubes can be a serious hazard.

Antibacterial activity

Sulphonamides are bacteriostatic but have a wide spectrum of activity against Gram-positive and negative-cocci and many Gram-negative bacilli. Sulphonamides have been successful in the treatment of acute streptococcal infections, pneumococcal pneumonia, gonorrhoea, meningococcal meningitis, some infections of the gut and many urinary tract infections. Many organisms, however, have now become resistant.

Toxic effects

Renal blockage. This was at one time a major complication made worse by low urinary output and an acid urine. The risk has now been greatly reduced, especially by longer acting sulphonamides such as sulphamethoxazole which are excreted very slowly and by highly soluble sulphonamides. Nevertheless, sulphadiazine (one of the most potent of the sulphonamides) can cause crystalluria and needs to be taken with a high fluid intake.

Hypersensitivity. Sulphonamides can act as haptens and when protein bound act as antigens. The risk varies widely according to the compound used and sulphathiazole, for example, is much more liable to cause reactions than others.

The most common reactions are rashes. Other types of reactions are infrequent.

Stevens-Johnson syndrome, bullous erythema multiforme (p. 211).

Contact dermatitis. Applications of sulphonamide preparations on the skin can cause intractable dermatitis and should not be used. Sulphacetamide eye drops, on the other hand, are useful for many infections.

Blood dyscrasias. Sulphonamides occasionally depress white cell formation and cause agranulocytosis.

Clinical applications

The main uses of sulphonamides are for urinary tract infections and for chronic bronchitis.

In patients with maxillofacial injuries causing leakage of CSF fluid, and therefore at risk from meningitis, sulphadiazine has traditionally been recommended for prophylactic purposes because sulphonamides cross the blood–brain barrier and produce considerably higher concentrations in the CSF than most other antimicrobials. Unfortunately, sulphadiazine is available only as an injection and, moreover, very many strains of meningococci are resistant. Rifampicin is probably, therefore, a better choice for prevention of post-traumatic meningitis. Rifampicin readily crosses the blood–brain barrier and is also effective against staphylococci which may reside in the nose and can cause meningitis.

The use of sulphonamides greatly declined after the introduction of the antibiotics but with the introduction of co-trimoxazole there was a considerable revival in their use.

Co-trimoxazole

Co-trimoxazole is a 5 to 1 mixture of sulphamethoxazole with trimethoprim.

Trimethoprim acts on the same sequential pathways of folic acid metabolism, as do the sulphonamides, but at a later stage, namely the synthesis of folinic acid from folic acid.

This combination of drugs is synergistic (in the true pharmacological sense) in vitro and they may together be bactericidal. Many bacteria which had become resistant to the sulphonamides are (or were) sensitive to co-trimoxazole.

One important limitation of this compound is that optimum levels for synergistic activity may not be achieved in the tissues, sputum or, particularly, in the urine. In some conditions therefore only the trimethoprim component is active.

Toxic effects

These can be caused by the sulphonamide component but although uncommon could be any of those described above.

The main side-effect of co-trimoxazole that might be expected after prolonged administration is induction of folic acid deficiency and macrocytic anaemia. Large doses of co-trimoxazole are needed to produce this effect which is readily reversed by giving folic acid. The risk is slight and patients have been kept on co-trimoxazole for 4 or more years for recurrent urinary infection without ill-effect.

On the other hand, co-trimoxazole can occasionally cause marrow depression and fatal agranulocytosis. The elderly, particularly women, are most at risk.

Clinical applications

Co-trimoxazole is mainly used for respiratory and urinary tract infections. It is effective in suppurative infections and in view of its broad spectrum of bactericidal activity is probably effective for severe infections of dental origin.

Co-trimoxazole has been shown to be more effective than other broad spectrum antibiotics such as ampicillin for a variety of purposes and has also been shown to be effective in some outbreaks of typhoid fever. Clinical trials have also shown that co-trimoxazole or trimethoprim alone are effective in reducing the frequency and severity of attacks of traveller's diarrhoea in high-risk areas such as Mexico. Co-trimoxazole is considered to be the treatment of choice for dysentery (shigellosis) and the prophylactic of choice in severely immunodeficient patients.

Although the introduction of co-trimoxazole largely overcame the problem of resistance to sulphonamides alone, the combination drug has become decreasingly useful for very many purposes because of the increasing frequency of resistance to it. Further, use over the years has made it clear that the incidence of serious adverse effects is approximately twice as great as those caused by amoxycillin, an antibiotic with a broadly similar spectrum of activity and similar applications.

An important recent indication for co-trimoxazole is for *Pneumocystis carinii* pneumonia which is particularly common in patients with AIDS. Although toxic effects are frequent and severe in these patients as a consequence of the high doses that have to be used, they are no greater than with the only other effective alternative, pentamidine.

Trimethoprim without sulphonamide (Ipral) is used for urinary and respiratory tract infections instead of combinations because of the higher incidence of sulphonamide rashes and other allergic responses in long-term use. Trimethoprim may also be effective in the treatment of enteric fever.

Metronidazole

Metronidazole is a synthetic antimicrobial, introduced for and highly effective against trichomoniasis, a common vaginal infection.

Metronidazole is given by mouth, is well absorbed and is active only against bacteria and protozoa which are obligate anaerobes. It is not active against aerobic bacteria or fungi. Metronidazole is highly effective against the organisms causing ulcerative gingivitis, and against other spirochaetes such as that causing syphilis, but less so than penicillin.

Metronidazole is mainly excreted in the urine and also appears in the saliva.

Toxicity

The toxicity of metronidazole seems very low but minor complaints such as nausea or a metallic taste are common. Rashes occasionally develop but are transient. There is interaction with alcohol causing flushing, sweating, palpitations and nausea which is severe enough for metronidazole to be used for the treatment of alcoholism. This may or may not be regarded as an undesirable reaction according to the reader's views. Patients should however be warned against taking alcohol when given metronidazole.

Clinical applications

Metronidazole is the drug of choice for the treatment of acute ulcerative gingivitis. It is at least as effective as penicillin and does not carry with it the dangers of allergic reactions. The narrow spectrum of activity of metronidazole is also an advantage as it does not cause disturbances of the normal oral microflora with the risk of superinfection. Recurrences are probably less common after treatment with metronidazole than with penicillin.

Metronidazole is one of the most effective and widely used drugs for severe anaerobic infections such as may follow escape of bowel contents into the peritoneum, or septic abortion. These infections may become disseminated and metronidazole is often given intravenously in such cases. In addition to its use for acute ulcerative gingivitis, metronidazole can be effective for the treatment of pericoronitis and other dental infections, which are often caused by anaerobes. It must be emphasised, however, that metronidazole is not completely effective against all anaerobic bacteria. Most other antibiotics, apart from the aminoglycosides, are effective against many anaerobes and may therefore be more effective than metronidazole or be used in combination with it for some infections.

THE PENICILLINS

The first antibiotic to be discovered has proved to be one of the safest and, after more than 30 years, still the most generally useful. In the early 1950s it was gloomily prophesied that penicillin would soon become obsolete. The threat by penicillin-resistant organisms was overestimated and penicillins, which include the newer penicillinase-resistant penicillins remain one of, if not the most, widely used group of antibiotics.

The term penicillin when unqualified refers to benzyl penicillin. The many other penicillins will be described with emphasis on their common features with and differences from benzyl penicillin.

The penicillins all act by interfering with bacterial cell wall synthesis and are bactericidal. Most of the penicillins except ampicillin and its analogues have a narrow spectrum of activity. This is not necessarily a disadvantage and penicillin remains the first choice for the treatment of dental infections, the vast majority of which are sensitive.

The chief problem with the penicillins is that of allergy; a patient who is allergic to one form of penicillin reacts to any of them. It must be remembered that many antibiotics with quite different names, such as ampicillin, and Distaquaine are also penicillins. These are all dangerous to the hypersensitised patient.

Mode of action

The cell walls of Gram-positive bacteria consist largely of a mucopeptide. The mucopeptide is synthesised in a series of stages from acetylmuramic acid and other amino sugar molecules to form glucans. These are laid down as long strands in layer upon layer and united by cross linkages until the cell wall consists of a single continuous giant bag-shaped molecule. Penicillins and the closely related cephalosporins inhibit the final crosslinking stage, a process aptly described as 'causing bacteria to drop stitches in the knitting of their overcoats'. This failure of cell wall formation makes the bacteria vulnerable to osmotic damage and leakage of electrolytes.

Bacteria are therefore attacked by penicillins and the cephalosporins at a particular stage in their life cycle (when actively dividing) so that other antibiotics which are bacteriostatic (depress reproduction) may theoretically impair or antagonise this action. This consideration is usually of little practical clinical importance but penicillin and tetracycline are antagonistic and should not be used together.

The main groups of penicillins are:

1. Penicillinase-sensitive penicillins
2. Penicillinase-resistant penicillins
3. Broad spectrum penicillins
4. Antipseudomonal and other special-purpose penicillins

Important features of the main penicillins are summarised in Table 3.1.

Penicillinase-sensitive (natural) penicillins

Benzyl penicillin (Penicillin G). Benzyl penicillin was the first to come into general use. It is mostly destroyed by gastric acid and must be given by injection. This together with the fact that it is also destroyed by bacterial penicillinases are among its few limitations. The fact that it is not effective against many Gram-negative bacilli is not wholly a disadvantage in that in many sites, such as the mouth, these organisms are not important. Further, the relatively narrow spectrum of activity makes superinfection (due to widespread destruction of the mucosal flora) less likely.

After intramuscular injection benzyl penicillin is absorbed within a few minutes, reaches a peak concentration in the blood within half to one hour and is then as rapidly excreted. Most of the excretion is by the kidney and within about 4 hours the blood level is negligible. Penicillin is therefore given in heavy dosage to compensate for this rapid and wasteful excretion.

Penicillin diffuses rapidly into all vascular tissues but poorly into glandular secretions (including saliva) and the CSF. However, penicillin is present in the exudate when tissues are acutely inflamed and hence is effective (for example) in acute ulcerative gingivitis. Penicillin diffuses poorly into fibrotic areas caused by chronic inflammation. In any case with the exception of actinomycosis and syphilis, the organisms causing chronic infections are rarely sensitive to penicillin.

With the exception of penicillinase-producing staphylococci (which are most often found in hospitals), penicillin is highly effective against most Gram-positive and -negative cocci, namely non-penicillinase-producing staphylococci, streptococci, pneumococci and gonococci. *Treponema pallidum*, actinomyces and clostridia among others, are also sensitive.

Phenoxymethyl penicillin (Penicillin V) is resistant to gastric acid and is taken orally. Its activity is almost the same as that of benzyl penicillin and can be used for most of the same purposes. It is usually reliably absorbed particularly from an empty stomach. The main limitations of penicillin by mouth are first that very high serum levels cannot be attained so quickly or so easily as with benzyl penicillin. Second, vomiting may prevent absorption and third, as with any other orally administered drug, reliance has to be placed on the patient to continue to take the drug. This is by no means as certain as might be expected.

Other more highly absorbed semi-synthetic penicillins have been introduced but generally speaking, are more highly protein bound. Small differences in their range of activity also make them less useful than phenoxymethyl penicillin. They have virtually passed out of use.

Clinical uses

Penicillin (in the absence of allergy) is the initial treatment of choice for any severe dental infection. The great majority of these bacteria are sensitive but whenever possible the precise cause of the infection should be determined bacteriologically. Alternatively, complete lack of response after 2 or 3 days of full dosage suggests that another antibiotic may be more effective.

Submaxillary cellulitis (Ludwig's angina) requires immediate large doses of intramuscular penicillin. Acute osteomyelitis of the jaws is another important indication but both of these conditions are now rare. Occasionally it may be justifiable to give penicillin to a patient with an acute alveolar abscess, but *only* if extraction has unavoidably to be delayed or when the patient's resistance is seriously impaired by (for example) immunosuppressive treatment.

Actinomycosis is a chronic infection caused by a filamentous bacterium sensitive to penicillin, but the fibrous reaction characteristic of the disease tends to protect the organism. Penicillin treatment has therefore to be continued for 6 or more weeks. Other antibiotics such as clindamycin appear to be better able to penetrate the poorly vascular tissue and may be more quickly effective.

Since the introduction of metronidazole, penicillin has become obsolete for the treatment of acute ulcerative gingivitis.

Adverse reactions

Penicillin given by the usual routes is virtually non-toxic and in the past enormous doses have been given over long periods without serious ill-effect. Penicillin is toxic to the central nervous system when injected into the CSF and the dose must be greatly restricted when this route is used.

As a result of destruction of part of the flora of the mouth or gut penicillin can lead to superinfection. In the past, use of penicillin lozenges in the mouth was often followed after a few days by redness and soreness of the tongue and buccal mucosa due to superinfection by *Candida albicans*. This form of treatment is not only obsolete but had no rational basis at any time.

The chief adverse effect of all the penicillins is

Table 3.1   The main features of some important antibiotics

	Special properties	Limitations	Useful activity examples	Side-effects of individual agents	Side-effects of the group	Comments
THE PENICILLINS						
Acid-labile penicillins (must be given by injection)						
Natural: Benzyl		Destroyed by penicillinases (especially from staphylococci)	Staphylo-, strepto-pneumo-, gonococci Actinomyces *Trep. pallidum* Clostridia			The most generally useful antibiotic in dentistry
Semi-synthetic: Methicillin	Resistant to staphylococcal penicillinase	Much less active than benzyl penicillin against most pathogens other than staphylococci	Staphylococci	Marrow depression (rarely)	Hypersensitisation common to all penicillins which all show cross-allergy to each other	Little application; replaced by cloxacillin etc.
Acid-resistant penicillins (can be given by mouth)						
Natural: Phenoxymethyl			Similar to benzyl penicillin			The most generally useful oral penicillin in dentistry and other uses
Semi-synthetic: Ampicillin	Broad spectrum	Destroyed by penicillinases	Many Gram-negative (gut) bacilli also sensitive	Rash common		
Amoxycillin	Ditto but better absorption and higher blood levels		Similar to benzyl penicillin	Rash common		Replaces ampicillin as a general-purpose broad spectrum antibiotic
Cloxacillin and flucloxacillin	Penicillinase resistant	Much less active than benzyl and other penicillins against pathogens other than penicillinase-producing staphylococci			Hypersensitisation common to all penicillins which all show cross-allergy to each other	Valuable for infections by penicillinase-producing staphylococci for which it should be reserved

THE CEPHALOSPORINS

			Risk of renal damage / Hypersensitisation less common than to penicillin but sensitivity to both occasionally	
Cephaloridine	Broad spectrum. **Fairly resistant to penicillinase**	Acid labile	Similar to the broad spectrum penicillins	Cross-resistance to both penicillin and cephalosporins e.g. by viridans streptococci, may develop
Cephalexin	Ditto but acid resistant			

OTHER ANTIBIOTICS AND ANTIBACTERIAL AGENTS

Erythromycin	Acid resistant. Hypersensitivity rare	Fairly rapid development of resistance	Similar to benzyl penicillin but also legionella	GIT disturbances — Often second choice for patients allergic to penicillin
Lincomycin	Good penetration of bone and fibrous tissue		Similar to benzyl penicillin but especially effective in bacteroides infections	Diarrhoea common. Occasional cases of colitis — Useful second choice for patients allergic to penicillin
Clindamycin	Good penetration of bone and fibrous tissue, but also better absorbed from the gut than lincomycin		Similar to benzyl penicillin but more active than lincomycin against many organisms	Diarrhoea common. Occasional cases of colitis — Possible second choice for patients allergic to penicillin
Tetracyclines	**Broad spectrum Absorbed from the gut**	Bacteriostatic only. Development of resistance by many pathogens	Widest activity of all	GIT upsets common. Superinfection. Raises the blood urea. Bound to calcium and iron in the diet. Staining of developing teeth — Largely replaced by the broad spectrum bactericidal antibiotics for general purposes. Still the drug of choice for certain exotic infections
Co-trimoxazole (Sulphamethoxazole and trimethoprim)	Broad spectrum. Absorbed from the gut. Bactericidal		At least as wide a range of bactericidal activity as the broad spectrum penicillins	GIT upsets and rashes. Agranulocytosis (rarely) — Broad spectrum bactericidal drug but increasingly widespread resistance
Metronidazole	Absorbed from the gut. Low toxicity. Allergy unknown		Obligate anaerobes including 'Vincent's' organisms	Nausea occasionally. Interaction with alcohol — The drug of choice for ulcerative gingivitis and many other anaerobic infections

that of allergy (hypersensitivity), usually in the form of rashes but occasionally causing fatal anaphylaxis.

Hypersensitivity to the penicillins

The most troublesome and dangerous complication of penicillin treatment is allergy, which probably develops in about 10% of patients but is usually mild.

The most common type of reaction is an irritating rash which may be maculopapular, erythematous or urticarial. A serum-sickness-like reaction with fever and joint pains is less common.

The most dangerous complication is an anaphylactic reaction. This may happen very quickly, within a few minutes after an intramuscular injection of penicillin in a susceptible patient. The patient may notice paraesthesia of the face, feel coldness of the hands and feet, and typically starts to wheeze due to bronchospasm. The face may become obviously oedematous. In a severe case peripheral circulatory failure (shock) with a rapid and severe fall in blood pressure causes pallor, sweating, coldness of the skin, fast thready pulse and loss of consciousness. The patient may not merely become unconscious and virtually pulseless but also cyanotic from inadequate oxygenation of the blood and die within 5 minutes of the onset of the reaction. Although this is a rare reaction to penicillin, the drug is given on so vast a scale that over the years it has caused many deaths.

Generally speaking the faster the onset of the reaction the more severe the reaction is likely to be. Penicillin by mouth hardly ever causes severe anaphylatic reactions, and these are delayed in onset as a result of the slower absorption of the drug.

Mechanisms of penicillin allergy

Reactions are the result of previous exposure to the drug, although the patient may not be aware of having had penicillin in the past. Traces of penicillin are often present in milk for instance as it is used for treatment of bovine mastitis.

Most patients who develop anaphylactic reactions have had a previous reaction to penicillin such as a rash.

The major antigenic determinant appears to be the penicilloyl group which forms as a result of metabolic cleavage of the beta-lactam ring. This product acts as a hapten and binds to body proteins to become antigenic.

Most persons receiving penicillin develop IgG or IgM antibodies but only a small minority have, by a variety of mechanisms, reactions. Specific IgE antibodies to penicillin form rarely, but are the cause of anaphylactic reactions, by binding to mast cells and causing release of mediators. Contrary to traditional belief and surprisingly, there appears to be no association between penicillin anaphylaxis and the common types of IgE-mediated allergies (atopic disease) which result from the same mechanisms.

On the rare occasions when no other antibiotic than a penicillin is likely to be effective for a life-threatening infection, it may be possible to predict the possibility of an IgE-mediated response and an anaphylactic reaction by skin testing with benzyl-penicilloyl polylysine, which gives a wheal and flare reaction within 10 minutes. Only about 10% of those who claim to be allergic to penicillin react positively in this way. Anaphylaxis is virtually unknown in those who give negative reactions to this test. However, even skin testing is not entirely safe, has caused occasional deaths and should only be carried out in expert hands with adequate precautions for dealing with emergencies.

Knowledge of penicillin allergy is somewhat fragmentary as anaphylactic reactions are rare: their incidence is reported to be only 0.01–0.05% in patients receiving penicillin. Moreover from the practical viewpoint, reliance will generally have to be placed on the history and an alternative given when the patient claims to be allergic to penicillin. In practice, therefore, the only reasonably safe lines of action are:

1. Make sure there is no history of previous reactions by asking patients whether they have had any ill-effects of any sort from penicillin.

2. Even when the history is negative, make sure that emergency drugs are handy.

The reason for this latter precaution is that, *very rarely*, a patient with a completely negative history or who has had penicillin on several previous occasions without ill-effect, has an anaphylactic reaction as the first manifestation of penicillin allergy.

Anaphylactic reactions to penicillin during the course of general anaesthesia have been described but the problems of recognising and managing such a situation are easier to imagine than to effect.

It is important, incidentally, not to give penicillin (or any other drug) by injection with the patient standing. Fainting after injection is considerably more common than loss of consciousness caused by anaphylaxis, but either can cause the patient to fall and be injured.

All these warnings sound as if penicillin should be avoided altogether, but in practice the rarity of severe reactions is such that, provided a few simple precautions are taken, they are unlikely to be seen.

The management of anaphylaxis is discussed in Chapter 19.

Long-acting penicillins

Procaine penicillin is a stable salt which when injected intramuscularly releases penicillin over 12 to 24 hours but achieves a low plateau blood level. Procaine penicillin with benzyl penicillin (fortified procaine penicillin) is used to get a higher peak level. Benethamine penicillin is much less soluble and a single intramuscular dose will provide a low concentration of penicillin in the blood for 4 or 5 days. Proprietary preparations use a mixture of soluble and 'insoluble' penicillins to try to get the best of all worlds. An example is Triplopen which is benzyl, procaine and benethamine penicillin.

The sole purpose of such preparations is to save repeated injections when there is any doubt whether oral penicillin will be taken regularly. But if a patient is allergic to penicillin then long-acting penicillins have worse effects from the continued release of the allergen over a long period.

The semi-synthetic penicillins

The isolation of the penicillin nucleus (6-amino penicillanic acid) was followed by the synthesis of several thousand different semisynthetic penicillins. This remarkable effort however yielded only a few agents with important advantages, but which nevertheless have greatly broadened the usefulness of the penicillins as follows:

Penicillinase-resistant penicillins

The first of these was methicillin; this is destroyed by gastric acid and has to be given by injection. Cloxacillin and its many congeners (the oxazolyl penicillins) are resistant to acid and can be given orally. Flucloxacillin is more completely absorbed and has a more prolonged action than cloxacillin. These penicillins help to overcome the problem caused by penicillinase-producing staphylococci.

It must be emphasised that the range of activity of these penicillinase-resistant penicillins is narrow and they are less effective against other common pathogens such as streptococci than benzyl penicillin. Therefore, there is rarely any indication for the use of cloxacillin in dentistry. It should only be used when there is clear bacteriological evidence that the infection is due to penicillinase-producing staphylococci. This is so uncommon in dentistry as to be an almost non-existent problem. However, bacterial (ascending) parotitis is sometimes caused by penicillinase-producing staphylococci, in which case flucloxacillin may be the drug of choice.

Broad spectrum penicillins

Ampicillin. This is acid stable (is active orally) and is effective against many Gram-negative bacilli in addition to those susceptible to benzyl penicillin. Ampicillin has a spectrum of activity almost as wide as that of tetracycline but with the additional advantage that it is bactericidal. Like benzyl penicillin, ampicillin and its relatives are destroyed by penicillinase. Ampicillin is somewhat less active against organisms sensitive to benzyl penicillin.

The main uses of the broad spectrum penicillins are in the treatment of respiratory and urinary infections.

Amoxycillin (Amoxil) has almost identical properties to ampicillin and a similar antibacterial spectrum when given by mouth. However, the peak blood levels reached are twice as high and food does not significantly interfere with absorption.

In dentistry, amoxycillin is suggested as the drug of choice for the prophylaxis of infective endocarditis as discussed later.

For urinary tract infections, a simple regimen of treatment is to give two large (3 g) doses of amoxycillin at intervals of 12 hours.

Side-effects. Ampicillin and amoxycillin carry with them the same risks of allergy as other penicillins but cause other rashes more frequently. These rashes are particularly common in those with infectious mononucleosis or with disordered antibody production from any other cause, but are not apparently associated with any increased risk of anaphylactic reactions.

Clavulanate

Clavulanate has little anti-bacterial activity but inhibits most of the β-lactamases which degrade many penicillins. Clavulanate with amoxycillin (Augmentin) is useful for penicillin-resistant staphylococci, gonococci and many strains of *E. coli*.

Unfortunately, penicillin resistance by viridans streptococci depends on a different mechanism and Augmentin does not appear to be of value for those who harbour resistant strains of viridans streptococci in the mouth.

Antipseudomonal and other special purpose penicillins

Increasing numbers of special-purpose penicillins such as piperacillin and mecillinam have become available particularly for use in pseudomonas and other Gram-negative bacilli such as severe salmonella infections. These penicillins have virtually no use in dentistry.

THE CEPHALOSPORINS

The cephalosporins have a chemical nucleus somewhat similar to that of penicillin and a similar mode of action. The first useful member of the group – *cephaloridine* – is destroyed by acid and has to be given by injection. It has been followed by a succession of acid-resistant analogues.

Although cephalosporins can often be given safely to patients allergic to penicillin, they are no longer regarded as suitable alternatives, as a result of the increasing prevalence of sensitivity to both groups of drugs. About 10% of patients allergic to penicillin are also allergic to the cephalosporins.

The main differences in the range of activity of the cephalosporins when compared with penicillin are therefore that cephalosporins are effective (a) against many penicillinase-producing staphylococci and (b) against many Gram-negative (gut) bacilli. The range of activity of the cephalosporins is somewhat similar to that of ampicillin – they are bactericidal to the common Gram-positive and Gram-negative cocci and to many Gram-negative bacilli. Unlike ampicillin, the cephalosporins are relatively resistant to penicillinase and are effective against many penicillinase-producing staphylococci. Nevertheless, there are few occasions when cephalosporins are the antibiotics of first choice.

Cephradine

Cephradine can be given by mouth or by injection. The latter might, rarely, be of use in a severe dental infection such as osteomyelitis where the causal bacteria had been shown to be sensitive. There are few occasions, therefore, when this antibiotic would have any advantages.

Other injectable cephalosporins such as cefuroxime and cephazolin are available for specific indications. Cefuroxime, for example, is more effective against *Haemophilus influenzae* and *N. gonorrhoeae*.

Cephalexin

Cephalezin is acid stable, is usually well absorbed and is subject to a very low degree of protein binding. It is more effective against certain Gram-negative gut bacilli than either cephaloridine or ampicillin but, apart from specific infections, the advantages of cephalexin are not such that it should be regarded as a 'general purpose' antibiotic.

Side-effects of the cephalosporins

The risk of hypersensitivity to the cephalosporins has already been mentioned. These agents are also more prone than the penicillins to cause superinfections, especially by *Candida albicans*.

Some of the newer cephalosporins can also interfere with haemostasis (see Ch. 12) to cause haemorragic tendencies.

Cephalosporins versus penicillins for dental use

The range of activity of the cephalosporins is not particularly relevant to dental infections.

When there is allergy to penicillin it is better to use agents whose structure differs more completely from penicillin, such as erythromycin. The latter also has the advantage of being unlikely to provoke hypersensitivity at all and certainly shows no cross sensitivity to penicillin.

Another possible limitation of the cephalosporins in relation to penicillin is that organisms may show cross-resistance. Viridans streptococci resistant to penicillin are also resistant to cephalosporins which are not therefore an appropriate alternative choice for the patient who has recently had penicillin.

In summary, a cephalosporin should only be given on the rare occasions when there is a specific bacteriological indication.

THE AMINOGLYCOSIDES

Streptomycin

Streptomycin is a bactericidal antibiotic which acts by interfering with bacterial protein synthesis. It is one of a large group of *aminoglycoside* antibiotics.

Streptomycin is poorly absorbed from the gut and is usually given by intramuscular injection. Its main use is for the treatment of tuberculosis and it has contributed to the low incidence of this disease in many countries today. Streptomycin is also effective against many Gram-negative bacilli and some staphylococci.

The management of tuberculosis is an example of controlled and effective combined antimicrobial chemotherapy that minimises toxicity and prevents emergence of resistant strains. The currently recommended initial phase treatment is with isoniazid and rifampicin supplemented by ethambutol or streptomycin.

Streptomycin is synergistic with penicillin which together form a highly effective bactericidal combination. This is valuable for the management of some dangerous infections such as infective endocarditis.

Toxic effects

Streptomycin and other aminoglycosides have a peculiarly specific and disabling toxic effect on the eighth nerve. The individual aminoglycosides vary in whether hearing or vestibular function is first affected. In some cases deafness or loss of balance is permanent. The severity of the effect depends both on the particular drug and individual susceptibility, but in general is determined by the overall dosage and age – the larger the overall dose and the older the patient, the greater the risk.

Another toxic effect of the aminoglycosides is that of mild neuromuscular blockade – this may be sufficient to potentiate the effect of curare and similar agents during anaesthesia.

Many aminoglycosides can also cause renal damage. This is made worse by the fact that excretion is then impaired and the concentration of the antibiotic in the body increases correspondingly.

Hypersensitivity. Rashes or drug fever affect a few patients but are typically mild. Among those who handle streptomycin frequently, particularly nurses and pharmacists, sensitisation of the skin is common and there may be severe contact dermatitis.

Dental applications of the aminoglycosides

Streptomycin itself has no important dental application. Neomycin has been used with bacitracin as a root canal paste, but with no proven advantages. Gentamicin is currently recommended for prophylaxis against infective endocarditis in dental patients for use in combination with intramuscular amoxycillin when the dental operation has to be performed under a general anaesthetic (p. 223). Only a relatively small dose of amoxycillin can be given by intramuscular injection, and in such circumstances gentamicin provides a valuable bactericidal supplement.

ERYTHROMYCIN

Erythromycin has a narrow spectrum of activity closely similar to that of penicillin. It is bactericidal in adequate concentrations and acts on growing organisms by interfering with protein synthesis.

Erythromycin is usually given by mouth but its activity is reduced by gastric acid. It is therefore given as enteric-coated tablets or as the stearate or estolate.

Erythromycin ethylsuccinate is used in place of the stearate in erythromycin mixture. The absorption of all forms of erythromycin from the gut is however highly variable so that adequate plasma levels may not be achieved.

Toxic effects

Toxicity of the basic agent is minimal but there may occasionally be nausea or vomiting. Erythromycin estolate by contrast can, after about 10 days' treatment, cause liver damage with pain, fever and often jaundice. If the drug is then stopped there is complete recovery.

Apart from this hepatotoxic effect of erythromycin estolate other preparations of erythromycin are among the most harmless of the antibiotics.

Clinical applications

The applications are essentially the same as for penicillin for which erythromycin is the main alternative to penicillin but it is also effective for legionnaire's disease. Erythromycin is used in dentistry, in prophylaxis against bacterial endocarditis.

The main drawback to more prolonged courses of erythromycin is the relatively rapid emergence of resistant strains. This applies not merely to staphylococci but even to haemolytic streptococci.

CLINDAMYCIN AND LINCOMYCIN

These related agents are completely unlike any other antibiotic in chemical structure. Their spectrum of activity generally resembles that of erythromycin or penicillin, although there are variations. Streptococci in general and many staphylococci are highly sensitive to clindamycin as are bacteroides species (Gram-negative anaerobic bacilli) and veillonella (anaerobic cocci) which may possibly be important in periodontal disease.

Clindamycin is for most purposes more effective than lincomycin and generally therefore replaces the latter. However, both are absorbed when given by mouth but clindamycin is remarkably well absorbed even from a full stomach or by patients with malabsorption syndrome and attains substantially higher blood levels.

Clindamycin and lincomycin appear to diffuse unusually effectively through all tissues (although the concentration in the CSF is low) and particu-

larly into bone and fibrous connective tissue. The toxicity of these compounds is low and enormous doses of lincomycin have been given to some patients without significant ill-effects.

Toxic effects. Hypersensitivity to either compound appears to be no more than a theoretical risk so far and attempts to induce it artificially have failed.

The most common side-effect of these drugs is diarrhoea.

The main danger of lincomycin and clindamycin is the risk of pseudomembranous colitis and, although overall the incidence of this complication is small, it is considerably higher than with other antibiotics. The cause of antibiotic-induced colitis is the proliferation of relatively resistant, toxigenic clostridia, particularly *C. difficile*. If pseudomembranous colitis develops it usually responds to oral vancomycin or metronidazole. Colitis can however be hazardous, especially to elderly and debilitated patients, particularly when under treatment with a variety of drugs. In other cases colitis seems to be self-limiting if the drug is stopped at the first sign, i.e. abdominal pain or passage of watery stools and mucus. It would be unreasonable therefore to withhold what seem to be very effective agents where needed, since the level of risk appears to be low in most patients. It must also be appreciated that colitis has occasionally followed the use of a wide variety of antibiotics including the penicillins.

Clinical applications

Clindamycin may have considerable advantages because of the effectiveness of absorption and its ability to get into bone and through fibrous tissue. There is no problem of cross-allergenicity or cross-resistance of bacteria to penicillin and these too are advantages.

The risk of pseudomembranous colitis, however, has lead to the recommendation that clindamycin be used only where there are specific bacteriological indications such as staphylococcal bone or joint infections or anaerobic infections, particularly by bacteroides species.

Despite this risk of pseudomembranous colitis, clindamycin is recommended in other parts of Europe as an alternative to penicillin for the prevention of endocarditis. Diarrhoea may be a nuisance even for short courses of treatment.

THE TETRACYCLINES

These agents, for which the term 'broad spectrum' was coined, have the widest range of activity of all antibiotics. They are effective against virtually all common groups of pathogenic bacteria (whether Gram-negative or -positive), mycoplasma, rickettsias, chlamydia, and even have some activity against tuberculosis and the malaria parasite. The only major group which is completely resistant are the fungi and viruses.

Tetracyclines are bacteriostatic, and may be antagonistic to bactericidal drugs, particularly penicillin.

Many bacteria, particularly strains of staphylococci and coliforms, have become resistant to the tetracyclines however.

Absorption

Tetracyclines are absorbed from the gastrointestinal tract and are usually given by mouth.

Absorption is never complete, and residual drug can cause some adverse effects in the gut. Tetracyclines combine with (chelate) divalent metals such as calcium or iron salts and these impede absorption of each other.

Tetracyclines are excreted in the urine, bile and faeces.

Mode of action. Tetracycline interferes with protein synthesis by bacteria and also to some extent by the host.

Toxic effects

Gastrointestinal disturbances

Minor effects such as discomfort, diarrhoea, nausea or vomiting are common especially with large doses and seem to be due to direct irritation.

Superinfection

Proliferation of *Candida albicans* or staphylococci is the result of the broad spectrum of activity of the tetracyclines and suppression of the greater part of the mouth or gut flora.

Candidal infection usually appears as oral thrush, acute antibiotic stomatitis, or sometimes as pruritis ani.

Tetracyclines are often used topically in the mouth quite empirically for the treatment of various types of ulceration. In susceptible patients this can lead to *C. albicans* infections (antibiotic stomatitis or thrush) sometimes within 48 hours (see Ch. 18).

The most severe type of superinfection is staphylococcal enterocolitis where swarms of antibiotic-resistant staphylococci invade the gut mucosa causing widespread superficial necrosis, diarrhoea, dehydration, circulatory collapse and often death. This complication mainly follows gastrointestinal surgery and the cause having been recognised has become rare.

Renal and metabolic complications

Tetracyclines interfere with protein synthesis and have an anti-anabolic effect. This causes increased excretion of nitrogen and a rise in blood urea even in otherwise normal patients. If the patient has pre-existing renal disease, renal failure can be precipitated. *Minocycline* and *doxycycline* do not however aggravate renal dysfunction.

Excessively high dosage of tetracyclines can cause liver damage.

Staining of the teeth

Since tetracyclines bind calcium salts they are incorporated into bones and teeth if given during calcification. The effect on the teeth is visible since tetracycline is laid down along the incremental lines of deposition of both enamel and dentine. If more than a minimal dose of tetracycline is given the teeth appear yellow when they erupt but gradually change to grey, brown or intermediate shades. The staining is permanent and if it affects the anterior teeth can be surprisingly disfiguring. The only way to prevent this effect is to avoid the use of tetracyclines during the last third of pregnancy and for at least the first 6 years of infant life. Calcification of the teeth extends over a longer period but these suggested guidelines will prevent any conspicuous effect.

The nature of this staining can be confirmed by

examining a ground section of tooth under ultra-violet light which causes the tetracyline to fluoresce a brilliant yellow. Intact teeth fluoresce under ultraviolet light only if exceptionally heavily stained.

It is now widely accepted that there are exceedingly few specific indications for using tetracycline in children under 8 and that, apart from some rare and exotic infections, other antibiotics are at least as effective.

Binding of divalent metals

Calcium or magnesium salts taken for peptic ulcer or indigestion are bound by tetracycline to form insoluble complexes which are not absorbed. The effect can be avoided by spacing out the times when the different drugs are taken.

Iron salts (taken for anaemia) are also chelated by tetracycline to form insoluble complexes.

Clinical applications

There is little to choose between the different tetracyclines and tetracycline itself or oxytetracycline is usually used. *Demeclocycline* is longer acting and needs only to be given 12-hourly.

Minocycline has a somewhat broader spectrum of activity and is active against the meningococcus.

The exceptionally broad spectrum of activity of tetracyclines has led to their widespread use for immediate treatment of all types of infection where (as is often the case) the precise bacteriological diagnosis has not been established, or as a second choice to penicillin.

This has proved effective for many respiratory and urinary infections but the increasing number of resistant organisms and the advent of broad spectrum antibiotics which are also bactericidal, such as ampicillin and co-trimoxazole, have greatly reduced the need to use tetracyclines.

There are some absolute indications for tetracycline but these are mainly exotic infections such as typhus or trachoma due to rickettsia and chlamydia, respectively. In infective diarrhoea replacement of fluid and electrolytes is the first essential. Antibacterials may also prolong the carrier phase.

There are few if any strong indications for tetracyclines in dentistry since most infections are either sensitive to penicillin or, where this is contraindicated, other bactericidal agents are used.

The use of tetracycline mouth rinses for oral ulceration has been mentioned and relief from symptoms or accelerated healing has been claimed for herpetic ulceration, recurrent aphthae and erosive lichen planus. The effectiveness of tetracycline for this purpose has been demonstrated in double blind trials both in the UK and the USA, even though the mechanism of its effect remains problematical. Since tetracycline used topically in this way is particularly prone to cause superinfection and candidosis, it should be given in combination with an antifungal agent. A convenient preparation is Mysteclin elixir which contains tetracycline and amphotericin in a syrup.

The broad spectrum of activity of tetracycline, particularly its activity against many anaerobes and Gram-negative species, and its binding to or etching of hard tissues has led to its use against severe periodontal disease. For this purpose it can be given orally or, in minute doses, directly into pockets in special slow-release preparations.

CHLORAMPHENICOL

Chloramphenicol was the second of the broad spectrum antibiotics to be introduced. Like tetracycline, chloramphenicol is bacteriostatic but although it is active against a slightly narrower range of microorganisms it has the outstanding advantage that it was, and for a long time remained, the only drug effective against *Salmonella typhi* and is useful for some anaerobic and other specific infections.

Chloramphenicol is resistant to gastric acid and is adequately absorbed when given by mouth.

Mode of action and activity

Choramphenicol is a potent inhibitor of bacterial protein synthesis.

Choramphenicol is at least as effective as tetracycline against the commoner Gram-positive cocci and Gram-negative bacilli but has no special advantages except in the treatment of typhoid fever and some anaerobic infections.

Toxic effects

The outstanding danger of chloramphenicol is its toxic action on the bone marrow. This complication is so dangerous (being often irreversible and fatal) and the range of alternative antibiotics available is so wide that its use is justifiable only for severe infections when no more effective drug is available.

The mechanism of chloramphenicol's toxicity to the marrow is not known. It was at one time believed to be the result of prolonged treatment but fatal cases have followed a few grams so that it has been suggested that in some way the marrow may be sensitised to the drug or that there is a genetically determined susceptibility.

Clinical applications

The only occasion when chloramphenicol should be used is for a life-threatening infection which has been shown not to be sensitive to any other antibiotic, for example, for typhoid fever. Since this is such a dangerous infection the risks associated with chloramphenicol have to be accepted.

Chloramphenicol is also valuable for intracranial infections such as meningitis caused by *H. influenzae* because of its ability to cross the blood–brain barrier and enter the CSF.

Chloramphenicol has no indications in dentistry. Nevertheless it has been, and in some quarters continues to be used as a component of root canal pastes. The reason for this appears largely to be its physical properties of stability and lack of colour. The value of antibiotic-containing root canal pastes is anyway highly questionable since surgical debridement of the canal and complete filling are more important. Neither chloramphenicol nor any other antibiotic is a safeguard against faulty technique, and however slight the risks may be in this application it seems peculiarly pointless to use a dangerous drug where its value is so doubtful.

VANCOMYCIN

Vancomycin is a bactericidal drug effective only against Gram-positive bacteria and has limited but important clinical uses. It is not absorbed from the gut, but is intensely irritant when injected. Vancomycin has, therefore, to be given greatly diluted by slow intravenous infusion.

Thrombophlebitis and fever are common. Rashes and reversible marrow depression are other possible complications but the most serious toxic effect, especially with high doses, is damage to hearing.

Vancomycin is used for severe staphylococcal and streptococcal infections such as some cases of infective endocarditis and is recommended for special risk patients in danger of developing the latter (Appendix I).

Vancomycin by mouth is usually effective in controlling antibiotic-associated pseudomembranous colitis (p. 32).

RIFAMPICIN

Rifampicin is a potent anti-tuberculous agent but is effective against many other pathogens. It is the recommended prophylactic agent against post-traumatic meningitis and for those exposed to meningococcal infection.

Rifampicin affects liver function; it is a potent hepatic enzyme inducer and accelerates the metabolism of many drugs such as anticoagulants and oral contraceptives, reducing their effectiveness. In prolonged courses rifampicin can cause liver damage, particularly in those with pre-existing liver disease. Among many other possible side-effects, rifampicin colours the saliva and urine orange.

PREVENTION OF INFECTIVE ENDOCARDITIS

Infective endocarditis is a serious infection that can occasionally follow dental treatment. Predisposing factors are the presence of a cardiac valvular defect or a prosthetic heart valve, and a bacteraemia. Historically, the first identified cause of bacteraemias in otherwise healthy persons was dental extractions, but there are many other possible causes ranging from invasive medical procedures to intravenous drug addiction. Dental operations can be incriminated in only about 15% of cases of infective endocarditis.

Most cases of infective endocarditis, when of dental origin, are caused by viridans streptococci which are usually sensitive to penicillin. Patients at risk from infective endocarditis should be given an antibiotic prophylactically, particularly before dental extractions or scaling. Those who are not allergic to penicillin should take 3 g of amoxycillin orally 1 hour before the operation, in the presence of the dentist or dental nurse. The recommendation to use amoxycillin is based on the fact that this drug is rapidly and reliably absorbed. Further, 3 g of amoxycillin produce higher and more prolonged bactericidal blood levels than can be readily produced by an acceptable regimen of injected antibiotics.

Those who are allergic to penicillin should take 1.5 g of erythromycin under supervision 1–2 hours before operation and 0.5 g 6 hours later. The reasons for this divided dose regimen is that erythromycin is less well absorbed than amoxycillin and in doses over 1.5 g may occasionally cause severe nausea.

Almost any dental procedure – even toothbrushing – can cause bacteraemia, but only extractions and scaling appear to offer a significant risk of infective endocarditis.

In all cases (whether or not antibiotics have been given) it is essential to warn all patients at risk to report any illness that has no obvious cause and which develops within 3 months after a dental operation. Infective endocarditis typically has an exceedingly insidious origin and late diagnosis significantly increases both the morbidity and mortality.

For full details of the currently recommended antimicrobial regimens for prevention of infective endocarditis, see Appendix I.

Risks versus benefits of antibiotic prophylaxis for infective endocarditis

The need for antibiotic cover in the prevention of endocarditis has been questioned by some. Many patients at risk have had no trouble after dental extractions without antibiotic cover. It has, as a consequence, been suggested that giving antibiotics in this way may be unnecessary and the risks might, overall, be greater than the hoped-for benefits.

Although in theory it might be desirable to cover other procedures such as endodontics, there is little evidence of any need to do so and, in addition, use of prophylactic antibiotics on too many occasions increases both the risk of producing penicillin-resistant bacteria* and of inducing hypersensitivity in the patient.

---

*Some penicillin-resistant viridans streptococci emerge within 24 hours and are not submerged for at least a month.

It is also clear that dental operations are increasingly uncommon antecedents of infective endocarditis and in some large American series have accounted for only 6–10% of cases. Since non-dental procedures are now more important, the peak age-group at risk has also steadily risen until it is now in the sixth decade. The persistently high mortality (30%) is mainly therefore a consequence of infections with pathogens such as *S. aureus* or *C. albicans* in patients who are elderly or debilitated.

It is notable that before the introduction of penicillin, rheumatic heart disease was more common, no prophylaxis was available for dental extractions, extractions were even more frequently carried out then, and infective endocarditis was always fatal. Nevertheless, even in those days infective endocarditis was a rare disease and apparently no more common than today.

On the other hand, the risks associated with bacterial endocarditis are so high that an attempt must be made to protect these patients. Further, it would not be feasible but obviously unethical to carry out the necessary clinical experiments to determine the optimal measures to be taken.

One has therefore to accept that, on the one hand, both the necessity for and the efficacy of conventional antibiotic regimens are unproven but, on the other hand, it is mandatory to give antibiotic cover to patients at risk, particularly before a dental extraction.

Other prophylactic uses of antibiotics in dentistry

Penicillin may also be given prophylactically before dental operations on patients whose resistance is impaired (by blood dyscrasias for instance) and to patients with severe maxillofacial injuries or who have had major oral surgery. Co-trimoxazole or rifampicin are preferable if the cranial cavity has been broken into, as penicillin does not cross the normal blood–brain barrier.

ANTIFUNGAL AGENTS

Fungal infections fall into two main categories. There are the common superficial infections of the skin such as ringworm or athlete's foot caused by organisms collectively known as dermatophytes.

The other group are the systemic or deep mycoses which are often dangerous and difficult to treat. They are increasingly important as a complication in many situations where the patient's defences are severely impaired. An obvious example is in transplant surgery or any other situation where immunosuppressive drugs are used.

Candida albicans is one of the most common causes of systemic mycoses but is unusual in that it can also cause superficial infections particularly of the mouth, vagina and skin.

These two types of fungal infection also differ in their response to antifungal agents; most drugs effective against the dermatophytes are ineffective against the systemic mycoses and vice versa.

Fungal infections, particularly the systemic mycoses, are difficult to overcome and, although the various antifungal agents are specific and often fungicidal, they are rarely as quickly or reliably effective as the antibiotics for bacterial infections. It is true that fungal infections tend to become established in patients with impaired defence mechanisms, but even superficial infections due to dermatophytes are often remarkably persistent for no very clear reason.

Nystatin

Nystatin and amphotericin, which are chemically similar *polyenes*, act by linking themselves to the fungal cell membrane. In so doing, 'holes' form in the membrane which becomes unable as a result to protect the normal fluid and electrolyte balance of the cell contents. *C. albicans* does not become resistant to nystatin (or amphotericin) in clinical use.

Nystatin is both almost insoluble and toxic when injected. It can as a result only be used topically, particularly in the gastrointestinal tract. Since the solubility is so low, nystatin is not absorbed to any significant extent; under these circumstances it is non-toxic and does not cause hypersensitivity. It has a bitter and unpleasant flavour and may for this reason occasionally cause nausea or be intolerable to the patient.

Clinical applications

Nystatin is effective against a number of fungi, of which the most important is *C. albicans*, the causative organism of thrush, denture stomatitis and of the several varieties of mucocutaneous candidosis.

Since it is not absorbed, nystatin tablets have to be allowed to dissolve in the mouth if they are to have any effect on oral infections. Since dentures also seem to provide an environment favourable to the growth of *C. albicans* these should be removed during treatment and disinfected.

Amphotericin

This is similar to nystatin in chemical structure and mode of action but is absorbed from the gut to a small degree. Amphotericin is somewhat less toxic systematically than nystatin and can be given intravenously for systemic fungal infections such as candidal endocarditis.

Toxic effects

Intravenous injection may be followed by unpleasant effects such as nausea, vomiting and fever. Renal damage is the most serious problem; it is an inevitable complication once a minimal dosage is exceeded and can cause irreversible renal failure. These risks are only acceptable in the treatment of severe fungal infections which are otherwise lethal and obviously such a drug should only be given when the diagnosis is absolutely certain. Hypersensitivity may also force treatment to be stopped.

Clinical applications

Amphotericin can be used in the same way as nystatin for superficial candidal infections and has the advantage of a less unpleasant flavour. Used in this way, it is a safe drug. The use of amphotericin for systemic mycoses has been described above.

Antifungal agents are often used prophylactically before transplant surgery as *C. albicans*, for example, from the patient's own mouth could be the source of disseminated infection under these circumstances. While the organisms are confined to the gastrointestinal tract there is a reasonable chance of controlling them at least temporarily, without risk.

Flucytosine (Alcobon)

Flucytosine is an antifungal agent which has considerably less systemic toxicity than amphotericin for systemic fungal infections. It is well absorbed from the gastrointestinal tract but has a narrow spectrum and is effective mainly for urinary candidosis. Resistance to flucytosine emerges relatively readily and as a result this drug seems ultimately less effective for systemic infections (candidal septicaemia or endocarditis) than drugs such as amphotericin which are more toxic. Nausea, vomiting, rashes and occasionally leucopenia have been reported but resolved when the drug was stopped.

Imidazole antifungal agents

The *imidazole* antifungal agents are unusual in that, unlike the polyenes, they are effective against superficial dermatophytes as well as many deep or systematised mycoses. In addition, the imidazoles are effective against some bacteria and are well absorbed from the gut. Examples are miconazole, ketoconazole and (for topical application on the skin) clotrimazole.

For systemic fungal infections such as candidal endocarditis the imidazoles are considerably less toxic than amphotericin but there is some doubt as to whether they are as effective. Miconazole is available as tablets and as an oral gel which can be used for oral candidal infections. Ketoconazole is available in tablet form and is useful in otherwise intractable candidal infections such as chronic candidal leukoplakia or candidosis in immunosuppressed patients.

The chief toxic effect of ketoconazole is liver damage which is occasionally severe, particularly after prolonged heavy dosage.

Miconazole may also be useful for angular stomatitis when there is a mixed candidal and staphylococcal infection.

ANTIVIRAL AGENTS

Antiviral agents are a development of little more than the last decade. The problem is peculiarly difficult in that viruses have no enzyme systems which can be blocked and for purposes of reproduction colonise the host's cells whose nucleic acid metabolism becomes perverted to suit the virus.

The antiviral agents proper are all synthetic. Their effectiveness is somewhat limited.

Idoxuridine

Idoxuridine closely resembles thymidine in structure and acts as a thymine antagonist. It is as a consequence active against DNA viruses, particularly superficial infections by the herpes group.

Idoxuridine has been chiefly used for ocular infections by herpes simplex (herpetic keratitis) which endangers eyesight. It is used in the form of eye drops for this purpose and is effective.

Idoxuridine seems to be less effective for recurrent herpes (herpes labialis), but this may be because the standard (0.1%) solution is too weak.

Herpes zoster may also respond to idoxuridine as eye drops when the first division of the trigeminal nerve is affected or as a cutaneous application for other sites. For the latter purpose it is available as a 5% solution (Herpid) in a vehicle (dimethyl sulphoxide) which enables it to penetrate the skin. This can also be used for herpes labialis. The main disadvantage is the high cost.

Idoxuridine has been replaced by acyclovir, which is more effective and less toxic, for many clinical indications.

Acyclovir

Acyclovir (Zovirax) is an analogue of a natural nucleoside and is effective against herpes simplex and zoster.

Action of acyclovir

The herpes simplex virus has a core of DNA of which deoxyguanosine is a building unit, while acyclovir is a deoxyguanosine analogue which readily enters human cells. When such cells contain herpes virus, viral thymidine kinase rapidly converts acyclovir to its monophosphate. This process is remarkably rapid since acyclovir binds strongly to and is phosphorylated more than a million times faster by viral thymidine kinase than by the comparable host enzyme. Once phosphorylated, acyclovir is unable to escape from the cell and is progressively converted to the triphosphate.

Viral DNA polymerase takes up acyclovir

triphosphate and incorporates it into viral DNA, in mistake for normal deoxyguanosine triphosphate. Thereafter, viral DNA production is blocked because no further units can be joined to the terminal acyclovir compound.

Host cell DNA polymerase, by contrast, will not incorporate acyclovir triphosphate; as a consequence there is no interference with host DNA production and acyclovir has an unusual degree of selectivity of action against herpes viruses. Also unlike most antiviral agents, acyclovir has unusually low toxicity, because of its highly specific action.

Unlike most antiviral agents, acyclovir because of its low toxicity can also be given intravenously for severe infections such as herpetic encephalitis.

Clinical applications

Acyclovir cream is used as a topical application for herpes labialis but has to be applied in the initial, prodroma, stage. Thereafter when blistering starts, viral damage has extended through the epithelium and the best that can be expected of an antiviral drug then is to limit the development of new crops of lesions. Acyclovir is moderately well absorbed from the gastrointestinal tract and is available as tablets or a mixture for oral administration and to achieve a systemic effect for more serious infections such as herpes zoster. Trigeminal herpes zoster which can cause intense pain as well as a facial rash, stomatitis and sometimes ocular damage can be a disabling disease especially in the elderly for whom large doses of oral acyclovir are indicated. Unfortunately acyclovir has no effect on latent herpes viruses, but if given long term will suppress recurrences. However this is not often feasible.

Intravenous acyclovir is mainly used for severe herpetic infections in immunodeficient patients and is now used prophylactically for these high-risk patients. As a consequence the incidence, as well as the morbidity and mortality from such infections has been significantly reduced.

Resistance to acyclovir can develop but does not appear to limit the usefulness of the drug in clinical use.

The chief toxic effects of acyclovir are raised blood urea or liver enzyme levels but these are reversible and only likely to cause concern when large doses of acyclovir are given intravenously.

Vidarabine is also an effective antiherpetic agent but has to be given by slow intravenous infusion. It is also more prone to cause troublesome toxic effects than acyclovir and does not appear to have any compensating advantages.

Amantadine

This antiviral agent is an effective prophylactic against influenza A_2 and has been approved for this purpose in the USA. It also has a therapeutic effect on the infection in the early stages. The severity of an attack of influenza may be diminished.

Amantadine has the advantages that, unlike a vaccine, it is not substrain specific. It can therefore be used when a major outbreak of influenza is anticipated but the substrain is unknown or unusual.

Amantadine can be given to those for whom vaccine is contraindicated. It is also of value to those with chronic respiratory disease who have just acquired the infection when it may improve respiratory function.

Amantadine has also been claimed to be of value in the treatment of herpes zoster but this has not been widely confirmed.

Strangely, amantadine is also used in the treatment of Parkinson's disease.

Zidovudine

This drug, formerly known as azidothymidine (AZT), is the only antiviral drug as yet which has been shown to be of clinical benefit in AIDS by its action on the human immunodeficiency virus (HIV).

Zidovudine is a synthetic nucleoside which is phosphorylated by intracellular enzymes to the 5'-triphosphate form. This inhibits viral reverse transcriptase and viral DNA chain formation is thus terminated.

Zidovudine raises the helper lymphocyte count, reduces the frequency of opportunistic infections in AIDS and prolongs life for a time. However, it is by no means curative and its toxic effects frequently limit the duration of treatment.

The adverse effects of zidovudine are muscle pains, headaches, nausea and insomnia. More important, it depresses the bone marrow and is toxic to both red and white cell precursors. Anaemia is usually the first sign and irreversible bone marrow failure has been reported.

Other antiviral drugs used in AIDS

A variety of other drugs with antiviral activity are being tested in AIDS. These include *ganciclovir* (for severe cytomegalovirus infections), *ribavirin* (which inhibits a wide variety of DNA and RNA viruses), alpha interferon (particularly in combination with zidovudine) and others. However, it will be some time before their usefulness can be established.

Treatable aspects of AIDS

While it is obviously desirable to eliminate the human immunodeficiency virus from the body, it must be remembered that the great majority of these patients die from other infections, secondary to the immunodeficiency. Treatment of these bacterial, fungal and other infections is currently therefore the major aspect of management of AIDS and can prolong life to a variable degree.

THE INTERFERONS

Interferons are a group of substances with antiviral activity produced by several different types of body cells. The interferons are species specific but not virus specific. Thus, only human interferons are effective in humans but, once produced against one type of virus, are effective against any other. Cells can also be induced to produce interferons under the influence of various non-specific stimuli.

More than three decades after their discovery interferons have become available for clinical use. As yet only alpha interferons have been licensed and their indications are for the treatment of a rare type of leukaemia (hairy cell leukaemia), which is associated with an HTLV virus, and as ancillary treatment for AIDS.

Experimentally, interferons appear to be effective in the treatment of chronic hepatitis B, either alone or in combination with other antiviral drugs. Toxic effects are severe however, and include a prolonged and unpleasant 'flu-like' illness or oc-

casionally bone marrow depression. It is thought that the unpleasant symptoms of influenza and some other viral infections may be due to endogenous production of interferon. So far only limited clinical trials have been carried out and the effectiveness of interferon in potentially lethal viral infections has not yet been firmly established. However, in one trial prolonged low-dose interferon was shown greatly to reduce cytomegalovirus infections and also opportunistic infections in renal transplant patients.

There is also interest in the possible anticancer effects of interferon as a result of its regulatory actions on normal cell division and on other cell functions such as the immune response. However, the value of interferon for this purpose has not yet been established.

'COLD CURES'

The common cold syndrome is caused by so many different viruses that production of a vaccine is not feasible and, until the day when an effective broad spectrum antiviral drug is produced, specific treatment is also unavailable.

So-called cold cures therefore aim to give symptomatic relief, particularly to clear the stuffy nose or control cough. Nasal decongestants depend on a sympathomimetic effect on the nasal mucosa which as a consequence becomes less vascular and swollen. Ephedrine is therefore a common ingredient and may be combined with aromatic oils such as menthol. These may have a small contributory effect of the same kind, but also give a 'fresh' smell to the preparation and to the breath.

The cough caused by many minor, viral upper respiratory infections can be suppressed by antitussives, particularly antihistamines or codeine preparations. Some of these over-the-counter preparations which contain both an antihistamine and codeine are therefore potent sedatives. This may be an advantage when an unproductive cough interferes with sleep, but can leave an undesirable hangover the following day.

The effectiveness of massive doses of vitamin C for prevention of colds has not lived up to the claims made for it. Some clinical trials have failed to demonstrate any significant effect.

SUGGESTED FURTHER READING

Anon 1987 Topical antibiotics and antiseptics for the skin. Drugs and Therapeutics Bulletin 25: 97

Cawson R A 1986 Update on antiviral chemotherapy: the advent of acyclovir. British Dental Journal 161: 245

Donowitz G R, Mandell G L 1988 Beta-lactam antibiotics. (First of two parts.) New England Journal of Medicine 318: 419

Donowitz G R, Mandell G L 1988 Beta-lactam antibiotics. (Second of two parts.) New England Journal of Medicine 318: 419

Dorsky D I, Crumpacker C S 1987 Drugs five years later: acyclovir. Annals of Internal Medicine 107: 859

Drouhet E, Dupont B 1987 Evolution of antifungal agents; past present and future. Reviews of Infectious Diseases 9 (suppl 1): S4

Faltynek C R, Oppenheim J J 1988 Interferons in host defense. Journal of the National Cancer Institute 80: 151

Finch R 1988 Anti-infectives. British Medical Journal 296: 261

Finegold S M, Wexler H M 1988 Therapeutic implications of bacteriologic findings in mixed aerobic-anaerobic infections. Antimicrobial Agents and Chemotherapy 32: 611

Franklin R, Cockerill III, Randall S E 1987 Trimethoprim-sulfamethoxazole. Mayo Clinic Proceedings 62: 921

Geddes A M 1988 Antibiotic therapy – a resume. Lancet i: 286

Gold D, Corey L 1987 Acyclovir prophylaxis for herpes simplex virus infection. Antimicrobial Agents and Chemotherapy 31: 361–367

Hay R 1985 Ketoconazole: a reappraisal. British Medical Journal 290: 260

Hay R 1987 Recent advances in the management of fungal infections. Quarterly Journal of Medicine 64: 631

Hermans P E, Cockerill F R 1987 Antiviral agents. Mayo Clinic Proceedings 62: 1108

Hermans P E, Wilhelm M P 1987 Vancomycin. Mayo Clinic Proceedings 62: 1116

Holgate S 1988 Penicillin allergy: how to diagnose and when to treat. British Medical Journal 296: 1213

Hoofnagle J H 1987 Antiviral treatment of chronic type B hepatitis. Annals of Internal Medicine 107: 414

Morris A G 1988 Interferons. Immunology (suppl 1): 43

Randall S E, Terrell C L 1987 The aminoglycosides: streptomycin, kanamycin, gentamicin, tobramycin, amikacin, metilmicin, and sisomicin. Mayo Clinic Proceedings 62: 906

Rosenblatt J E, Edson R S 1987 Metronidazole. Mayo Clinic Proceedings 62: 1013

Sandstrom E G, Kaplan J C 1987 Antiviral therapy in AIDS. Clinical pharmacological properties and therapeutic experience to date. Drugs 34: 372

Sattler F R, Weitekamp M R, Ballard J O 1986 Potential for Bleeding with the new beta-lactam antibiotics. Annals of Internal Medicine 105: 929

Saxon A, Beall G N, Rohr A S, Adelman D 1987 Immediate hypersensitivity reactions to beta-lactam antibiotics. Annals of Internal Medicine 107: 205

Shanson D C 1987 Antibiotic prophylaxis of infective endocarditis in the United Kingdom and Europe. Journal of Antimicrobial Chemotherapy 20 (suppl A): 119

Sperber S J, Hayden F G 1988 Chemotherapy of rhinovirus colds. Antimicrobial Agents and Chemotherapy 32: 409

Surbone A, Yarchoan R, McAtee et al 1988 Treatment of the acquired immunodeficiency syndrome (AIDS) and AIDS-related complex with a regimen of 3′-azido-2′, 3′-dideoxythymidine (Azidothymidine or Zidovudine) and acyclovir. Annals of Internal Medicine 108: 534

Terrell C L, Hermans P E 1987 Antifungal agents used for deep-seated mycotic infections. Mayo Clinic Proceedings 62: 1116

Tyrrell D A J 1987 Interferons and their clinical value. Reviews of Infectious Diseases 9; 243

Wassilew S W, Reimlinger S, Nasemann T, Jones D 1987 Oral acyclovir for herpes zoster: a double-blind controlled trial in normal subjects. British Journal of Dermatology 117: 495

Whitley R J 1988 Ganciclovir – have we established clinical value in the treatment of cytomegalovirus infections? Annals of Internal Medicine 108: 452

Wilson W R, Cockerill III F R 1987 Tetracyclines, chloramphenicol, erythromycin and clindamycin. Mayo Clinic Proceedings 62: 906

Wise R 1987 Antimicrobial agents: a widening choice. Lancet ii: 1251

Wood M J, Geddes A M 1987 Antiviral therapy. Lancet ii: 1189

Young L S 1987 Treatable aspects of infection due to Human Immunodeficiency Virus. Lancet ii: 1503

4. Antiseptics, anti-caries agents and related drugs used in routine dentistry

In the lay mind, Victorian concepts about spread of infection die hard and it still seems to be believed that bacteria leap out of drains and lavatory pans to attack anyone nearby. This strange belief enables the manufacturers of antiseptics to achieve what must be the purest and most complete apotheosis of capitalism. Advertisements therefore exhort the housewife to protect her family by pouring an antiseptic (literally) down the drain and as a corollary to rush out to buy more in order to repeat the process *ad infinitum*. The benefits from this cycle of events come, of course, solely to the manufacturers and their advertising agents.

Historically, antiseptics played a crucial role in the early victories against infection but only because there was no appreciation of how infection was transmitted. Thus, the first example was the insistence, by Semmelweiss, in nineteenth century Vienna, that students who had attended autopsies should wash their hands in antiseptic before assisting in the labour ward. Needless to say this innovation was carried through in the teeth of opposition and ridicule. Its effectiveness in reducing puerperal mortality brought Semmelweiss neither success nor popularity.

The name of Lister is inseparably associated with his introduction of antiseptics into the operating room and his success in reducing postoperative sepsis.

Antiseptics must be clearly distinguished from antibiotics and their synthetic analogues. Antiseptics have a relatively crude toxic effect on living cells but in high concentration, and *given enough time*, can kill a variety of accessible bacteria when circumstances are favourable.

Antibiotics, by contrast, act in exceedingly low concentrations and have selective actions which interfere with the metabolism of microorganisms in such a way as to have bacteriostatic or bactericidal effects. Antibiotics (unlike antiseptics) are effective and generally innocuous when given systemically.

Disinfectants and antiseptics

There is no real difference between antiseptics and disinfectants. Disinfection refers to the *cleansing* of any item and implies the removal of bacterial contamination, particularly by antiseptics. However, the latter will only kill a proportion of these contaminants and are generally ineffective against bacterial spores. Antiseptics are often little more effective than thorough mechanical cleansing with soap and water, and should in general only be used in conjunction with the latter.

Antiseptics poison living tissues, whether human or bacterial, and their limitations are as follows:

1. They are non-selective in their action on cells and need to be used in relatively high concentrations.

2. They require considerable time (usually many hours) to destroy significant numbers of bacteria.

3. They are usually inhibited by organic matter such as blood or pus.

4. They are usually ineffective against bacterial spores and will not necessarily destroy viruses.

As a consequence of these limitations, antiseptics are only of value in assisting the disinfection of contaminated surfaces. They are ineffective or poisonous if given internally and their differences from antibiotics and related antimicrobials have been described in the previous chapter. Antiseptics will also not sterilise instruments; this can only be achieved by autoclaving. However, it may sometimes be acceptable to store *sterilised* instruments in an antiseptic solution temporarily.

Mode of action of antiseptics

Antiseptics can act in a variety of ways including:

a. Coagulation and precipitation of cell proteins. Phenols are an example.

b. Damage to cell membranes. This allows leakage of cell contents, particularly electrolytes, and cell death. Detergents in particular affect cell membranes.

c. Oxidation of thiol (SH) groups. Many cell enzymes are dependent on free SH groups. When these are oxidised by agents such as the halogens, cell damage is severe and the cell usually dies.

Antiseptics are therefore toxic to cells in general. These effects are not specific to microorganisms but severe damage to host cells can be limited by restricting the use of antiseptics in man to superficial application where the intact epithelium is protective, or to hard dental tissues which are resistant to chemical damage. Some antiseptics can be used to irrigate wounds but must be used in dilute solution and only if they have no toxic effect if absorbed.

The effectiveness of an antiseptic depends upon:

1. The properties of the agent itself.
2. The degree of dilution.
3. The time it is allowed to act.
4. The degree of interference by other materials, either organic contaminants such as blood or pus or chemicals such as soap.

Some antiseptics are relatively unstable and after a time break down; antibacterial power is then lost or the solution will actually support bacterial growth.

Uses of antiseptics

Antiseptics should only supplement and are not a substitute for adequate mechanical cleansing. They can be used for two main purposes, namely:

1. Disinfection of non-living surfaces – often termed 'environmental disinfectants'.
2. For use on living surfaces, namely skin, mucous membranes and teeth.

Typical applications of antiseptics in hospital are therefore:

1. Disinfection of surfaces in high-risk areas such as operating areas.
2. Disinfection of faecally or other heavily contaminated articles.
3. Disinfection of food preparation areas.
4. Preoperative cleansing of surgeons' and patients' skin.

INDIVIDUAL ANTISEPTICS

Phenolics

Phenol derivatives such as Sudol or Hycolin are cresols in soap solution used for environmental disinfection of such things as floors or bedpans. They are cheap and effective, have a wide range of antibacterial activity, are not easily inactivated but tend to be irritant or caustic.

Cresols of various sorts, beechwood creosote (which contains cresols) and other phenolics such as paramonochlorphenol are used as dressings to disinfect root canals. They are strongly antiseptic but agents such as paramonochlorphenol nevertheless seem to do little harm and (surprisingly) do not appear to irritate periapical tissues.

Alcohols

Ethyl and isopropyl alcohol are effective and rapidly active. At the optimal concentration of 70%, alcohol is useful for preparing clean skin for injections. It is, however, ineffective on the oral mucosa.

Surgical spirit (a mixture of methyl and ethyl alcohol) is used for wiping down surfaces such as trolley tops or bracket tables.

Halogens

Hypochlorites have a wide range of antibacterial activity by releasing chlorine. Their action is rapid but they are inactivated by organic matter. Strong solutions (e.g. Chloros) have a characteristic smell and bleaching power. Milder compounds such as Milton (1% sodium hypochlorite) are often used for irrigation of root canals to wash out infected debris after reaming and for disinfecting dentures in patients with denture stomatitis (candidosis).

Two per cent sodium hypochlorite is also recommended for cleaning working surfaces where there is a risk of contamination by hepatitis viruses. Hypochlorites are effectively virucidal (if allowed sufficient time), but have the disadvantage of being corrosive and may blunt some stainless steel instruments.

Iodine. 2.5% iodine in 70% alcohol is a strong and rapidly acting bactericidal agent, and will kill some spores and viruses in addition to most bacteria and fungi. It is not greatly inhibited by organic matter and is effective for surgical preparation of clean skin. It stains the skin and can, rarely, cause sensitisation or severe rashes in an already sensitised person.

Organic halogen compounds

Iodophors. Iodophors are combinations of iodine and surface active detergents which act together to have a cleansing and enhanced germicidal effect. Iodine is slowly released and the action is prolonged. These preparations are non-irritant, are said not to cause sensitisation and are non-staining. Povidone iodine (Betadine) is widely used for preparation of patients' skin and operators' hands before surgery.

Chloroxylenols. Chloroxylenols have a pleasant smell but are greatly inactivated by organic matter. Their antibacterial activity is relatively weak and unreliable. Dettol is the best-known example. This is so ineffective against one opportunistic pathogen (*Pseudomonas aeruginosa*) that it is used in culture media as a selective agent to encourage the growth of this organism.

Hexachlorophane. Hexachlorophane is effective mainly against Gram-positive cocci particularly *Staph. aureus*. It is non-irritant and rarely causes sensitisation. In babies systemic absorption through the skin can be toxic. Hexachlorophane leaves a germicidal residue to the skin and is an effective

preparation widely used for disinfection of patients' skin and surgeons' hands before operation. For this purpose hexachlorophane is incorporated into soap or used as a detergent cream (e.g. Phisohex). Disinfection is slower than with chlorhexidine and hexachlorophane must be applied repeatedly to get a useful effect by its cumulative action. Despite its antiseptic properties hexachlorophane can became contaminated and permit the growth of bacteria.

Chlorhexidine (Hibitane). Chlorhexidine, a biguanide, is a highly effective antiseptic with a wide and rapid antibacterial action especially when in alcoholic solution. It is as effective as iodine in alcohol, both of which when rubbed firmly on to the skin on gauze for 2 minutes remove about 80% of skin organisms. Chlorhexidine is non-irritant and non-toxic. It is inactivated by soap but cationic detergent preparations such as Hibiscrub are available.

Chlorhexidine 0.5% in 70% alcohol and Hibiscrub are both widely used for preoperative skin preparation of both patient and surgeon. It is non-corrosive so that it can be used for storing sterile instruments or burs and is an effective and useful general purpose antiseptic for dental purposes.

The effectiveness of chlorhexidine in aqueous solution is enhanced by the cationic detergent cetrimide. This preparation known as Savlon can be used for a wide variety of purposes from irrigation of wounds to the cleansing of instrument trolleys.

Chlorhexidine in alcohol also has a rapid antiseptic action on the oral mucosa and in aqueous solution inhibits dental plaque formation. It has, however, an unpleasant flavour and does not, of course, remove existing plaque.

Aldehydes

Aldehydes are potent bactericidal agents, but *formaldehyde* is little used now.

Glutaraldehyde is more potent, more rapidly acting and less irritant and lacks the unpleasant smell of formaldehyde.

A useful preparation of glutaraldehyde is a 2% alkaline solution in 70% isopropyl alcohol which may be used for so-called 'cold sterilisation' of delicate instruments such as glass-fibre optics endoscopes. Many bacteria are killed after 30 minutes' exposure and many spores are destroyed after 7–10 hours. Full sterilisation is not achieved, however, and the action of glutaraldehyde against *M. tuberculosis* for example, is weak.

Glutaraldehyde 2% is recommended for treatment of articles such as impressions contaminated by hepatitis B virus, but which cannot be autoclaved. Exposure to 2% glutaraldehyde for this purpose should be for at least 1 hour, but preferably for 12 hours.

Glutaraldehyde should not be used on body surfaces as it is irritant and allergenic.

Dyes

Aniline dyes such as crystal (gentian) violet and brilliant green are active against some Gram-positive organisms but are easily inactivated by organic matter. Application of gentian violet was a traditional treatment for infantile thrush, but it is potentially irritant and its use on mucous membranes or unbroken skin is no longer advised. In any case it is also so messy as to be obsolete.

Acridine dyes, particularly acriflavine and proflavine, have a wider range of antibacterial activity than the aniline dyes, are bactericidal and are not appreciably inactivated by organic matter. They can be used for application to superficial wounds or burns.

Quaternary ammonium compounds

Benzalkonium chloride (Roccal) and *cetrimide (Cetavlon)* are examples. They are good detergents but poor antiseptics. Their action is mainly bacteriostatic and is against only a narrow range of microorganisms. They also support the growth of *Ps. aeruginosa*. They are inhibited by organic matter and completely inactivated by soap.

DISINFECTION POLICIES

Policies determining the choice and uses of antiseptics vary from one hospital to another but a typical current example would be as follows:

1. *Environmental disinfectants*
   (i) Hycolin 2% for routine use apart from food preparation surfaces.

   (ii) Sodium hypochlorite 1% (must be freshly prepared). Especially indicated for clearing up blood or other discharges from hepatitis or AIDS patients.
2. *Staff handwashing*
   (i) The hands should be washed thoroughly in liquid soap and water.
   (ii) Povidone iodine 7.5% (Betadine) surgical scrub or, especially by those sensitive to iodine, chlorhexidine 4% surgical scrub (Hibiscrub) should be used.

The hands cannot be sterilised, but scrubbing up in this way will significantly reduce the bacterial count on the skin surface for a limited period. Surgical gloves give added protection, but microbes readily leak out through minute perforations. For extra protection, in high-risk situations, two pairs of gloves may need to be worn.

3. *Preoperative preparation of patients' skin*
   (i) Thorough washing with soap and water.
   (ii) Paint with povidone iodine 10% in alcohol OR chlorhexidine 0.5% in alcohol.
4. *Skin cleaning before injections*
   Wipe with 70% isopropyl alcohol.

USES OF ANTISEPTICS IN DENTISTRY

The main occasions when antiseptics are used in dentistry can be summarised as follows:

1. For storing sterilised surgical instruments and operating equipment.
2. For preparation of the skin before surgery.
3. For preparation of the surgeon's hands.
4. For preparation of the skin before venepuncture and other injections.
5. For preoperative preparation of the oral mucous membrane.
6. For superficial infections of the mouth in lozenges or mouth washes.
7. In dentifrices.
8. For inhibition of bacterial plaque (chlorhexidine).
9. In endodontic treatment.
10. For irrigation of infected areas, such as pericoronitis or infected sockets.

These uses will not all be discussed in detail but the role of antiseptics will be considered in relation to other measures used in the management of some of the more important infective diseases affecting the mouth and teeth.

Instruments and operating equipment

Antiseptics should not be used in an attempt to sterilise instruments. Sterilisation should be by physical means, preferably autoclaving (134°C for 3 minutes). Antiseptics can often, however, be used for short-term storage of heat-sterilised instruments.

Antiseptics can be used for cleaning the surface of bracket tables or operating trolleys. But even then an operating trolley should be covered by a sterile towel on which the instruments lie.

Preparation of surgeons' hands

Surgeons' hands often also carry pathogens. The wearing of surgical gloves gives partial protection to the patient but microbes can nevertheless manage to get through minute perforations.

'Scrubbing up' for surgery involves thorough washing followed by the use of antiseptics, and similar methods are used as for preparation of the skin of the operating site.

As discussed earlier a typical regimen would be to wash the hands thoroughly with running water and a detergent preparation containing hexachlorophane, chlorhexidine or povidone-iodine followed by applications of 10 ml of 0.5% chlorhexidine in alcohol rubbed on the hands until dry. In spite of extreme care and the use of potent antiseptics, the patient's skin and the surgeon's hands cannot be sterilised. The best that can be achieved in practical terms is a significant reduction in the resident bacteria for a limited period.

Preparation of the skin for surgery

Before a skin incision is made, the patient's own dermal bacteria must be eliminated as far as possible from the field of operation. The usual skin flora often includes staphylococci and other pathogens but these tend to be deeply entrenched, particularly in hair follicles.

Adequate skin preparation requires thorough washing, for which purpose an antiseptic soap (such as *Hibiscrub–chlorhexidine* in a detergent) can be used followed by applications of powerful (but not irritant) antiseptics. This can be done by firm swabbing with alcoholic chlorhexidine for several minutes. When the skin is deeply contaminated or the risks of infection are high (as in poorly vascular tissue) repeated compresses of an *iodophor (povidone-iodine)* for 30 minutes at a time will give better clearance of skin bacteria. Where applicable the skin must be shaved just before antiseptic preparation.

Preparation of skin surfaces for injection or venepuncture

It is traditional to cleanse the skin with 70% isopropyl alcohol.

Preparation of the oral mucous membrane

The oral mucosa represents a much less severe problem than the skin. Virulent pathogens such as *Staphylococcus aureus* are uncommon, the bacteria are superficial and accessible to antiseptics, and local immunity is high. Teeth are, as a result, extracted with minimal aseptic or antiseptic precautions, leaving a large bony wound which, with rare exceptions, heals remarkably rapidly. Infected sockets are usually due to other causes.

It may be considered desirable to prepare the oral mucosa before injecting a local anaesthetic but if this is to be anything more than a gesture, the antiseptic must (a) act very quickly (within 30 seconds) and (b) have a drying effect on the mucosa to prevent recontamination with saliva. The only preparations which are at all effective are therefore those in alcoholic solution such as iodine or (better) 2% chlorhexidine. Seventy per cent alcohol which is effective as a skin antiseptic is ineffective on the oral mucosa.

Preparation of the oral mucosa for surgery is not a practical proposition as contamination with saliva is inevitable.

Superficial infections of the mouth and throat

Antiseptic lozenges. These lozenges contain antiseptics such as cetyl pyridinium or benzalkonium chloride and are popular over-the-counter preparations used for conditions ranging from aphthous stomatitis to sore throats. There is no evidence that these lozenges are of any benefit and they can cause harm by chemical irritation or inducing superinfection if used persistently.

Worse still, diagnosis of serious diseases, especially cancer, can be delayed if the patient chooses to treat himself rather than get expert help.

Mouthwashes and antiseptic lozenges. Mouthwashes have a mechanical cleansing effect. Any antiseptic that they contain has little effect since it is in the mouth for so short a time. The warmth of a mouthwash may also be comforting and is traditionally thought to improve the local circulation. Again any such effect is transient.

Antiseptic lozenges are unlikely to have any function other than freshening the mouth. If the concentration of antiseptic is such as to have any effect on pathogens, then the lozenges are likely to cause mucosal damage. Prolonged use may also cause mucosal irritation.

PRECAUTIONS AGAINST TRANSMISSION OF SERIOUS INFECTIONS IN THE DENTAL SURGERY

The two most serious infections from which the dental surgeon is currently at risk are hepatitis B and AIDS. Vaccination against hepatitis B is particularly important, and gives adequate protection to most (but not all) of those that receive it. Although as yet only one dentist appears to have developed AIDS as a result of his occupation, the infection can be acquired via needlestick injuries and at least one general surgeon has died from this disease. The possibility of its transmission to or from a dental patient cannot therefore be dismissed. The following are recommended precautions to lessen these hazards, but it must be borne in mind that carriers of these viruses will frequently be treated unknowingly.

1. The patient should be treated at the end of the working day
2. Dental staff should wear gloves (preferably two pairs), goggles, mask, gown and plastic apron. Any skin wounds should be adequately protected.
3. Disposable instruments should be used wherever possible and all non-disposable instruments should be autoclaved (121°C for 20 minutes or

134°C for 3 minutes) after decontamination in fresh 1% sodium hypochlorite.
4. Air-turbines and ultrasonic scalers should not be used, because of the risk (though unproven) of aerosal spread of infection.
5. Needles should not be resheathed (except into a special receiver), broken or bent, or removed from disposable syringes.
6. All disposable instruments should be put in puncture-proof boxes, double wrapped in plastic bags which are clearly labelled as a biohazard, for transmission to the incinerator.
7. All working surfaces should be covered with plastic sheeting.
8. Any spilt blood or other discharge, should be quickly wiped up using fresh 1% sodium hypochlorite.
9. Instruments and impressions which cannot be autoclaved should be soaked in 2% glutaraldehyde for at least an hour but preferably overnight.

Hepatitis B vaccines

Hepatitis B is more readily transmitted than the human immunodeficiency virus and once acquired, can be fatal, although less frequently than AIDS. Dental surgeons are at high risk for infection by the hepatitis B virus and for the even more dangerous delta agent. Active immunization is therefore advisable as it protects against both agents.

The vaccines consist of alum-adsorbed inactivated hepatitis B surface antigen. The latter is obtained from human carriers (H-B-Vax) or made biosynthetically (Engerix B) by recombinant DNA technology. Three doses are given over 6 months and a booster dose may be given later. Adverse effects are uncommon and mild but include soreness at the injection site, headache, malaise or joint pains.

If there has been exposure or suspected exposure to the virus, as a result for example of a wound, specific hepatitis B immune globulin (HBIG) should be given for immediate passive protection and followed by active immunization.

PREVENTION OF DENTAL CARIES

Dental decay is an infective process. It is the result of a localised attack on the enamel and dentine by bacteria concentrated within a persistent plaque and mediated by acids produced by the metabolism of sugar from the diet.

Bacterial plaque is a complex adherent deposit formed on the teeth. Its formation is probably initiated by deposition of protein from saliva but the main components are bacteria and polysaccharides (polyglucans) synthesised particularly by *Streptococcus mutans* which is usually regarded as playing the main role in dental caries. Filamentous organisms are also present in large numbers but their role is not clear.

Essential properties of cariogenic bacteria appear to be both an ability to produce acid and to synthesise polysaccharides. The latter serve to give the plaque its adhesive properties. They prevent dilution or neutralisation of bacterial acid by saliva and also form a reserve food supply for the bacteria.

Plaque forms on all surfaces of the teeth, but caries develops only in stagnation areas where plaque can form thickly and remain undisturbed. The main factors necessary for caries to develop are as follows:

1. Cariogenic bacteria.
2. Bacterial plaque.
3. Substrate (dietary sugar) for acid production.
4. Stagnation areas on the teeth.
5. Susceptible dental tissues.

Prevention of dental caries may as a consequence be based (in theory at least) on the following measures alone or in combination:

1. Antibacterial (antibiotics or vaccines).
2. Restriction of substrate (limitation of frequency of sugar intake).
3. Obliteration of stagnation areas (fissure sealants).
4. Increasing the resistance of the dental tissues (fluorides).
5. Other measures.

While these and other possibilities exist, they are not all practical propositions. Many have various drawbacks or are not widely acceptable.

In fact, by far the most effective and certainly the safest single measure – limitation of frequency of sugar and sweet intake which can virtually abolish dental caries – is unacceptable to the general public.

The next most effective, proven measure is fluoridation of the water supply. But this too has failed to gain general acceptance.

And there the situation remains at the moment.

There are other ways of using fluorides as described later and some of the other anticaries measures have yet to be fully evaluated. Nevertheless, no dramatically effective and acceptable caries preventive agent seems likely to appear in the near future.

Antibacterial measures

Antibiotics

Long-term penicillin therapy is associated with a reduced incidence of dental caries but this can hardly be justified for such a minor condition. In the long run it is likely that complications would be more serious than the disease.

Vaccination

There is evidence from animal studies that a vaccine against *Streptococcus mutans* gives protection against caries. Natural immunity to caries probably does not exist in man and hence the bacterial preparation has to be given with an adjuvant to enhance the immune response.

The mode of action of such vaccines is ill-understood but the most obvious possibility is that the vaccine would stimulate antibody production. Nevertheless, the only immune globulin reaching the mouth in appreciable quantities is IgA in the saliva. IgG and IgM are present in the exudate from the gingival crevice but the amounts are so small that it is exceedingly difficult to obtain measurable samples. The exudate from the gingival crevice naturally increases in amount as the gingivae become more inflamed. However, it seems, to say the least, unacceptable to suggest that gingivitis should be encouraged in order to lessen the risk of dental caries.

Nevertheless, when all is said and done, it can be argued that if the vaccine works it hardly matters what the mode of action is.

Other problems associated with the production of an effective anticaries vaccine include the following:

Safety. All vaccines can cause side-effects, some of which are dangerous and occasionally fatal. Since caries is not a dangerous condition it is essential that the vaccine has no ill-effects worse than the disease itself.

Effectiveness. Vaccines are never 100% effective and in general are used only where there are no other preventive measures available for dangerous or untreatable infections. There are, by contrast, simple methods of prevention of dental caries of proven effectiveness. Even if these fail or are neglected, restorative procedures are not totally ineffective and, although tedious and unpleasant for the patient, are not particularly hazardous. .

Specificity. Vaccines are highly specific. Elimination or inactivation of *Strep. mutans* from the mouth in man might lead to other organisms taking over the cariogenic role.

Acceptability. There has been increasing resistance by the general public to immunisation and the vaccination rates for the important childhood fevers have fallen progressively. This may be partly because of apathy, but also anxieties about encephalitis following the use of whooping cough vaccine has increased public antipathy (however ill-informed) towards immunisation of all kinds.

These points possibly present an over-pessimistic assessment. At the same time, in view of the efforts being put into the development of an anticaries vaccine, it is important to have some idea of the nature and extent of the difficulties involved.

Antiseptics

Chlorhexidine mouthrinses have been shown to inhibit plaque formation and if used regularly this effect is maintained. Nevertheless the usefulness of this action in depressing caries activity has not been established clinically. In a trial carried out in Scandinavia where a relatively high concentration of chlorhexidine (0.4%) was used, the effect on dental caries was barely detectable.

It is probable that the limitation of chlorhexidine in this role is due to its poor penetration into stagnation areas.

Fissure sealants

Fissure sealants are plastics which are either bonded to dental hard tissue by the so-called acid-etch technique (to form a submicroscopic mechanical key) or by direct (chemical) adhesion to the tissues. Examples include methacrylate and polyurethane compounds, some of which also incorporate fluoride salts.

These agents seal the pits and fissures with a protective layer resistant to acid attack. They cannot be used on interproximal surfaces but the occlusal pits and fissures are the most vulnerable zones and the first to be attacked in children. These areas are also least well protected by fluorides and, apparently, by vaccines under experimental conditions.

A drawback to the use of fissure sealants is that if the technique of application is less than perfect, leakage under the sealant allows caries to develop undetected.

Fluorides and their actions on the dental tissues

Fluoride was detected in human dental enamel in 1805 and waterborne fluoride was detected by Berzelius in 1822. By 1897 it had not merely been hypothesised that fluoride would make teeth more caries resistant but it was postulated that this effect might be mediated by an antienzymic or antibacterial effect. Fluoride-containing dentifrices became available at least as early as 1902. Then the whole matter was more or less forgotten.

Prevention of dental caries

Dental caries is an infective process and although there is a variety of possible approaches to prevention, the only drug of firmly established value is fluoride compounds.

Absorption and distribution

Fluorides are rapidly absorbed from the gut. They have a strong affinity for calcium salts particularly calcium phosphate and become incorporated into the bones and teeth during dental development. Fluoride not immediately incorporated in hard tissues is rapidly excreted in the urine.

Fluorides continue to enter bone after development is complete but, after the teeth have been fully formed, negligible amounts of fluoride are incorporated by continued apposition of cementum.

Fluorides enter the hard tissues by replacing hydroxyl groups to form calcium fluorapatite.

Effects of fluorides on the teeth

The most closely studied effect of fluoride is on dental caries. The optimal effect is achieved when the drinking water contains about 1 part per million (p.p.m.) of fluoride and is ingested throughout the period of dental development. These subjects have about 50% less dental caries than those from non-fluoride areas. This finding has been confirmed on so vast a scale in many parts of the world that all other variables that might affect these results can reasonably be excluded.

Inhibition of dental caries by fluorides

Mechanism of action. The means by which fluoride reduces dental caries are not clear but the main possibilities are as follows:

1. By a direct effect on the development of dental enamel. Fluoride can replace hydroxyl groups to form calcium fluorapatite and can have the following effects:
   a. Fluorapatite is more resistant to solution by acid than hydroxyapatite. It is, however, suggested that the initial rate of dissolution of these two compounds is similar but there is secondary precipitation of insoluble calcium fluoride from fluorapatite on the surface of the enamel crystallites, and this reduces the rate of movement of hydrogen ions into the crystals and slows further dissolution.
   b. Larger crystallites are formed. These have fewer imperfections. The crystalline lattice is more stable and a smaller surface area per unit volume is accessible for attack by hydrogen ions.
   c. The enamel has a lower carbonate content. This also reduces solubility.
   d. When enamel is attacked calcium phosphates are reprecipitated and fluoride enhances the possibility of their crystallising as apatite. Remineralisation of enamel after attack is therefore favoured.
2. Effects on the enamel surface. It has been suggested (but not generally accepted) that fluorides reduce the tendency of the enamel surface to adsorb proteins. In this way plaque may not build up so quickly.
3. Effects of fluoride on bacterial plaque. Fluoride is incorporated into bacterial plaque in relatively high concentrations but is mostly bound to organic material. Were the fluoride in plaque mainly unbound, that is in ionised form, it has been postulated that the concentrations might be high enough to affect bacterial metabolism, and possibly inhibit acid production, or synthesis of polysaccharides. It is questionable, however, whether the small proportion of free fluoride in plaque is sufficient to have any of these effects.

When fluorides are applied topically the local concentration is very high; the majority believe that plaque should be removed before topical application of fluoride to ensure that an adequate concentration of the ion reaches the enamel surface.

Although this action of fluorides may possibly play a part by depressing bacterial metabolism, it would appear that the main effect is on the enamel itself.

Methods of using fluorides

Fluorides can act systemically or locally on the teeth. Both effects can be achieved when fluoride salts are ingested after the teeth have erupted. Methods of using fluorides are:

1. *Ingestion*
   a. In drinking water, other fluids or foods.
   b. Fluoride tablets.
2. *Local applications*
   a. Toothpastes.
   b. Mouth rinses.
   c. Topical application.

Fluoride in drinking water

Fluorides are most effective when ingested throughout the period of dental development. This is most conveniently, effectively, reliably, economically and safely achieved by the addition of sodium fluoride to the water supply to maintain a concentration of one part per million ($= 1$ mg/l). In addition to its effects on the development and maturation of enamel, fluorides ingested in the drinking water can also have a topical effect on the teeth.

No effort is needed on the part of the recipients and since daily fluid intake is relatively constant, the daily dosage level is equally constant. Overdose is practically impossible, since about 2500 litres of water would have to be swallowed in a short period to cause acute poisoning. Chronic overdose is almost equally difficult to achieve.

Fluoride taken in this way reduces dental caries by about 50%.

Unfortunately organised opposition to fluoridation of drinking water is strong and only about 5 million out of 55 million of the population of Britain receive artifically fluoridated water. About 0.5 million others receive water containing natural fluoride at or near the optimum level.

In the USA many more areas and a higher proportion of the population receive fluoridated water. Studies in these and control areas have continued for many years. The benefits have been confirmed and no ill-effects have been reported.

Fluorides in food

One of the expressed objections to fluoridation of water is that adults who are at a level of risk from dental caries continue to take in fluorides unnecessarily. Although there is no evidence of any harmful effect, it can still be argued that after long-term exposure there might be effects that are as yet unrecognised.

Fluoride salts can therefore be added to school milk or to table salt. Both are effective, but both are less reliable than when fluoride is added to the water, as the intake can vary widely.

Fluoride tablets

These contain 0.25 mg to 1 mg fluoride, usually in a lactose base. When taken by the mother during pregnancy, the fetus benefits little, however, as the placenta acts as an effective barrier to the fluoride ion and, even more important, the fluoride is taken up in maternal bone.

Mottling of the enamel can be a complication even of conventional dosage of fluoride tablets, especially as a fluoridised dentifrice is likely also to be used. Because of the wide individual susceptibility to mottling, therefore, a balance has to be struck between adequate protection and the risk of

discoloration of the teeth. At present the *suggested* regimen is as follows:

1. To be used where fluoride in the drinking water is less than 0.3 p.p.m.
2. Should be taken as soon as teeth start to erupt.
3. Tablets should be chewed to get a local effect also.
4. Dosage:

Birth to 6 months	0.25 mg F/day
6–18 months	0.25–0.5 mg F/day
18–24 months	0.25–0.75 mg F/day
over 24 months	0.5–1.0 mg F/day.

The reduction in dental caries is less than when the water is fluoridated. This benefit is decreased even further if the tablets are not taken consistently over a long period.

The other disadvantage is, as with other tablets, that of a child taking a handful of tablets and receiving a dangerous overdose.

Recent work suggests that the most effective way of using fluoride tablets is to get the child slowly to dissolve a tablet of fluoride in the mouth at night just before going to sleep. This has several effects. It produces a very high (up to 1000 p.p.m.) concentration of fluoride locally; it also allows the fluoride a long period to act. Pleasantly flavoured fluoride tablets are available and by this means reductions in caries of up to 90% or greater have been reported. If this work is substantiated then this would be the most effective preventive measure available. It is probable however that supervision would be essential to ensure that tablets are taken regularly.

Fluoride toothpastes

Dentifrices might be expected to be a highly effective method of applying fluoride. If the teeth are brushed regularly and efficiently then the fluoride salt is brought by a mildly abrasive vehicle into intimate contact with the enamel once or twice daily.

Several problems have arisen in formulating these toothpastes. Fluoride salts tend to become rapidly bound to calcium carbonate (the commonly used abrasive) and a satisfactory alternative abrasive was not easy to find. Some fluoride salts, notably stannous fluoride, stain the teeth and some fluoride toothpastes have an unplesant flavour.

Most of the problems have been overcome.

Current fluoride toothpastes contain sodium fluoride and sodium monofluorophosphate with a relatively inert abrasive. Nevertheless, the amount of available fluoride declines gradually during storage as the active agent reacts with other components.

Fluoride toothpastes can reduce caries experience by 20–30%.

Some doubt is still expressed as to whether infants should use fluoride toothpastes because a significant amount of fluoride is swallowed. The worst effect that might be expected from this small amount of ingested fluoride is mild mottling of the enamel. On the other hand, increased resistance to caries might result from incorporation of the ingested fluoride into the forming enamel.

However, virtually only fluoride-containing dentifrices are currently available and following their introduction there has been a general decline in the prevalence of dental caries in children. Admittedly sceptics point out that there are other possible explanations for this phenomenon but it seems likely that the widespread use of fluoride dentifrices, encouraged by persuasive advertising, has had a major effect.

Fluoride mouth rinses

Trials have shown that this method can also be effective. The best results have been obtained from daily use of a 0.05% sodium fluoride solution rinsed round the mouth for 1 or 2 minutes.

Supervision is needed to ensure that the rinse is used for an adequate period and to see that the rinse is not swallowed. The effort needed is therefore considerable and the procedure may be too extravagant in manpower to be practical on a large scale.

Fluoride salts for topical application

1. Sodium fluoride. This was the first to be used. Sodium fluoride was used originally in a 1% solution but it is now more usual to apply it as a 2% solution. The advantages of sodium fluoride are: (a) it is stable chemically but has to be stored in plastic containers as glass may be attacked; (b) the taste is not too unpleasant; (c) it is not irritating to the gingivae and it does not cause staining of the teeth.

2. Stannous fluoride. Stannous fluoride is used in a 2% to 8% solution. Clinical studies have suggested that it is more effective than sodium fluoride (2%) in reducing caries. In vitro stannous fluoride apparently also reduces the rate of solution of enamel by acid. The greater effectiveness of stannous fluoride clinically must be regarded as yet to be proved as more recent studies have not confirmed the earlier favourable findings.

Disadvantages of stannous fluoride are: (a) it is unstable in aqueous solution. Its effectiveness is rapidly reduced and a fresh solution must be made up on each occasion; (b) it has an unpleasant and astringent flavour; (c) it sometimes causes gingival irritation and blanching; (d) it often stains the teeth. This might also mask caries and so confuse the findings in clinical trials.

Although the early reports of the greater protective activity of stannous fluoride were not confirmed in later reports, some still believe it to be the most effective agent for topical application. For this purpose a stable. 0.4% stannous fluoride gel (Omnigel) is available.

3. Acidulated phosphate fluoride (APF). APF is a solution of sodium fluoride in weak phosphoric acid. Laboratory studies suggest that APF increases the uptake by enamel of fluoride when compared with a stannous or neutral sodium fluoride.

Clinical trials have shown that APF gives a greater reduction in caries than other topically applied fluorides that have been discussed. As seems to be usual, the striking improvements noted in the initial trials have not been entirely repeated in later trials but it does seem that APF may have a significantly better effect than sodium or stannous fluoride.

Fluoride gels. APF has been incorporated into a gel which is applied to the teeth in specially designed trays.

Fluoride gels applied in commercially made trays have also been proposed for home use by parents of caries-prone children, However, unsupervised application of fluorides in this way can lead to undesirable amounts of fluoride being ingested and this may also cause nausea. Home use of fluoride gels in this way should therefore be discouraged – or as one group of investigators quaintly expressed it, 'Home gelling should not be undertaken'.

In several areas of the country also, the prevalence of caries in children has declined so greatly that there now is little need for topical application of fluorides. The chief indications for these agents are therefore:

1. Highly caries-susceptible children, not responsive to other preventive measures.
2. Patients with xerostomia, particularly those who have been irradiated for cancer.

Patients whose salivary glands have been destroyed by irradiation are not merely highly susceptible to dental caries but also to osteoradionecrosis of the jaws and osteomyelitis secondary to infection from the teeth or to extractions. Prevention of caries and periodontal disease is therefore essential.

In such circumstances as these, where topical application of fluorides is indicated, APF gel is probably most widely favoured.

Adverse effects of fluorides

Ingestion of an overdose of sodium fluoride can cause acute poisoning. This is rare. More commonly there is continued intake of relatively large amounts of fluoride either as an occupational hazard or as a result of high natural fluoride content of water. This last condition is known as chronic endemic fluorosis.

Acute fluoride poisoning

Sodium fluoride has been used as a rat poison and an insecticide. It is white powder which can be mistaken for such foods as flour or powdered milk. Acute poisoning has resulted from addition of sodium fluoride powder into food. The lethal dose of fluoride for man is not known, but is probably about 2.5 g. Sodium fluoride in high concentrations is strongly irritant and some of the main effects of ingestion of large amounts of this compound are nausea, vomiting, diarrhoea and bleeding from the gut.

In fatal cases death has usually been ascribed to poisoning of enzyme and transport systems. With massive overdose the blood has been noticed to be uncoagulated at autopsy. This presumably is due to calcium binding by fluoride which would also lead to tetany and cardiorespiratory failure.

Chronic endemic fluorosis

Chronic endemic fluorosis affects the teeth, the skeleton and to a lesser extent other organs.

Dental fluorosis – mottled enamel. When the fluoride content of the drinking water exceeds 2–4 p.p.m. characteristic defects are seen in the teeth. The mildest form of dental fluorosis is shown by chalky white patches in the enamel though the surface is intact and of normal texture. These white patches become stained a brownish colour.

With more severe fluorosis the enamel becomes rough or pitted and brittle. In spite of these defects the teeth retain an increased resistance to dental caries.

The teeth are generally the most sensitive index of fluorosis since they are easily seen and because defects show up at low levels of fluoride intake (between 2 and 4 p.p.m.) when changes in the skeleton may be difficult to detect. At the level of 1 p.p.m. when fluorides have a significant (but invisible) effect on the teeth the skeleton shows no detectable change.

Skeletal fluorosis. Skeletal fluorosis develops when the fluoride content of the drinking water is high (between 4 and 14 p.p.m.) as happens in some parts of the world, particularly North India and North and South Africa. The main features are excessive calcification. Osteophytes form at the margins of joints, tendons, ligaments, and fascia become calcified and joints become fused. The vertebral column in particular can become completely rigid. Radiologically the bone is dense, the structure is indistinct but in spite of the increased density, fractures are common.

The clinical effects are stiffness of the back and legs and limitation or slowing of movement. The progressive osteosclerosis of the spine leads to narrowing of the neural canal and compression of the spinal cord. This can cause neurological complications of which the most severe is paraplegia.

Fluorides and osteoporosis

In non-fluoride areas osteoporosis is common. Osteoporosis is probably part of the ageing process. It is almost universal and is characterised by progressive loss of osseous tissue from the skeleton.

There is a constant turnover of bone but after about the age of 35 bone begins gradually to be lost and this accompanies a comparable loss of muscle, and age changes in eyes, viscera and other organs.

Osteoporosis is characterised by progressive thinning of trabeculae, increased radiolucency of the skeleton and weakening of bones. Common complications are collapse of vertebrae or fractures of the neck of the femur in the elderly with delayed healing.

In areas where the water contains at least 4 p.p.m. fluoride osteoporosis is uncommon and the skeleton is of greater density than in non-fluoride areas.

Beneficial versus adverse effects of fluoride

The known toxic effects of fluorides in excessive dosage have been used by antifluoridationists as 'evidence' that since large doses of fluorides are poisonous therefore *any* dose of fluoride is poisonous. This sort of extrapolation is not justified as, of course, it is possible to have toxic effects from any substance, even water, if taken in sufficiently large quantities.

All that can reasonably be said against fluoridation is that (as with other drugs) adverse effects may not become apparent for years. Nevertheless, in areas where the natural level of fluoride in the water is 1 p.p.m. there is no evidence that there is any excess morbidity or mortality that could in any way be attributed to the fluoride in the water. There is no reason to think that addition of fluoride artificially to the water in the same concentrations is likely to have any other adverse effect. This has been confirmed in areas of the USA where fluoridation of the water supply was started as long ago as 1944.

The beneficial effects of fluorides are to all intents and purposes solely by enhancing the resistance of the teeth to dental caries. At somewhat higher levels of fluoride in the drinking water there is reason to believe that increased density of the skeleton protects against the effects of osteoporosis but at these levels dental mottling becomes severe.

Although fluoridation of water supplies has not been widely adopted in Britain, there has been a striking decline in the prevalence of this disease, to the extent that it is now common to see children with caries-free mouths. This change must largely be attributed to the virtually universal use of fluoridized toothpastes.

Note: Although the value of the fluorine ion is well known in dentistry, its importance in pharmacology is less obvious. It is an essential element in all modern inhalational anaesthetic agents where it confers the valuable property of noninflammability without the toxicity of other halogens. There is even a case on record of an American nurse who developed skeletal fluorosis and nephrocalcinosis, as a result of addiction to methoxyflurane (a discontinued alternative to halothane) which is significantly metabolised to release fluoride. Fluoride is also an important component of many other drugs such as benzodiazepines and the benzodiazepine antagonist *flu*mazenil.

DENTIFRICES

Toothpastes are the usual form in which dentrifices are used. Tooth powders are still available but their use has declined.

Functions

These may be summarised as:

1. To remove bacterial plaque.
2. To reduce dental caries.
3. To prevent gingivitis.
4. To achieve other effects, e.g. desensitisation of exposed dentine.

Toothbrushing with a dentifrice will remove plaque, but only from accessible surfaces of the teeth (not from pits, fissures, or interstitial surfaces) and only if carried out carefully and conscientiously.

Toothbrushing alone will effectively remove plaque but a dentifrice aids the process and makes the whole dull business considerably more pleasant. Long-term comparative trials of toothbrushing with and without dentifrices have in fact proved not to be feasible because volunteers will not willingly forego the use of a dentifrice for more than a few days. Flavouring agents are therefore one of the most important components, as without them a dentifrice is unlikely to be used.

Thorough and regular toothbrushing with a dentifrice will control or prevent marginal gingivitis. It has little or no effect on dental caries unless a fluoride toothpaste is used.

Composition

The basic components of toothpastes are:

1. Abrasives.
2. Soap or detergent.
3. Binding agents.
4. Flavouring agents.
5. Humectant.
6. Preservative.
7. Colouring.

In addition there may be ingredients with some pharmacological activity such as:

8. Fluoride salts.
9. Antiseptics and antacids.
10. Agents to desensitise exposed dentine.

Abrasives. These, with a detergent, materially assist in the removal of plaque. Abrasive is essential for the removal of stains from the teeth.

The abrasive must be hard enough to remove deposits, but not so hard as to cause excessive wear of the enamel surface. Calcium carbonate (precipitated chalk) is satisfactory and has been the most widely used. With the advent of fluoride toothpastes other abrasives have had to be found since fluoride is bound by calcium carbonate. Dicalcium phosphate, calcium pyrophosphate and other materials – including chemically inert plastic particles – have been used to overcome this problem.

The mechanical effect of the abrasive on the teeth depends on several variables. The amount of abrasive trapped among the toothbrush filaments depends both on the amount used and the effectiveness of the binding agent. The effect is enhanced by the stiffness of the filaments and the muscular effort put into the operation. Finally, once dentine is exposed, it is worn away more quickly than enamel.

Soaps and detergents. In the past simple soaps were used, but synthetic detergents such as sodium lauryl sarcosinate are now more general.

Binding agents. A common example in present use is carboxymethyl cellulose. This compound (widely used in commodities as diverse as wallpaper adhesive, purgatives and ice cream) forms a mildly adhesive gel by imbibition of water, but this is slow and the gel does not take up more moisture in the mouth so quickly as to wash away. This gel helps to keep the toothpaste in the toothbrush.

Flavouring agents. The importance of these agents, which make a tedious process more pleasant, have been emphasised. Flavouring agents are chosen to give a subjective sensation of 'freshness' or even 'tingling freshness'. Essential oils, particularly peppermint or spearmint, are common examples.

Non-fermentable sweeteners such as saccharine or sorbitol are also included. Sucrose for obvious reasons should not be used, although it has been in the past.

Humectants. These are hygroscopic or moisture-retaining agents, such as glycerine or sorbitol, to keep the paste soft and prevent it from solidifying.

Preservative. This is a non-toxic antiseptic, such as sodium benzoate, to inhibit bacterial proliferation in the preparation. It has no useful antibacterial action in the mouth.

Colouring. The dentifrice should look attractive, especially if children are to be encouraged to use it. Appropriately chosen colours also have a strong subjective effect in convincing the user how much 'good' the preparation is doing. And what could be better than a striped toothpaste.

Fluoride salts. The use of fluorides in the inhibition of caries has been discussed. They are probably the only pharmacologically effective agent used in toothpastes.

Antiseptics and antacids. Antiseptics in toothpastes and mouthwashes have too weak an action and are too transiently in the mouth to have any significant effect. Chlorhexidine, which has been shown to inhibit plaque and which tends to persist in the mouth, may possibly have a useful effect, but there is as yet no positive evidence of this when it is incorporated in a dentifrice.

Antacids such as magnesium oxide or hydroxide are incorporated in some dentifrices. The idea, of course, is that the alkali neutralises acid produced on the surface of the teeth and so inhibits decay. Plaque is however very resistant to external changes in pH and is unaffected by momentary changes in its immediate environment.

Desensitising agents. These are more or less irritant compounds which are designed to promote secondary dentine formation. If used in a dentifrice, however, they must not be so irritant as to damage the adjacent tissues. One commercial preparation contains 10% strontium chloride and another, 1.4% formalin for this purpose.

Other desensitising agents are applied directly to the area after it has been isolated with cotton wool rolls. These include silver nitrate, formalin, zinc chloride, fluoride salts and corticosteroids. The variety of agents recommended suggests perhaps that there is some uncertainty as to their effectiveness.

ANTIBACTERIAL EFFECTS OF TOOTHPASTES

The antiseptics present in toothpastes are not generally expected to have any significant effect on dental disease. More important is the role of toothpastes in assisting mechanical removal of plaque and as a vehicle for fluorides. Often any antiseptic present seems to serve merely as a preservative but some have been shown to reduce the numbers of bacteria in the saliva for a short time.

Chlorhexidine and its derivative hexetidine are now however available in dentifrices. These have a more persistent effect. Chlorhexidine 1% gel had the greatest effect and depression of salivary bacteria persisted for up to 5 hours. A hexetidine-containing, commercially available toothpaste had a lesser effect than chlorhexidine gel, but still significantly greater than that of conventional antiseptics. Whether this effect is of any clinical value has not been shown.

Chlorhexidine

Chlorhexidine has proved to be a useful, effective and safe antiseptic with many applications. As mentioned earlier, it is one of the few agents which have been shown to clear the oral mucosa of bacteria as a preparation for injections.

Aqueous chlorhexidine has also been shown to inhibit dental bacterial plaque formation. It is active against oral streptococci, is adsorbed on to enamel and may also bind to the polysaccharides of the plaque.

Chlorhexidine will not remove plaque but if the teeth have been carefully scaled and polished, a mouthrinse of 0.1 or 0.2% chlorhexidine, preferably used at least twice daily, will diminish the amount of plaque formed. As long as chlorhexidine is used this effect is maintained and trials have shown this measure to be effective for 2 or more

years. On the other hand, plaque formation quickly reverts to normal as soon as chlorhexidine is stopped.

Staining of the teeth may discourage some from using chlorhexidine but the stain can usually be removed by toothbrushing with a conventional dentifrice. In many cases, however, it is the patient's failure to use a toothbrush and dentifrice effectively which has created the need to use chlorhexidine. If chlorhexidine is used, silicate cement restorations are likely to be permanently ruined by staining.

Although chlorhexidine can be shown to have a plaque-inhibiting effect, it is not as effective as toothbrushing. If the patient is an efficient and regular toothbrusher chlorhexidine brings no additional benefits. Some trials have not confirmed the effectiveness of chlorhexidine in reducing plaque or gingivitis. The quantitation of plaque and gingivitis is notoriously subjective and it is not too surprising therefore that findings have not been consistent.

Chlorhexidine is available commercially as a gel (1%) and as a 0.2% mouthwash. The gel has the advantage of having a more pleasant flavour but its effectiveness in the control of plaque seems not to have been convincingly established. The mouthwash appears to be more effective but is probably best regarded as an aid to toothbrushing when the latter is substandard.

Before a course of chlorhexidine is started all dental plaque and calculus should be removed to allow the drug a fair start.

An important limitation of chlorhexidine is that it does not penetrate into subgingival pockets or into stagnation areas in general. Hence it seems to have little effect on periodontal pockets, even though it may mitigate supragingival plaque formation.

The effect of chlorhexidine on dental caries seems to be no more than marginal, as mentioned earlier.

Hexitidine

Hexitidine is an analogue of chlorhexidine and has similar antibacterial activity in vitro. Clinically, hexitidine has a lesser antiplaque effect than chlorhexidine when the same (0.1%) concentration is used, but a similar effect when the concentration of hexitidine is raised to 1.4%. Hexitidine has been reported to have a shorter duration of action in the mouth, but testing of this drug has been on only a small scale compared with chlorhexidine.

PERIODONTAL DISEASE

Drugs have little place in the routine prevention of management of chronic periodontal disease.

Acute ulcerative gingivitis predominantly affects neglected mouths and it is important to clean up the mouth and remove plaque, calculus and debris which harbour vast number of organisms. This should be started at the earliest opportunity, preferably at the first visit. These oral hygiene measures are important since anaerobes typically depend on other bacteria to maintain a low local oxygen tension. Oral hygiene can therefore be effective alone and antimicrobials may be unnecessary.

A suitable course of treatment with metronidazole is three 200 mg tablets a day for 3 days. In addition, efforts must be made to improve the patient's standards of oral hygiene in the hope of preventing recurrences.

Acute ulcerative (Vincent's) gingivitis responds quickly to metronidazole but this infection does not play any important role in the aetiology of periodontal disease in general.

The most important measure in the management of periodontal disease is the control of bacterial plaque. This depends on regular conscientious toothbrushing. Regular use of chlorhexidine as a mouth rinse (or possibly in a dentifrice) seems to have a more specific effect by depressing dental plaque formation but this does not improve on effective toothbrushing.

Local application of antiseptics (such as iodine solutions) to the gum margins can do no more than transiently depress gingival flora, and astringent mouthwashes, to 'harden' the gums, are useless.

Many antibiotics, particularly tetracycline, have been tested, usually as topical applications, for control of pocket bacteria in periodontal disease in both humans and animals. Tetracycline may be effective for disease, such as juvenile periodontitis or suppurating pockets, unresponsive to conventional treatment. Long-term use of tetracycline, however, is likely to create a resistant bacterial population.

DENTIFRICES: SUMMARY

The main points about the role of toothpastes and toothbrushing in the management of both dental caries and periodontal disease can be summarised as follows:

1. Removal of bacterial plaque is important, particularly to control gingivitis, but 100% success is rarely achieved.

2. Almost the only means of controlling bacterial plaque is to remove it mechanically, soon after it forms, by regular toothbrushing.

3. Toothpastes aid this process by their detergent and abrasive components but probably at least as important is their role of making toothbrushing more pleasant and thereby encouraging the habit.

4. Toothpastes contain antiseptics, but their effect (if any) in the mouth is slight, transient and difficult to detect.

5. Dental caries is very little affected by toothbrushing itself as most cavities develop in totally inaccessible sites. Caries at the cervical margins is an exception and can be prevented by removal of plaque at the gingival margin by toothbrushing.

6. Fluoride salts incorporated in dentifrices reduce caries to a variable degree. Their effectiveness probably depends on the skill with which toothbrushing is carried out, the local concentration of fluoride that is achieved in stagnation areas, and the length of time for which it is in contact with plaque in these areas.

7. Toothbrushing has a more certain effect on gingival plaque, the removal of which will to a large extent control marginal gingivitis.

8. Regular chlorhexidine rinses have been shown to reduce bacterial plaque formation. The value of chlorhexidine when incorporated in a dentifrice in the long-term control of either marginal gingivitis or dental caries remains to be established.

Overall the effectiveness of dentifrices in themselves is limited and manufacturers' claims for them – not surprisingly – are generally exaggerated. At the same time the value of toothpaste advertisements should not be underestimated. They at least achieve the not inconsiderable feat of providing an appealing motive to the general public for maintaining the habit of toothbrushing. And that is more than can be said of most dental health education.

DRUGS USED IN ENDODONTICS

Drugs may be used in endodontics:

1. To preserve an exposed but vital pulp.
2. After extirpation of a vital pulp.
3. After the root canal has become infected following pulp death.

Pulpotomy and pulp capping

When this is indicated (an exposed pulp in a tooth with open apices) successful preservation of the vitality of the pulp depends on the following principles:

1. A good aseptic technique.
2. Use of a non-irritant pulp-dressing which encourages calcification.

Aseptic technique is essential (both here and in any other type of endodontic treatment) to prevent introduction of bacteria from the patient's mouth or (worse) from the operator's hands. The latter may carry *Staph. aureus* – a virulent organism to which the pulp may be highly susceptible. The operating field must also be disinfected.

Pulp dressings. If the pulp is healthy and especially if the apices are incomplete the aim is to keep the pulp alive at least until the apices are closed and to encourage the pulp to re-form a roof of hard tissue. Calcium hydroxide is widely used and overall offers a reasonable chance of success. Proprietary preparations based on calcium hydroxide are usually used for convenience.

The infected pulp. Very occasionally there is a need to preserve a pulp which is vital but so inflamed as to cause pain. One approach has been to use a dressing containing demethylchlortetracycline (which has a broad spectrum of activity and a prolonged action) with triamcinolone, a strongly anti-inflammatory corticosteroid. This is often effective in abolishing pain, but it seems that in most cases the pulp eventually dies. This preparation is therefore less popular than was at one time.

Root canal treatment

The basis of successful endodontic therapy is by surgical excision of infected tissue. The cavity thus made is then completely sealed to prevent seepage of tissue fluid into dead spaces where it can remain as a culture medium for bacteria.

Antibiotics versus surgical technique. At one time endodontic treatment was managed as an antibacterial therapeutic problem. Cultures were taken and antibiotic mixtures were used to 'sterilise' the canal.

However, removal of infected tissue is more important and antibacterial drugs are of secondary value. Infection in the root is removed by thorough reaming of the canal walls to remove inner infected dentine and leave a simple conical shape.

If infection has spread to cause an acute periapical abscess, it can be effectively drained through the open root canal. It is rarely necessary to give even a short course of systemic antibiotics to accelerate the healing of such an infection. This may have to be considered, however, if the patient's resistance is in any way impaired.

Use of antiseptics

Whether or not the pulp chamber is severely infected, asepsis should be maintained. The tooth should be isolated with rubber dam and the operation field (tooth crown and adjacent rubber dam) disinfected by swabbing with chlorhexidine in alcohol. Instruments must be heat sterilised. Preparation of the canal is assisted by 'lubricating' the reamers with a mild antiseptic such as hydrogen peroxide (10 vol.) or 1% sodium hypochloride. The canal can also be irrigated with 1% hypochlorite (or Milton) or hydrogen peroxide, then normal saline. The danger that effervescent agents such as hydrogen peroxide can force infected debris through the apex by gas pressure is probably theoretical. It may be that irrigation fluids have no more than a mechanical washing function. Sterile normal saline may be just as effective, but most antiseptics have the advantage of being stable and should not need to be sterilised before use.

Root canal dressings

Between visits sterility is maintained (or re-infection prevented) by using an antiseptic dressing on a paper point. Commonly used antiseptics are paramonochlorphenol, formocresol or camphorated phenol or proprietary preparations based on similar agents. These do not seem to irritate the periapical tissue. The paper point is held in place with a temporary filling.

Antibiotic preparations. Polyantibiotic root canal pastes have fallen into disfavour in many quarters as having no tangible advantages, but sometimes having at least theoretical dangers. Penicillin mixtures should not be used, as even this minute amount can cause a severe reaction in a sensitised patient. Chloramphenicol mixtures have no advantages and might possibly be dangerous. A bacitracin-neomycin paste has at least the advantage of an exceptionally wide spectrum of antibacterial activity and less toxicity than chloramphenical. Polyantibiotic pastes retain some popularity, but it can be shown that careful aseptic surgical technique alone is the most important factor for success. It is also arguable that antibiotics should be given systemically if there is any case for giving them.

Root canal preparation and filling

The aims of surgical (mechanical) preparation of the root canal are:

1. Clearance of all tissue debris and exudate from the canal.
2. A sufficiently enlarged canal of simple conical shape.
3. Absence of symptoms.

The narrow space between the filling point and the canal walls is obliterated with a sealant of semiliquid zinc oxide in eugenol, or an equivalent proprietary preparation. The canal is then permanently filled with a well-fitting gutta-percha point. The crown of the tooth can be restored in the normal fashion.

PRE- AND POSTOPERATIVE USE OF DRUGS FOR DENTAL AND ORAL SURGERY

Pericoronitis

Pericoronitis is an infection of the blind pocket round a third molar which has started to erupt into the mouth.

Pericoronitis usually responds quickly to local measures, namely irrigation under the flap and frequent hot mouthwashes. Severe infection can, however, spread quickly and there may already be lymphadenitis when the patient is first seen. In this case metronidazole or penicillin (if there are no contraindications) should be given.

When the infection has subsided the tooth can, if necessary, be extracted.

Prophylactic use of antibiotics for oral surgery

The main applications have been considered in the previous chapter but antibiotics may also be used prophylactically:

1. For major jaw surgery.
2. For difficult disimpactions of third molars.
3. After severe maxillofacial injuries.

In the case of major surgery such as resections of the jaw followed by grafting or 'push back' operations for prognathism, it is vital to get vascularisation of the graft and union either of the graft to adjacent bone or between newly exposed bone surfaces. All this must happen in the presence of considerable amounts of blood clot. The consequences of bone infection are disastrous and treatment is more difficult than prevention.

In the case of third molar disimpactions, the prophylactic use of antibiotics is more controversial. Many believe that without them the incidence of painful infected sockets is much higher. Once a socket has become infected localised osteitis does not respond to antibiotics; their prophylactic use here is therefore possibly justifiable. On the other hand, evidence has been produced showing that good aseptic technique renders antibiotics unnecessary for this type of operation.

Maxillofacial injuries. Penicillin, 600 mg, is usually given as a routine measure to patients who have had severe maxillofacial injuries. In these patients there is a greater chance of infection of blood clot from the exterior by way of a periodontal pocket when this is in the fracture line.

If the cranial cavity has been opened by a fracture passing through the cribriform plate of the ethmoid, then rifampicin (p. 35) is probably the antibiotic of choice.

Infected sockets

These are generally spoken of as 'dry' sockets because of the absence of clot. The main predisposing factors may be (i) poor local blood supply, (ii) operative trauma and (iii) local fibrinolytic activity. The lower molar region is usually affected and infection was a common complication of disimpaction of third molars in the era before the introduction of antibiotics.

An infected socket is an area of localised osteitis where part of the bone of the lamina dura dies and eventually sequestrates. These sequestra are usually small, however, and are eventually shed unnoticed.

The clot having been destroyed, the socket fills with debris from the mouth and there is persistent low-grade infection. Once this has happened, antibiotics have no useful effect.

The usual measures are to:

1. Irrigate the socket thoroughly with warm dilute antiseptic or normal saline to remove debris.
2. Lightly pack the socket with Whitehead's varnish or bismuth-iodoform-paraffin-paste (BIPP) on ribbon gauze.
3. Repeat daily if pain remains severe and persistent.
4. Prescribe a hot mouthwash to keep the rest of the mouth clean.
5. Prescribe an analgesic such as aspirin.

Healing takes its own time and the socket eventually fills with granulation tissue. This may take 10 or more days, in its initial stages at least is very painful and there is so far no effective way of hastening resolution. Hence, where there is a strong chance of this complication – as after difficult disimpaction of third molars – prophylactic use of an antibiotic may be justified. Infected sockets are by contrast so uncommon a complication of ordinary dental extractions that the routine use of antibiotics is pointless and undesirable.

Various proprietary preparations both for the prevention and treatment of dry sockets have been introduced from time to time.

Postoperative oedema

After extensive oral surgery there is often – not surprisingly – considerable facial swelling. The main consideration is to make sure that there is no postoperative infection. Once the clot is firmly established, i.e. 24 hours after operation, frequent hot rinses will help to make things more comfortable and the oedema resolves in its own time. Proprietary preparations of proteolytic enzymes are intended to speed up this process but have never been shown to be of any significant benefit.

A short course of systemic corticosteroids taken with non-steroidal anti-inflammatory agents preoperatively can often abolish postoperative pain and swelling. However, the choice of drugs is largely empirical and the optimal regimen has yet to be worked out.

SUGGESTED FURTHER READING

Brennen T A (1987) The Acquired Immunodeficiency Syndrome (AIDS) as an Occupational Disease. Annals of Internal Medicine 107: 581

CDC 1987 Update on hepatitis B prevention. Annals of Internal Medicine 107: 353

CDC 1987 Recommendations for prevention of HIV transmission in health-care settings. Journal of the American Medical Association 258: 1293

Cottone J A, Molinari J A 1987 Selection for dental practice of chemical disinfectants and sterilants for hepatitis and AIDS. Australian Dental Journal 32: 368

Council on Dental Therapeutics 1988 Infection control recommendations for the dental office and the dental laboratory. Journal of the American Dental Association 116: 241

Forrest J O 1987 Stannous fluoride gel in preventive practice. Dental Practice March 5: 13

Grenby T H, Saldanha M G 1984 The antimicrobial activity of modern mouthwashes. British Dental Journal 157: 239

Moran J, Addy M, Newcombe R 1988 The antibacterial effect of toothpastes on the salivary flora. Journal of Clininal Periodontology 15: 193

Porter S R Scully C, Cawson R A 1987 AIDS: update and guidelines for general dental practice. Dental Update Jan/Feb

Seymour R A, Heasman P A 1988 Drugs and the periodontium. Journal of Clinical Periodontology 15: 1

Shaw J H 1987 Causes and Control of Dental Caries. New England Journal of Medicine 317: 996

Sim A J W, Dudley H A F 1988 Surgeons and HIV. British Medical Journal 296: 80

Stephen K W, McCall D R, Tullis J I 1987 Caries prevalence in northern Scotland before, and 5 years after, water defluoridation. British Dental Journal 163: 324

Turnidge J D 1988 A reappraisal of co-trimoxazole. Medical Journal of Australia 148: 296

Zacherl W A, Pfeiffer H J, Swancar J R 1985. The effect of soluble pyrophosphates on dental calculus in adults. Journal of the American Dental Association 110: 737

5. The nervous system
I. The neuromuscular junction and the autonomic nervous system

Most activities of the body are under the control of the nervous system. In simple terms (taking no account of minor exceptions) there are:

1. *The Voluntary Nervous System.* This mediates conscious control of muscular activity.

2. *The Involuntary or Autonomic Nervous System.* This controls in an automatic fashion the function of such structures as the heart and blood vessels, intestines and glands.

The arrangement of nerve connections in the efferent (outflow) fibres is different in the voluntary and autonomic nervous systems. The neuronal outflow from the spinal cord illustrates these differences (Fig. 5.1)

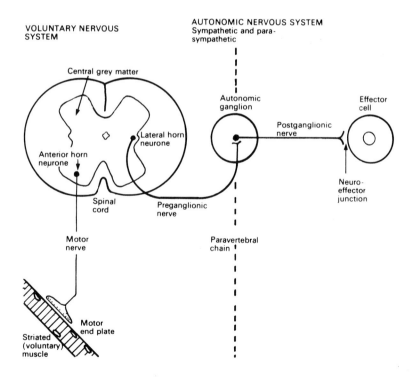

Fig. 5.1 Outflow of nerve fibres from the spinal cord in the voluntary and autonomic nervous system

THE VOLUNTARY NERVOUS SYSTEM AND THE NEUROMUSCULAR JUNCTION

The pharmacological basis of muscular contraction and the activation of the neuromuscular junction by chemical agents is of considerable practical importance, particularly in general anaesthesia.

For many kinds of operation it is essential to have muscular relaxation. In the past, this was obtained simply by inducing very deep anaesthesia with its attendant dangers. However, it is possible to achieve any degree of muscular relaxation by blocking the chemical processes involved in muscular activity. Under these circumstances, the anaesthetic agent is required only to keep the patient unconscious, in a light plane of anaesthesia.

Mechanisms

The efferent nerve fibres in the voluntary nervous system are the axons of the motor nerve cell bodies in the anterior grey horn. The bundles of axons are called motor nerves. These travel without interruption to supply striated (voluntary) muscle. These motor nerve fibres carry the nerve impulses from the central nervous system to the muscles whenever a voluntary movement is initiated.

On the surface of the muscle the axon splits up into several fine nerve branches. These do not quite touch the muscle fibres, but are separated from them by a minute gap of about 20 nm. The region of the termination of the motor nerve on the surface of the muscle fibre is called the motor end-plate.

Electrical excitation spreads down the motor nerve, into its terminal branches, and then produces electrical excitation in the muscle fibres; this is followed by contraction of the muscle. There is no electrical continuity across the motor end-plate, but the terminals filaments of the motor nerve contain vesicles of acetylcholine. When an action potential passes down to the end of the nerve fibre, these vesicles empty into the gap between the nerve ending and the surface of the muscle fibre. Acetylcholine then diffuses across the gap to stimulate receptors on the surface of the muscle. This results in a wave of electrical excitation passing along the muscle fibre. The electrical excitement in the muscle fibre is followed in turn by contraction.

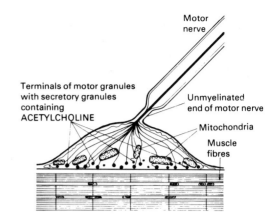

Fig. 5.2 Diagrammatic representation of the motor end-plate

The junction between a motor nerve ending and the adjacent region of a voluntary muscle fibre is represented diagrammatically in Fig. 5.2.

In electrical terms, when an excitable cell such as a nerve or muscle is in its resting, non-stimulated state, it is not conducting waves of electrical activity. Under these conditions there is a negative charge within the cell relative to the outside. This is called the polarised (resting) state. When the cell is stimulated, electrical excitement takes the form of a wave of depolarisation which passes along the cell. Depolarisation means that the membrane allows a positive charge to pass from the outside of the cell membrane to the cell interior. Thus, the potential difference between the inside and outside of the cell is abolished during electrical excitation. The chemical and electrical similarities to the process of neural transmission (see Ch. 9) will be obvious.

In the muscle fibre, therefore, when acetylcholine reaches cholinergic receptors on its surface the muscle becomes depolarised. Electrical excitation of a muscle fibre is, therefore, a wave of depolarisation. This spreads along the length of the fibre which, as a consequence, contracts.

One short burst of nerve impulses in the motor axon leads to a brief release of acetylcholine over the muscle fibre. The subsequent contraction of the muscle which follows is short-lived because the acetylcholine is rapidly removed (hydrolysed) by an enzyme – acetylcholinesterase – to form acetate and choline. Acetate is oxidised to form carbon dioxide and water. Some of the choline is taken up again into nerve endings for re-synthesis of acetylcholine. Stimulation leads only to a single contraction. Even when the muscle is kept in a depolarised state it relaxes after the initial contraction.

To recapitulate, the sequence of events in the initiation of muscular contraction, therefore, appears to be that:

1. The motor nerve cell body or its dendrites are stimulated (by another neurone) in the central nervous system.

2. The wave of excitation travels along the axon of the motor neurone and leaves the central nervous system in the motor nerve. This terminates on the surface of striated muscle fibres of a voluntary muscle.

3. The excitation in the nerve is in the form of a wave of depolarisation moving from the central nervous system to the motor end-plates.

4. At the nerve terminal in the motor end-plate, the zone of depolarisation causes acetylcholine to be released into the gap between nerve and muscle. This chemical transmitter diffuses across the gap to reach cholinergic receptor areas on the surface of the muscle.

5. The stimulation of these areas by acetylcholine causes a wave of depolarisation in the muscle which travels from the receptors beneath the motor end-plate to spread over the entire muscle.

6. Depolarisation of muscle is followed by contraction. The depolarisation is short-lived because acetylcholine is hydrolysed by cholinesterase.

Muscle relaxant drugs

Paralysis of muscles during general anaesthesia can be produced by drugs which interfere with the normal stimulation of the acetylcholine receptor on the surface of the muscle.

During treatment with these paralysing drugs, the muscles of respiration are as severely affected as other striated muscle. The patient therefore has respiratory paralysis and respiration must always be maintained artificially.

The term 'muscle relaxants' is euphemistically applied to these drugs but in fact they are muscle *paralysing* agents.

Muscle relaxants are divided into two groups: (a) non-depolarising and (b) depolarising drugs.

Non-depolarising muscle relaxants

The non-depolarising muscle relaxants act by binding to the cholinergic receptors on the surface of the muscle in the region of the motor end-plate. They therefore prevent access of acetylcholine to the receptors and thus prevent depolarisation in the muscle. Since a wave of depolarisation must pass over the muscle to produce contraction, the muscle does not contract and remains in the relaxed state. This type of drug effect is known as *competitive antagonism* because the muscle relaxant is competing with acetylcholine for access to the receptor on the muscle. A substance (such as acetylcholine) which binds to a receptor and then stimulates it is called an '*agonist*', while a substance which binds to a receptor and then has no action (except to prevent agonists from reaching the receptor) is called an '*antagonist*'.

The action of these neuromuscular blockers can in turn be antagonised by a cholinesterase inhibitor (such as neostigmine) which increases the concentration of acetylcholine around the cholinergic receptor.

Examples of non-depolarising muscle relaxants are tubocurarine and pancuronium. Tubocurarine is an extract of curare, a South American arrow poison. Tubocurarine is given by injection, starts to act within 3–5 minutes and is effective for about 30 minutes. Tubocurarine is a weak ganglion blocker and thus produces hypotension. It often also causes erythematous rashes probably as a result of inducing histamine release. Pancuronium does not have these disadvantages to any significant degree and has, therefore, largely replaced tubocurarine as a muscle relaxant for major surgery.

Depolarising muscle relaxants

These agents, of which suxamethonium is an example, act in an unusual way. They have some agonist activity – that is, they bind to the muscle receptors and cause depolarisation. However, unlike acetylcholine, which produces very short-lived depolarisation, the depolarising muscle relaxants cause depolarisation of the muscle beneath the motor end-plate which persists for several minutes. During this time, the muscle cannot be further depolarised and cannot respond to acetylcholine.

Depolarising agents produce more rapid and complete muscle relaxation than the non-depolarising group, but unlike the latter their action cannot be terminated by giving an anticholinesterase or any other drug.

When suxamethonium is given there is initial twitching of the muscles as depolarisation spreads over the muscle fibres. As mentioned earlier, muscle can only contract once following a single wave of depolarisation and, even when depolarisation is maintained, the muscle then relaxes. A single intravenous injection of suxamethonium produces muscular paralysis for about 5 minutes. The effect of the drug is terminated by the action of plasma *pseudocholinesterase*. This enzyme hydrolyses the drug and abolishes its pharmacological activity.

The action of suxamethonium is greatly prolonged – often for many hours – in patients who have an inherited deficiency of plasma pseudocholinesterase. During this period of paralysis, respiration must be maintained artificially until the respiratory muscles recover. An anticholinesterase (which blocks hydrolysis of acetylcholine) will not accelerate recovery and could theoretically slow it by increasing depolarisation at the motor end-plate.

Clinical applications of muscle relaxants

Since paralysis of voluntary muscle is always accompanied by respiratory paralysis, it is inevitably terrifying. Muscle relaxants are therefore usually given under general anaesthesia and always accompanied by assisted (intermittent positive pressure) respiration.

Their uses include:

1. Relaxation of laryngeal muscles to aid endotracheal intubation.

2. Relaxation of abdominal muscles, to gain access to the viscera, or of limb muscles when a joint has to be manipulated.

3. To relax persistent spasm of the larynx (rarely).

4. To counter the violent convulsions of electroconvulsive therapy used in the treatment of severe depression (p. 92).

5. Suppression of the patient's efforts to breathe when mechanically assisted ventilation is carried out. Without a muscle relaxant there is a tendency to fight the action of the respirator.

6. Relaxation of muscle spasm in tetanus to allow assisted ventilation to be given.

THE AUTONOMIC NERVOUS SYSTEM

The axons of nerves which leave the spinal cord to form the autonomic nervous system have their cell bodies in the lateral grey horns. These efferent axons then terminate in autonomic ganglia where they excite the nerve cells of the autonomic nerves to supply most of the structures in the body which are not under voluntary control. These include digestive and sweat glands, the heart and blood vessels, and the smooth muscle of the alimentary and genitourinary systems.

There are two peripheral junctions in the autonomic outflow:

1. A nerve–nerve junction in the autonomic ganglion.

2. A neuroeffector junction at the point of nerve supply to the organ.

At both of these junctions there is a gap of about 20 nm with no electrical continuity.

The chemical transmitter at the nerve–nerve junction (the synapse)—both *sympathetic and parasympathetic*—in the autonomic ganglia is acetylcholine.

At the neuroeffector junction of the parasympathetic system, the transmitter is acetylcholine.

At most neuroeffector junctions of the sympathetic system the transmitter is *noradrenaline.*

SYMPATHETIC AND PARASYMPATHETIC SYSTEMS

The autonomic nervous outflow is divided into two functional divisions: the sympathetic and parasympathetic nervous systems. Activation of the sympathetic system is associated with increased physical and emotional activity and brought into heightened function during fright, fight and flight. The parasympathetic system is brought into use during more sedate ('vegetative') activities such as digestion, sleep and contraction of the smooth muscle of the gut and bladder.

THE SYMPATHETIC NERVOUS SYSTEM

Nerve cells in the lateral grey horns of the spinal cord in segments Tl to L2 give off axons which leave the cord with each efferent nerve. The axons terminate in the sympathetic ganglia where they form a synapse with a nerve cell, the axons of which form the sympathetic nerves travelling to organs under sympathetic control (Fig. 5.3).

Another part of the sympathetic outflow is the nerve to the adrenal medulla, which has no synapse along its course. From a developmental point of view, the adrenal medullary cells are analogous to the nerve cell bodies in the sympathetic ganglion and, like them, are stimulated by nerves arising in the lateral horn of the cord.

The chemical transmitter substance in the sympathetic ganglia is *acetylcholine* but in most sites the transmitter in the neuroeffector junction is *noradrenaline.*

There are, however, exceptions: these are the nerves to the adrenal medullary cells and to the sweat glands which are cholinergic. The adrenal medulla secretes both adrenaline and noradrenaline.

Fight, fright or flight

The concept of the sympathetic nervous system as mediating the responses to an emergency is a useful one. When violent action is anticipated or carried out the cardiovascular, respiratory and skeletal muscle systems need to respond appropriately.

Important responses of the body as a result of sympathetic stimulation in response to an emergency therefore include:

1. Increased cardiac output to increase the blood supply to the muscles to enable them to act more vigorously.

2. Vasodilatation in the skeletal muscles which provide the action.

3. Dilatation of the bronchi and increased rate of respiration to maximise oxygen intake.

4. Central stimulation (sensations of anger or panic) and dilatation of the pupils.

To compensate for the diversion of blood to the more active parts, the blood flow to the skin and viscera is reduced by contraction of the smooth muscles of their arterioles. Digestive secretions

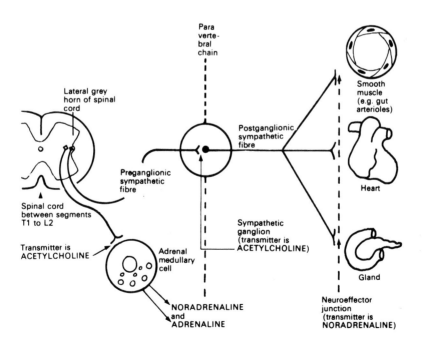

Fig. 5.3 Diagram of sympathetic nervous system to show the main connections and the sites of release of the different chemical mediators.

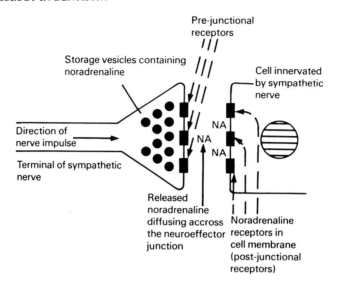

Fig. 5.4 This diagram of a sympathetic (adrenergic) nerve ending indicates the way in which noradrenaline released from the storage vesicles diffuses across the synaptic cleft to reach specific receptors on target cells, i.e. those innervated by the sympathetic nervous system. The stimulation of prejunctional noradrenaline receptors inhibits further release of transmitter.

(including salivation) and peristalsis also decrease and sphincters close.

Sympathetic activity therefore prepares the body for violent action and sympathomimetic drugs produce these effects to a greater or lesser degree and with varying degrees of selectivity.

The sympathetic nerve ending and its target organ are shown in Figure 5.4.

Sympathomimetic drugs

Sympathomimetic drugs are those which produce some or all of the effects of sympathetic activation. The main examples are the natural products *noradrenaline* (norepinephrine) and *adrenaline* (epinephrine).

At the neuroeffector junction the released noradrenaline diffuses across the gap and stimulates specific receptors in the target cells. The effects of sympathetic transmitter (adrenaline or noradrenaline) binding and then activating these post junctional receptors are:

1. Increased force and rate of the heartbeat.
2. Increased velocity of conduction down the atrioventricular bundle (bundle of His).
3. Increased excitability of the myocardium.

4. Vasodilatation in the myocardium and in voluntary (striated) muscle.
5. Vasoconstriction in skin and viscera.
6. Bronchodilatation.
7. Central stimulation.

Injected noradrenaline does not produce all these different effects with the same degree of intensity. Other sympathomimetic drugs also have selective actions to produce only a few of these effects.

The selective action of sympathomimetic drugs depends on the fact that there are three main groups of sympathetic (adrenergic) receptors. Sympathomimetic drugs can therefore act on one or several of these receptors at the same time. These different receptors can also be selectively blocked by another group of drugs, that is the adrenergic blocking agents described later.

One important aspect of these subdivisions of sympathomimetic activity is that many (e.g. vasoconstriction or bronchodilatation) are sometimes useful while others, e.g. increased myocardial excitability, can be dangerous to susceptible patients.

The three types of adrenergic activity are:

α_1 *actions:*
1. Vasoconstriction in the viscera.

2. Vasoconstriction in the skin.

β_1 actions:

1. Increased rate of beating of the heart.
2. Increased rate of conduction down the A–V bundle.
3. Increased myocardial excitability.
4. Increased force of contraction of the heart.

β_2 actions:

1. Bronchodilatation.
2. Vasodilatation in the myocardium.
3. Vasodilatation in the voluntary muscles.

Prejunctional (inhibitory) receptors. In addition to postjunctional alpha and beta receptors, which have the actions already described, there are also (to make things even more difficult) *prejunctional* (presynaptic, α_2) receptors within the cell membranes of those nerve endings which release noradrenaline. By a feed-back mechanism, the release of noradrenaline into the synaptic cleft stimulates the prejunctional receptor and this *inhibits* further release of noradrenaline and shortens its action. Blockade of prejunctional receptors therefore causes release of noradrenaline.

An alpha receptor blocking drug, such as phentolamine (which happens to block both pre- and postjunctional receptors), produces an initial dilatation of arterioles, but this action is quickly weakened or terminated because of the blockade of the prejunctional alpha receptors; this leads to an outpouring of noradrenaline which overcomes the initial dilatation of the blood vessels.

Phentolamine therefore has only a short duration of action as an antihypertensive drug. Prazosin, by contrast, is a selective postjunctional alpha receptor blocker and having no significant prejunctional receptor blocking action, has no effect on noradrenaline release. It therefore causes prolonged vasodilatation and is a useful antihypertensive drug (see also Table 5.2)

Adrenaline (one of the adrenal medullary hormones) injected subcutaneously produces α, β_1 and β_2 actions, all of similar intensity. There is tachycardia and increased force of contraction of the heart (causing increased systolic blood pressure), vasodilatation in muscles (which tends to cause a fall in the diastolic blood pressure) and bronchodilatation.

Large doses of adrenaline increase the excitability of the myocardium and can cause dangerous cardiac arrhythmias. Adrenaline is virtually never given intravenously, because a sudden increase in β_1 stimulation of the heart can produce ventricular fibrillation. Fibrillation means that there is no effective ventricular contraction and therefore total loss of cardiac output. If uncorrected this is followed by death in a few minutes.

Subcutaneous injection of *noradrenaline* produces all these actions, but the α_1 effects are much stronger than the β_1, and β_2 actions. Thus, noradrenaline causes mainly constriction of the arterioles in the skin and viscera. This raises the peripheral resistance in the vascular system and thus raises the blood pressure – particularly the diastolic component. The rise in blood pressure usually causes reflex slowing of the heart.

Other more selective drugs. Isoprenaline (isoproterenol) has only β_1 and β_2 effects and has no α activity. Since it stimulates β_1 and β_2 receptors only, isoprenaline produces tachycardia and increased force of contraction of the heart (β_1 effects) and bronchodilatation (β_2 effects). This has the danger that an overdose can increase the excitability of the myocardium and cause ventricular fibrillation.

Salbutamol is even more selective. It stimulates β_2 receptors only and has very little action on β_1 receptors. Thus, it produces bronchodilatation with little tachycardia or increase in excitability. There is therefore little danger of ventricular fibrillation.

Central effects of sympathomimetic agents

Sympathomimetic drugs cause central stimulation – an effect in keeping with the flight, fright and fight actions of the sympathetic system. Thus, adrenaline causes sensations of anxiety or panic. Amphetamines and more especially cocaine produce sensations of alertness or elation which, in the case of cocaine in particular, is so pleasurable as to make the drug highly addictive. Appetite suppressants such as diethylpropion have a similar but milder effect. All sympathomimetic agents induce wakefulness and amphetamines have been widely used in the past, for example, by students working (as usual) at the last moment for examinations or by truck drivers who want to complete a long journey without delay.

As a result of the pleasurable stimulation of mood

induced by cocaine, amphetamine and related drugs, they are prone to cause dependence. They are as a consequence controlled drugs.

Noradrenaline has no significant effects on mood.

Directly and indirectly acting sympathomimetic agents

Many of the drugs mentioned so far – noradrenaline, adrenaline, isoprenaline and salbutamol – act directly on α and/or β receptors. They are therefore called directly acting sympathomimetic agents.

Another group of drugs such as the amphetamines have an indirect sympathomimetic action. These do not stimulate α and β receptors but enter the storage vesicles to displace noradrenaline which then leaves the nerve ending. The transmitter crosses the gap and stimulates the α and β receptors. In this way, such drugs lead only indirectly to receptor activation.

Ephedrine is a drug which has both indirect and direct sympathomimetic activity.

The classification of sympathomimetic drugs is therefore as follows and is summarised in Table 5.1.

1. Directly acting:
   Noradrenaline: α activity stronger than β activity.
   Adrenaline: α, β_1 and β_2 activity.
   Isoprenaline: β_1 and β_2 activity.
   Salbutamol: β_2 activity.
2. Indirectly acting:
   Cocaine.
   Amphetamine (mainly stimulation of the CNS and only weak peripheral actions).
3. Mixed direct and indirect action:
   Ephedrine.

1. Directly acting sympathomimetic drugs

Noradrenaline. This produces visceral and cutaneous vasoconstriction. When given intravenously noradrenaline produces an almost immediate rise in blood pressure. For this reason it has been used in the treatment of shock but has the disadvantage that the intense vasoconstriction reduces the blood supply to vital organs. Most shocked patients with peripheral circulatory failure are not, therefore, treated in this way nowadays because the aim of treatment is to increase blood flow to vital organs such as the kidneys.

Noradrenaline is used in some local anaesthetic solutions to prolong duration of action by producing vasoconstriction around the site of injection, but it has no advantages for this purpose and is dangerous because of the risk of acute hypertension.

Adrenaline. This has been extensively used in the past as a bronchodilator in the treatment of asthmatic attacks. Following a subcutaneous injection (the correct route of administration in most cases), there is not only effective bronchodilatation but the systolic blood pressure and heart rate increase. As a result the use of adrenaline in asthma has ceased since the introduction of the selective β_2 agonists such as salbutamol. But adrenaline is still given for anaphylaxis.

Adrenaline should not be given intravenously because of the danger of cardiac arrhythmias.

Adrenaline is widely used as a vasoconstrictor agent incorporated with local anaesthetics to prolong their action and over many decades of use, has proved to be safe.

Isoprenaline is another powerful bronchodilator drug which is used in asthma. Isoprenaline is absorbed through the oral mucosa; the drug directly enters systemic capillaries and so avoids breakdown in the liver.

The preferred mode of administration of isoprenaline is by inhalation. The drug is given as an aerosol from a pressurised nebuliser giving a fixed dose. The main advantages of this route of administration are that the lungs receive a high concentration of the drug immediately while relatively little passes to the rest of the body. Nevertheless, some patients have given themselves greatly excessive amounts and died suddenly – probably because of ventricular fibrillation due to massive β_1, stimulation. The use of isoprenaline has therefore greatly declined.

Isoprenaline is also used in the treatment of arrhythmias of the heart when increased rate of initiation of the cardiac impulse or increased A–V conduction is needed. Isoprenaline may be used to treat loss of consciousness due to excessive bradycardia or heart block.

Salbutamol is one of the drugs of choice in the day-to-day management of bronchial asthma. Salbutamol is a selective β_2 stimulator – it produces

Table 5.1 Sympathomimetic drugs

Effect on	Noradrenaline (Norepinephrine)	Adrenaline (Epinephrine)	Isoprenaline (Isoproterenol)	Salbutamol	Receptors involved
Heart					
a. Rate	*Slowed* (reflexly due to BP rise)	*Increased* (direct action)	*Increased* (direct action)	Some stimulation with large doses only	β_1
b. Force of contraction	*Increased* (partly due to slowing but also some direct stimulation)	*Increased* (direct action) palpitations due to a + b	*Increased* (direct action) palpitations due to a + b		
c. Output	Insignificant change	*Increased*	*Increased*		
d. Excitability	*Increased*	*Much increased*	*Much increased*		
Blood vessels to:					
a. Muscle	No effect	Dilated	Dilated	Dilated	β_2
b. Skin and viscera	Constricted	Constricted	No effect	No effect	α_1
c. Heart	No significant effect	Dilated	Dilated	Dilated	β_2
Total peripheral resistance	*Increased*	*Increased*	*Decreased*	*Decreased*	
Blood pressure: Combined effects of changes in (i) cardiac output and (ii) peripheral resistance as shown above					
a. Systolic	*Rises*	*Rises*	*Rises* or little change	Slight increase	
b. Diastolic	*Rises*	*Falls*	*Falls*	Slight decrease	
Central nervous system	Insignificant effect	*Stimulation:* feelings of fear and anxiety, respiration increased, tremor	Stimulation	Insignificant	
Bronchioles	Insignificant effect	Dilatation	Dilatation	Dilatation	β_2

bronchodilatation without significantly increasing cardiac excitability.

Salbutamol is usually given by inhalation of an aerosol or of a powder from a special dispenser (Rotahaler). Salbutamol can also be given orally – and is absorbed from the upper part of the small intestine – or intravenously. Intravenous injection produces an almost immediate response and is useful in the management of acute asthmatic attacks, when the intense brochospasm prevents adequate inhalation of an aerosol.

Aminophylline is another drug often given intravenously for acute asthma, but has the disadvantage of stronger β_1 effects on the heart. Large doses of aminophylline, though effective, can therefore precipitate dangerous cardiac arrhythmias or even ventricular fibrillation. The risk of this is negligible with intravenous salbutamol which is probably, therefore, the drug of choice for the treatment of mild or severe asthmatic attacks. Aminophylline can also provoke nausea, vomiting, fits and circulatory collapse.

2. Indirectly acting sympathomimetic drugs

Sympathomimetic agents have a stimulant effect on the CNS (p. 69). Adrenaline causes sensations of wakefulness, anxiety or panic. Others, such as cocaine and amphetamine, produce wakefulness and elation.

Cocaine. This is the only local anaesthetic agent which is strongly sympathomimetic, having indirect α and β effects by displacing stores of noradrenaline at the sympathetic nerve endings and blocking their reuptake. Cocaine is therefore an effective vasoconstrictor and also has similar effects on the heart to adrenaline. Overdose may cause sudden death probably from ventricular fibrillation. Because of this risk cocaine is not given by injection.

Cocaine has an almost unique assortment of properties in that it is:

1. A potent, (indirectly acting) sympathomimetic agent, and hence a vasoconstrictor.
2. A potent local and surface anaesthetic.
3. A strong central stimulant.
4. A drug of addiction because of its euphoriant effects.

Amphetamine. Amphetamine has weak peripheral sympathomimetic activity. Amphetamine usually produces only slight bronchodilatation, tachycardia and hypertension. Its main action is on the brain. Amphetamine is a central stimulant and increases mental activity, decreases sensations of sleepiness and fatigue, and produces excitement, euphoria and anorexia.

The drug has been used in the past to suppress the appetite in the hope of controlling obesity. Unfortunately, the drug is powerfully addictive and the effect on appetite only transient. Because of its high addictive potential, amphetamine is used very little in clinical practice and it is a Controlled Drug.

Amphetamine has, however, been shown both to enhance the effect of morphine and to reduce the central nervous system depression that the narcotic causes. This may therefore be a valuable clinical use for this otherwise much denigrated drug. The use of psychoactive agents to enhance the effect of analgesics is also discussed in Chapter 7.

3. Sympathomimetic drugs with both direct and indirect actions

Ephedrine. Ephedrine has two actions: it displaces stores of noradrenaline from sympathetic nerve endings and it also stimulates α and β receptors, as does adrenaline.

Ephedrine can be used in the treatment of asthma and for this purpose is given orally. Ephedrine is occasionally given by injection to maintain the blood pressure during a spinal anaesthetic.

Ephedrine may be used in nose drops for hay fever and in dentistry, to reduce congestion and oedema of the nasal mucosa, and thus improve drainage from the maxillary antrum. This may be useful if, for example, the antrum is exposed to infection via an oro-antral fistula.

Adrenoreceptor (adrenergic) blockers

The idea of a division of the results of sympathetic stimulation into α and β effects was confirmed by showing that these effects could be selectively blocked by different drugs.

Drugs such as phentolamine and thymoxamine bind to and block α receptors, leaving β activity mainly unaffected. These agents are known as α blockers.

β-blocking drugs block β receptors, but some have other additional actions. Important examples are propranolol and oxprenolol.

α receptor blockers

Phentolamine binds reversibly to α receptors. This short-acting drug has been used in the diagnosis and management of phaeochromocytoma. This is a tumour of the adrenal medulla which secretes adrenaline and noradrenaline. These tumours cause hypertension which is reversed by phentolamine.

Phentolamine and other α blockers are used to try to increase blood flow in the tissues in peripheral obstructive vascular disease. In shock, α blockers may by themselves lower blood pressure, and in practice blood, plasma or dextran is also given intravenously to replace the circulating fluid volume and restore the blood pressure.

Thymoxamine is a long-acting α blocker which is used in the treatment of hypertension due to phaeochromocytoma.

Prazosin is a seletive, postjunctional α receptor blocker. It is widely used for the treatment of hypertension.

Uses of α adrenoreceptor blocking drugs

These include the treatment of:

1. *Hypertension* due to:
a. Phaeochromocytoma (a tumour producing adrenaline and noradrenaline).
b. Overdosage of noradrenaline or potentiation of pressor amines (particularly by tyramine in cheese) in patients receiving monoamine oxidase inhibitors (see Ch. 6).
c. Essential hypertension: the older α blockers were not usually suitable, as their hypotensive effects did not persist and side-effects were troublesome. Side-effects included tachycardia, postural hypotension and gastrointestinal actions such as diarrhoea, as a result of unopposed parasympathetic activity. However, newer drugs such as labetalol which possesses both α and β adrenoceptor properties are useful hypotensive agents. The pure α_1 adrenoceptor blocker prazosin has no action on prejunctional α receptors (Table 5.2). It is a very effective vasodilator and is also valuable in the treatment of essential hypertension.

2. *Peripheral vascular disease.* α blocking agents such as tolazoline may be used for the relief of spasm of peripheral vessels in Raynaud's disease and to promote the healing of chronic ulceration of the skin which is a complication of varicose veins for instance. However, little success usually comes from such treatment.

β receptor blockers

Propranolol blocks both β_1 and β_2 receptors. Because of its action on β_1 receptors, it diminishes sympathetic drive to the heart. Thus, the tachycardia and increased cardiac work of exercise are blocked – this is of benefit to patients with angina pectoris. Such patients have an impaired blood flow

Table 5.2 Drugs acting on pre- and postjunctional α receptors

Drug	Action on prejunctional α receptor	Action on postjunctional α receptor	Result of drug action
Phenoxybenzamine Phentolamine Talazoline	Blockade ∴ more NA released	Blockade ∴ vasodilatation	Weak vasodilator ∴ little or no hypotension
Prazosin	No effect	Blockade ∴ vasodilatation	Strong vasodilator Considerable antihypertensive action
Clonidine Methyldopa	Powerful stimulation ∴ reduced NA release	Weak stimulation ∴ tendency to vasoconstriction	Net result is vasodilatation and hypotension because NA not released

NA, noradrenaline.

to the myocardium, so that exercise which increases the oxygen needs of the myocardium, causes pain in the chest. Propranolol decreases the response of the heart to exercise and thus prevents the pain of angina.

Propranolol is also used to block background sympathetic tone which otherwise enhances the excitability of the heart. The ability of the drug to decrease myocardial excitability makes it useful for the treatment of cardiac arrhythmias such as atrial and ventricular tachycardias and extrasystoles.

Propranolol also blocks both β_2 receptors and background sympathetic tone which dilates the bronchi. Asthmatic individuals rely on such relaxation of the bronchial muscle to maintain a free airway and a β_2 blocker causes a dangerous degree of bronchospasm in such patients.

Atenolol and *metoprolol* are selective β_1 blockers and have similar actions and uses to propranolol in cardiovascular disease. Because they have relatively little β_2 blocking action they have less toxicity in asthmatic patients – but nevertheless enough to produce dangerous bronchospasm in some individuals.

Practolol is another selective β_1 blocker, but this can cause dry eyes, ocular damage which can culminate in blindness, rashes, stomatitis and peritoneal adhesions as side-effects and its use is now restricted to specialist emergency treatment.

The β blockers are also used in the treatment of hypertension. This is partly by decreasing the stroke volume of the heart, but there is also a central action on the nervous control of blood pressure, a reduction in renin output by the kidney and a reduction in the release of noradrenaline from sympathetic nerves.

Uses of β blocking agents

The main applications can be summarised as:

1. *Angina pectoris.* β blockers diminish sympathetic drive to the heart, particularly during exercise, and reduce cardiac effort.
2. *Cardiac arrhythmias.* β blockers reduce cardiac excitability. This may be useful during general anaesthesia with halothane which sensitises the myocardium to catecholamines such as adrenaline. β blockers may also be effective in controlling

arrhythmias after myocardial infarction and these drugs have been shown to improve survival by reducing the risk of reinfarction.

3. *Essential hypertension.* β blockers diminish sympathetic tone, decrease cardiac output, but possibly also have a central action on nervous control of blood pressure.
4. *Anxiety*, which is characterised by obvious sympathetic overactivity (dry mouth, palpitations, tremor), and which can disable speakers and musicians who are giving public performances, generally responds better to β blockers than to benzodiazepines.

In addition to these important applications, β blockers have a remarkable range of activities, a few of which are discussed in later chapters but are summarised here:

1. Arrhythmias.
2. Hypertension.
3. Angina pectoris.
4. Acute and secondary management of myocardial infarction.
5. Thyrotoxicosis.
6. Hypertrophic cardiomyopathy and some other heart diseases.
7. Migraine prophylaxis.
8. Essential tremor.
9. Anxiety states with strong sympathetic manifestations.
10. Open angle glaucoma.
11. Alcohol and narcotic withdrawal.
12. Portal hypertension.

They may also be effective contraceptive agents since they are potent spermatocides.

Note: Individual β blockers vary significantly in their effectiveness in these different applications.

Sympathetic blockade in the treatment of hypertension

Peripheral resistance, and hence blood pressure, can be lowered by reducing sympathetic tone, i.e. the vasoconstrictor action on the arterioles is diminished. This effect may be predominantly:

1. Central, e.g. clonidine and methyldopa act centrally but also have important peripheral effects (Table 5.2); β blockers may also act on the CNS.

2. At the arteriole, e.g. prazosin.

3. At the adrenergic nerve ending, e.g. guanethidine. β blockers possibly reduce transmitter release.

These are discussed in more detail in Chapter 10.

β blockers may also be used preoperatively to control excessive anxiety and arrhythmias which result from the latter and from other causes.

Appetite suppressants (anorectics)

Anorectics are drugs used to suppress appetite (i.e. induce anorexia) in order to help the obese lose weight. It is convenient to discuss them here as most of them are related chemically to the amphetamines.

Obesity is one of the current major problems in medicine, particularly because of its association with or contribution to hypertension, atherosclerosis and ischaemic heart disease.

Individuals vary widely in their ability to cope with a given calorie intake. Although the obese person may not necessarily have a greater calorie intake than a thin person, the only way by which he can safely and reliably lose weight is by eating (and drinking) less and by taking more exercise. This is more easily said than done since an uncommon degree of self-discipline is needed to remain persistently faithful to a restricted and boring diet.

Sympathomimetic agents, particularly the amphetamines, suppress appetite. Amphetamines and other somewhat similar drugs, such as diethylpropion (Tenuate), are addictive and are controlled drugs. They have very similar effects to the amphetamines. They may cause mild euphoria, insomnia, 'edginess' or tachycardia in some patients.

Fluorinated amphetamines such as fenfluramine (Ponderax) have the opposite side-effects. They have a sedative action on the CNS and their main disadvantages are drowsiness and sometimes depression. The main advantage of this different action is that patients are less likely to become dependent and insomnia is less likely to be a problem. In addition fenfluramine, unlike the amphetamines, does not antagonise antihypertensive therapy. This is important as obesity and hypertension are often associated.

The appetite suppressant effect of both these types of drugs is real, but most patients seem quite quickly to acquire tolerance and the effect is relatively transient. Needless to say, anorectics are completely ineffective when patients do not also restrict their diet.

The current view is that anorectics have little more than a temporary effect but they can be used for a short time to help with dietary re-education. Fenfluramine, however, has been used for periods of at least 6 months with significant and sustained loss of weight.

THE PARASYMPATHETIC NERVOUS SYSTEM

The general arrangement of neurones in the parasympathetic nervous system is similar to that in the sympathetic (Fig. 5.5).

The parasympathetic nerve fibres leave the CNS with some of the cranial nerves (e.g. the nerves to the ciliary muscle and iris travel with the third cranial nerve; the vagus mainly carries parasympathetic fibres to the thoracic and abdominal viscera) and with the sacral nerves from segments S2 and S3. The parasympathetic ganglia are generally closely associated with the organs which they innervate – thus the postganglionic nerve fibres are very short. The neurotransmitter chemical in both the parasympathetic ganglion and in the neuroeffector junction is acetylcholine.

Muscarinic and nicotinic effects

At the neuroeffector junction of the parasympathetic system acetylcholine is said to exert *muscarinic* actions because these sites are also stimulated by the toxin, muscarine (from the poisonous toadstool *Amanita muscaria*). The effects of acetylcholine at the sympathetic and parasympathetic ganglia and at the motor end-plate of voluntary muscle are called *nicotinic* because in low concentrations nicotine also stimulates these sites. In high concentration nicotine blocks transmission across these junctions. The importance of these distinctions is that, although acetylcholine is the chemical transmitter in these different situations, the muscarinic effects are blocked by atropine while the nicotinic effects are not.

At all sites under normal conditions the action of acetylcholine is brief because it is destroyed by the enzyme *acetylcholinesterase*. This is in contrast to

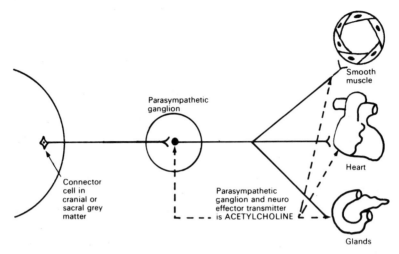

Fig. 5.5 The parasympathetic nervous system. This shows the main connections and that acetylcholine acts as the transmitter at both the ganglion and neuroeffector junctions.

the termination of the action of noradrenaline, which is actively taken up again into the sympathetic nerve endings and thus removed from the receptor targets.

Parasympathomimetic drugs

Acetylcholine is a parasympathomimetic drug, but is not used clinically because it is almost immediately destroyed by cholinesterase in the blood and tissues.

Anticholinesterases act by inhibiting the enzymes which normally destroy acetylcholine. Thus, the action of acetylcholine which has been physiologically released is greatly enhanced.

Physostigmine (eserine)

Physostigmine is a reversible inhibitor of cholinesterase and an important use for it (or one of its analogues such as pyridostigmine) is in the treatment of myasthenia gravis. The latter is characterised by increasing muscle weakness and excessive fatiguability as a result of loss of acetylcholine receptors in the motor end-plate. This in turn appears to be due to autoantibodies to these receptors. Anticholinesterases increase the concentration of acetylcholine in the region of the receptors and thus increase muscular power.

Physostigmine eye drops are used to constrict the pupil. When this happens, fluid can more readily drain from the anterior chamber and reduce intraocular pressure. Physostigmine is therefore used to lower the excessive intraocular pressure characteristic of glaucoma.

Anticholinesterases, such as pyridostigmine can also be used in an attempt to increase salivary secretion in diseases of these glands, such as Sjögren's syndrome. However, other cholinergic effects of these drugs (particularly physostigmine), such as nausea, diarrhoea and bradycardia are often troublesome.

Another use of anticholinesterases is to reverse the action of non-depolarising muscle relaxants such as tubocurarine.

The organophosphorus insecticides

Chemicals such as DFP (di-isopropylfluorophosphonate), are *irreversible* inhibitors of cholinesterase. They are quickly absorbed through the skin and mucous membranes. Even a small amount applied to the conjunctival sac can produce systemic effects. These include increased salivary and bronchial secretions, bronchospasm, colic and diarrhoea. Muscle twitching followed by paralysis is caused by the enhancement of the nicotinic action of acetylcholine and death results from respiratory paralysis.

Similar compounds form the basis of the chemical weapons known as nerve gases.

Carbachol

Carbachol has actions similar to those of acetylcholine but it is not destroyed by cholinesterase. When given by injection it increases the smooth muscle tone in the gut and bladder. It is used to initiate peristalsis after an operation and to treat an atonic bladder. Carbachol is also used to expel gas from the large intestine before an X-ray examination of the abdomen.

Acetylcholine and other cholinergic drugs – Summary

1. Acetylcholine is the chemical transmitter at all ganglia *and* endings of the autonomic nervous system with the single exception of adrenergic endings of the sympathetic system.

2. Acetylcholine has a wide variety of effects but it is too unselective in its actions and is too rapidly destroyed by cholinesterase to be useful clinically.

3. Cholinergic agents such as pilocarpine and its analogues have been used for such purposes as increasing salivary secretion, but their widespread unselective actions (direct cholinergic effects) make their use impractical.

4. Other choline esters such as carbachol are resistant to cholinesterase and have more selective actions. They may be used to stimulate bowel or bladder action after surgery, for example.

5. Anticholinesterases are used in medicine principally as antidotes to competitive neuromuscular blocking agents and in the treatment of myasthenia gravis.

Parasympathetic blocking drugs (anticholinergic agents)

Atropine

Atropine,* together with hyoscamine and hyoscine, is derived from solanaceous plants – particularly Deadly Nightshade, the berries of which are poisonous because of these substances.

The atropine group of drugs antagonises the actions of acetylcholine at *muscarinic* sites only. Thus, they block the action of acetylcholine on the heart, on glands and on smooth muscle, but do *not* affect synaptic transmission in the autonomic ganglia and at the motor end-plate of voluntary muscle.

Atropine-like drugs act by competing with acetylcholine for cholinergic receptors at *muscarinic* sites. This is therefore an example of a competitive type of drug antagonism (see Fig. 5.6).

The actions and uses of atropine (or atropine derivatives) are therefore as follows:

1. As premedication to diminish salivary and bronchial secretions during anaesthesia.

2. To diminish vagal slowing of the heart during induction of anaesthesia. The effectiveness or even the need for atropine for this purpose nowadays is questionable.

3. To reverse excessive slowing of the heart (sinus bradycardia), particularly after myocardial infarction (see Ch. 10).

4. To induce bronchodilatation in asthma. Atropine itself is little used for this purpose but isopropyl atropine (*ipratropium*) is an effective and useful bronchodilator with less drying effect on bronchial secretions than atropine.

5. To reduce bronchial secretions and bronchospasm in patients being treated with an anticholinesterase such as eserine for myasthenia gravis.

6. To dilate the pupil (by local instillation into the conjunctival sac) to facilitate ophthalmoscopic examination of the retina. This effect is produced by abolition of parasympathetic-mediated pupillary constrictor tone. At the same time, the ciliary muscle is paralysed (because this is also under parasympathetic control) and the patient cannot accommodate his lens for near vision.

These effects can be prolonged and a similar but shorter-acting drug – such as homatropine – may be preferred. Alternatively the action of atropine can be reversed in the eye by the local instillation of eserine eye drops.

---

* Atropine was used by sixteenth century ladies to dilate the pupils and produce 'sparking eyes'; hence its older name, Belladonna (lit. fair lady). Atropine was also valued as a poison and its name derives from Atropos (one of the Fates of Greek mythology) whose job was to cut the thread of life.

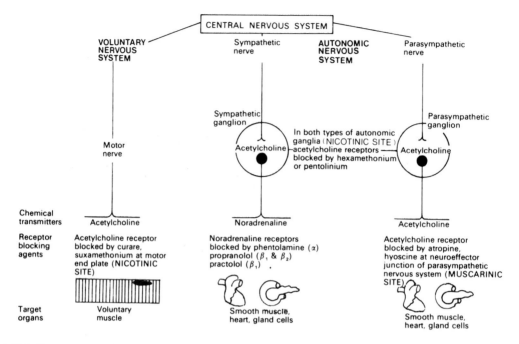

Fig. 5.6 This diagram summarises the types of chemical mediators released in both the voluntary nervous system and the autonomic nervous system. In addition the different blocking agents and their sites of action are shown.

Atropine and related drugs are contraindicated in glaucoma, since they block drainage from the anterior chamber of the eye and further increase intraocular pressure.

7. To moderate excessive central cholinergic activity and hence reduce muscle spasm in parkinsonism (Ch. 6).

8. To give symptomatic relief for peptic ulcer, possibly by diminishing motor activity ('spasm') in the alimentary tract and by blocking parasympathetically mediated acid secretion (see Ch. 17).

Hyoscine

Hyoscine has identical peripheral actions to atropine, but while atropine is a central stimulant, hyoscine is a depressant. It produces sleepiness and inhibits the vomiting centre. Hyoscine is thus a particularly valuable drug as a premedication before general anaesthesia. Not only does it reduce salivary and bronchial secretions (and therefore lessens the risk of pulmonary complications), but it lessens the apprehension of the patient while being brought to the anaesthetic room. This in turn reduces the amount of anaesthetic necessary to produce general anaesthesia and also the risk of vomiting.

The antiemetic properties of hyoscine also make it effective in preventing travel sickness.

Antihistamines, such as promethazine, cyclizine and diphenhydramine, happen also to have some hyoscine-like properties and hence are also useful in the management of motion sickness.

Anticholinergic drugs of this type and related synthetic substances are used in the symptomatic treatment of the pain of peptic ulcer – presumably by decreasing the amount of gastric acid secreted and abolishing spasm.

Atropine-like drugs also block muscarinic receptors in the brain and reduce the severity of parkinsonism (see Ch. 4).

Acetylcholine as an autonomic transmitter and acetylcholine blocking drugs – summary

Because acetylcholine is the transmitting agent at many different sites, it mediates a wide range of different effects. This is a difficult area of pharma-

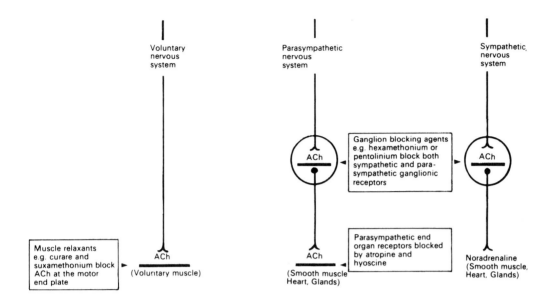

Fig. 5.7 Receptor blockade of acetylcholine (ACh) in different parts of the nervous system by different drugs.

cology and it may be useful to summarise these actions and the consequences of blocking them.

Acetylcholine is the chemical transmitter at:

1. *All autonomic ganglia*, whether sympathetic or parasympathetic.

2. *All parasympathetic nerve endings.* Also sympathetic nerve endings controlling sweat glands and vasodilator fibres.

3. *Neuromuscular end-plates.*

Unfortunately for the reader, drugs with an anticholinergic action do not block all these activities and different drugs act at the different sites in a selective fashion as follows:

1. Ganglion blocking agents. These block transmission at sympathetic ganglia and quickly lower blood pressure. Parasympathetic activity is also blocked so that there are effects such as depressed salivary secretion, constipation and retention of urine. An example is hexamethonium (see Ch. 10).

2. Anticholinergic agents. This term is somewhat arbitrarily used for agents which act at *post* ganglionic, cholinergic, i.e. (mainly) parasympathetic nerve endings. They include atropine and drugs with atropine-like actions. Such drugs have a muscarinic blocking effect. In other words, they block the muscarine-type actions of acetylcholine (Fig. 5.7).

Anticholinergic agents mainly therefore:

a. depress digestive secretions including salivation;

b. relax smooth muscle of the gut and bronchioles;

c. depress vagal activity and increase heart rate.

Some of these agents, such as hyoscine, depress the CNS and thus produce sedation and suppression of the vomiting reflex.

3. Competitive neuromuscular blocking agents. Acetylcholine is the chemical transmitter at the neuromuscular junction. This is one of the so-called nicotinic actions of acetylcholine and is *not* antagonised by atropine. Curare and related drugs, however, block this action of acetylcholine by combining with (competing successfully for) the specific receptors on the motor end-plate. The effect can only be reversed by promoting the build-up of a sufficient concentration of acetylcholine.

This is done by using an anticholinesterase to prevent the destruction of normally produced acetylcholine.

It is relatively easy perhaps to accept that acetylcholine should have such different functions as it is acting simply as a chemical transmitter in different sites with different effector organs. It is undoubtedly difficult on the other hand to understand how it is that all the actions of acetylcholine are not blocked by a single antagonist.

It has to be admitted that there is no simple and convincing explanation, but it is clear that the muscarinic and the nicotinic receptors at the motor end-plate have some minute structural differences in that they are antigenically distinct. Thus in the disease myasthenia gravis, there are autoantibodies to acetylcholine receptors. However, these autoantibodies appear to act only against nicotinic nerve endings and cause muscle weakness; they do not affect muscarinic nerve endings and, therefore, have no atropine-like action.

Effects of autonomic drugs on salivary function

Salivary secretion is stimulated by parasympathetic activity and inhibited by sympathetic stimulation, as exemplified by the dry mouth of acute anxiety. In addition, salivary secretion can be diminished as a result of dehydration (itself occasionally caused by drugs, particularly the potent diuretics) or disease of the glands themselves.

Causes of drug-induced xerostomia are listed in Chapter 18 but can be summarised as follows:

1. Drugs with anticholinergic effects such as:
   Atropine and its analogues.
   Tricyclic antidepressants.
   Phenothiazines and antihistamines.
2. Sympathomimetic agents such as:
   Ephedrine and other sympathomimetic drugs in cold cures.
   Decongestants and bronchodilators.
   Amphetamines.

Increased salivation is not a clinical problem as any excess is swallowed unless there is dysphagia or impaired neuromuscular function to cause dribbling. Drugs which increase salivary secretion (sialagogues) may be needed if the glands are diseased and the amount of functional tissue reduced. Unfortunately the only effective sialagogues are the cholinesterase inhibitors (physostigmine and its analogues) which also increase the activity of all organs with muscarinic nerve endings, such as the gastrointestinal tract, with diarrhoea as the main side-effect as discussed earlier. When such drugs are given (particularly for the treatment of myasthenia gravis), atropine or an analogue has therefore also to be given.

SUGGESTED FURTHER READING

Anon 1983 Atracurium. Lancet i: 394
Argov Z Mastaglia F L 1979 Disorders of neuromuscular transmission caused by drugs. New England Journal of Medicine 301: 409
Boakes A J, Laurence D R, Lovel K W, O'Neil R, Verrill P J 1972 Adverse reactions to local anaesthetic/vasoconstrictor preparations: a study of the cardiovascular response to Xylestesin and Hostacain-with-Noradrenaline. British Dental Journal 133: 137
Boakes A J, Laurence D R, Teoh P C, Barar F S K, Benedikter L T, Prichard B N C 1973 Interactions between sympathomimetic amines and antidepressant agents in man. British Medical Journal 1: 311
Feely J, De Vane P J, Maclean D 1983 Beta-blockers and sympathomimetics. British Medical Journal 286: 1043
Frishman W H 1981 β adrenoceptor antagonists: new drugs and new indications. New England Journal of Medicine 305: 500
Frishman W H 1982 Drug therapy. New England Journal of Medicine 306: 1456
Frishman W H 1982 The beta-adrenoceptor blocking drugs. International Journal of Cardiology 2: 165
Hoffman B B, Lefkowitz R J 1980 Alpha-adrenergic receptor subtypes. New England Journal of Medicine 302: 1390
James I M, Griffith D N W, Pearson R M, Newbury P 1977 Effect of oxprenolol on stage-fright in musicians. Lancet ii: 952
Lees G M 1981 A hitch-hiker's guide to the galaxy of adrenoceptors. British Medical Journal 283: 173
Mirakhur R K 1979 Anticholinergic drugs. British Journal of Anaesthesia 51: 671
Motulsky H. J, Insel P A 1982 Adrenergic receptors in man. New England Journal of Medicine 307: 18
Norman J 1979 Neuromuscular blocking drugs. British Journal of Anaesthesia 51: 471
Shepherd J T, Vanhoutte P M 1981 Local modulation of adrenergic neurotransmission. Circulation 64: 655
Snyder S H 1979 Receptors, neurotransmitters and drug responses. New England Journal of Medicine 300: 465

6. The nervous system
II. Depressants of cerebral function

Depressants of the CNS are among the most widely used drugs both medically and non-medically. Most of the drugs of dependence (apart from cocaine and amphetamine) are CNS depressants and conversely CNS depressants of any type are addictive in varying degree.

Alcohol is the archetype of all sedatives, hypnotics and general anaesthetic agents and is also the most widely used drug of addiction. The main action of alcohol, namely progressive, non-selective depression of the CNS, is essentially the same as that of barbiturates and of anaesthetic agents.

Alcohol as a general CNS depressant

The effects of alcohol illustrate well many of the actions of CNS depressants and since there is almost unlimited opportunity to observe them, it may be helpful to consider them in some detail.

The apparent differences between the effects of anaesthetic agents and sedatives such as barbiturates on the one hand and alcohol on the other depend mainly on dose and rate of uptake. When dosage is small, the social circumstances under which the drug is taken are also important. All, in large enough doses, cause unconsciousness and eventually respiratory depression and death. In smaller doses sleep is promoted if circumstances are favourable and alcohol is often spoken of euphemistically as a 'night cap'.

In moderate dosage both barbiturates and alcohol relieve anxiety – 'Dutch courage' is a nickname for this property of alcohol.* This relief of anxiety by alcohol, as with barbiturates, is at the cost of blunting other mental faculties. In favourable social circumstances anaesthetic agents, sedatives and alcohol have similar effects by depressing the higher centres.

Under appropriate circumstances (pubs or parties) small amounts of alcohol, by blunting anxiety and inhibitions, usually produce a pleasant brightening of mood and conversation – an almost essential requirement to alleviate the hideous boredom of most social occasions. Initially, at least, a congenial atmosphere develops and as more drink goes down, tongues are loosened and talk becomes noisier. For this reason, alcohol is widely regarded as a 'stimulant'. This however is a dangerous misconception since the unselective depressant action of alcohol on the CNS causes both rapid deterioration of skill and judgement, and also such loss of insight that the drinker believes his performance to be improved. As more drink goes down, therefore, speech becomes slurred due to deterioration of muscular control, moods become unpredictable (but generally worsen) and movements become unco-ordinated.

The consequences of these effects of alcohol in terms of motor accidents alone, have been disastrous. In many, aggression is released and expressed as violent arguments, fighting or lethal car driving. Eventually if enough drink is taken and if vomiting does not start first, the hypnotic action of alcohol becomes overwhelming and is marked traditionally by the guest (or host) sliding under the table.

Death due to acute alcohol overdose can happen when an enterprising individual decides to swallow

---

* The use of the term 'Dutch courage' does not, incidentally, refer to any lack of courage on the part of the Dutch, but was probably because of the introduction of Hollands, that is Dutch gin.

in quick succession (often for a bet or bravado) two or more bottles of neat whisky or gin – a bottle usually contains 750 ml of approximately 40% ethanol. Death can result from depression of the respiratory centre or more often from aspiration of vomit.

General anaesthetic agents are given rapidly, in relatively heavy dosage, and by a route (inhalation or intravenously) ensuring rapid absorption. Nevertheless, small doses of general anaesthetic agents are just as intoxicating as alcohol. Nitrous oxide (laughing gas) in particular can cause wild euphoria, as can ether. Both agents were used as intoxicants soon after the discovery of their anaesthetic properties and 'ether revels' were a remarkable feature of an otherwise puritanical social scene in the USA of the nineteenth century.

Chloroform was introduced as an anaesthetic agent by Sir James Simpson as a result of experiments with a wide variety of agents which he and his colleagues tried out on themselves in 1847. When chloroform was tried, 'Immediately an unwonted hilarity seized the party: they became bright-eyed, very happy and loquacious – expatiating on the delicious aroma of the new fluid. The conversation was of unusual intelligence and quite charmed the listeners . . .'. There was a sudden crash and the experimenters awoke later.

The similarities between the effects on Simpson and his friends of chloroform and those of alcohol will be only too obvious.

Alcohol can also be used as an anaesthetic agent but has severe limitations. It has a mild analgesic action and in the past, drunken stupor was the best provision that could be made against the pain of early surgery. The analgesic effect of alcohol often causes a drunk to be unaware of injuries and this analgesic effect is enhanced by the tranquillising effects of alcohol. Thus, the drunk may not feel the pain so much and is also less concerned about such pain as he feels.

When taken by mouth alcohol is too prone to cause vomiting to be useful as an anaesthetic. It is also insufficiently volatile to be used as an inhalational agent, but has been used experimentally as an intravenous anaesthetic. It has no special advantages and the anaesthetic dose is close to that which causes respiratory depression.

In view of its desirable properties, it is hardly surprising that alcohol is so heavily used and attempts at prohibition have generally failed – strikingly so in the USA in the period 1920 to 1933. Increasing and punitive taxation also does not discourage consumption, which steadily rises. Most governments have, therefore, taken advantage of the situation to use alcohol as a source of enormous revenue. The public cannot do without alcohol and the State cannot do without the revenue. So for these and other reasons alcohol is an almost inseparable feature of our culture.

Alcohol is a potent drug of addiction by virtue of its power to promote sociability (initially at least), to blunt anxiety and to induce a pleasantly stuporous state. The ready availability and social acceptability of alcohol also contribute to its wide use as a drug of addiction.

Withdrawal can have severe effects on the confirmed alcoholic and continued heavy consumption can damage health in various ways. Alcohol is nevertheless the only permitted drug of addiction, and addiction is on a huge scale.

Alcohol has virtually no uses in medicine, apart from being an effective skin antiseptic. Its 'strengthening' and 'tonic' properties are illusory, or no more than subjective. Belief in such effects is, however, widely held and sedulously encouraged by the brewers and distillers. 'Tonic' wine is itself a contributory cause of chronic alcoholism.

Terminology

Depressants of the CNS have varying degrees of selectivity of action on different aspects of brain function and are of the following types:

1. Sedatives and tranquillisers

The *anxiolytic agents* (*minor tranquillisers*) are used to alleviate anxiety, ideally without causing drowsiness. There is no sharp distinction between sedatives and tranquillisers. The most widely used minor tranquillisers are the benzodiazepines, such as diazepam.

The *neuroleptics* (*major tranquillisers*) such as the phenothiazines are used to suppress psychotic overactivity in the treatment of schizophrenia and other psychotic states.

2. Hypnotics

Hypnotics are used to induce sleep, but in smaller doses are often used as sedatives. Until recently barbiturates were the main hypnotics used, but have been largely replaced by the benzodiazepines which are safer in overdose and less addictive.

3. Narcotics (opioids)

Narcotics, strictly speaking, are drugs which induce narcosis (stupor). In conventional usage, however, the term narcotic is applied (for all practical purposes) only to the opioids and their synthetic analogues – the narcotic analgesics. These are the most powerful analgesics and are some of the most powerfully addictive drugs.

Unfortunately, since the narcotic analgesics are in some ways the most important drugs of addiction, the term 'narcotic' is sometimes loosely used – and officially used in the USA by the Federal Narcotics Bureau – to include all drugs of addiction. This is misleading, since some drugs of addiction, such as cocaine, are strong CNS stimulants and have a completely opposite effect to that of the narcotics.

4. Analgesics

Analgesics are drugs used to lessen the sensation of pain. Their effectiveness in this role is, however, limited and beyond a certain point toxic effects predominate.

5. General anaesthetics

These are agents that rapidly induce unconsciousness which is deep enough to prevent arousal by pain, however severe. Anaesthetic agents are not necessarily potent analgesics, but there are exceptions, such as nitrous oxide, which is strongly analgesic even though it is a weak anaesthetic.

6. Anticonvulsants

Anticonvulsants are drugs used to control or prevent epileptic fits.

HYPNOTIC DRUGS

Hypnotics are drugs which produce a state of sleep which is similar in depth to physiological sleep, in that the subject can be roused by external stimuli. However, the sleep produced is not the same as normal sleep – rapid eye movement (REM) sleep is suppressed and there is diminished dreaming. The physiological importance of REM sleep is not known.

There is no doubt that hypnotics are over-prescribed. Little harm can come to a patient from not sleeping; when the need for sleep is great, falling asleep should be irresistible. The use of a hypnotic may be justified during admission to hospital before an operation or before a stressful dental procedure, but once the anxiety-provoking situation has been resolved, the drug should be stopped. Depression and chronic anxiety states are also common and often interfere with sleep.

Hypnotics are not generally analgesic – and some of them, such as barbiturates, potentiate sensitivity to pain. If pain prevents sleep an analgesic should be given.

There are several different types of hypnotics in general use. These include:

1. Nitrazepam, temazepam and other benzodiazepines.
2. Chloral hydrate.
3. Chlormethiazole.
5. Antihistamines.

Benzodiazepines

The earlier hypnotics were non-specific depressants of the CNS and in overdose could cause medullary paralysis. The main action of benzodiazepines by contrast is to suppress anxiety and induce sleep largely by this means.

In addition to lessening anxiety and inducing sleep (in appropriate dosage and circumstances), benzodiazepines have varying degrees of anticonvulsant activity.

A great variety of benzodiazepines is now available but they differ mainly in their duration of action and to a slight degree in their other properties.

Mode of action. Benzodiazepines act on the

limbic system in the brain, where they potentiate the inhibitory neurotransmitter, gamma-amino-butyric acid (GABA), and there are GABA-benzo-diazepine receptor complexes in the brain.

Gamma-aminobutyric acid is released from neurones in the CNS into the synaptic cleft. It binds to the GABA receptor and reduces the excitability of the adjacent excitatory neurone by increasing its permeability to chloride ions.

Closely associated with the GABA receptor is the benzodiazepine receptor, where the action of benzodiazepines is to potentiate the inhibitory action of GABA by increasing permeability to chloride ions and further decreasing the excitability of the neurone.

The action of benzodiazepines can be reversed by the benzodiazepine antagonist, flumazenil. The latter acts by binding strongly to the benzodiazepine receptor and displacing benzodiazepine molecules from it. Potentiation of the inhibitory action of GABA is thus reversed.

Nitrazepam (Mogadon), like other benzodiaze-pines, is one of the hypnotics of choice. Its hypnotic action is enhanced by its ability to diminish anxiety, which is a common cause of poor sleep. It has a half-life of about 24 hours and thus its sedating action may persist well into the next day.

Diazepam (Valium) itself has a half-life of 20–50 hours and also has active metabolites which may persist longer. As a hypnotic, diazepam can cause more prolonged hangover than nitrazepam.

Flurazepam (Dalmane) is widely used as a hyp-notic. Even though it has a short half-life, it has (like diazepam) a metabolite which is a powerful hypnotic and has a very long half-life.

Temazepam (Euhypnos, Normison) has a short half-life and no active metabolites, and is therefore increasingly widely recommended as a hypnotic.

Temazepam was widely used by aircrew to enable them to sleep, whenever off duty, during the Falklands campaign. They were able to fly 6 hours after taking the hypnotic without any evidence of impaired performance.

Benzodiazepines have the following advantages over the barbiturates:

1. Respiratory depression is slight. It is only important in patients with chronic respiratory disease with impaired oxygen exchange.

2. Overdose does not cause severe progressive depression of respiration. Hence, the risk of suc-cessful suicide is so slight as to have raised doubts as to whether it is even possible. Enormous amounts of benzodiazepines are prescribed and attempts at suicide are made with almost any tablets (especially 'sleeping tablets') that are handy. Most deaths ascribed to benzodiazepines have either been in patients with chronic lung disease or who have been taking other drugs or alcohol at the same time.*

3. The addictive potential is much less. How-ever, benzodiazepine dependence may be seriously disabling for many weeks.

4. In the elderly, benzodiazepines are less likely to cause nocturnal confusion.

5. After-effects ('hangover') tend to be less. Many patients experience no subjective after-effects, but most have slightly depressed mental acuity for a few hours after waking and careful testing shows that reaction times, for example, are usually prolonged for several hours after waking especially when the longer-acting benzodiazepines have been taken.

The effects may come on very quickly and benzodiazepines should be taken immediately before going to bed – not in the bath and certainly not in the car while driving home in the evening.

Chloral hydrate and trichloroethanol

Chloral hydrate has been in use since the nine-teenth century. It was the first synthetic hypnotic and relatively safe, since in normal doses it does not cause respiratory depression. It has a very unpleas-ant taste and can cause gastric irritation. This reduces the chances of overdosage, but is otherwise a disadvantage.

Large doses of chloral cause depression of respi-ration, of the heart and of the vasomotor centre.

Chloral is quickly absorbed from the gastrointes-tinal tract and converted into trichloroethanol which is the active metabolite. *Triclofos* is an ester of trichloroethanol and has similar actions to and

---

* One person, with suicidal intent, took 2000 mg of diazepam but remained responsive and not disorientated. He was discharged apparently none the worse for wear after 48 hours but the metabolite, desmethyldiazepam, was still being excreted 2 weeks later.

the advantages of chloral hydrate. Triclofos has the additional advantages over chloral of not causing gastric irritation and is a tablet not a liquid.

Another tablet form of chloral is *dichloralphenazone* (Welldorm) which (as the name indicates) includes the analgesic phenazone, which is otherwise little used. A fruit-flavoured syrup is also available for children.

Chloral is mainly used as a hypnotic for children. It is not a hepatic enzyme inducer.

Chlormethiazole

Chlormethiazole (Heminevrin) is an effective hypnotic with a short duration of action. It can cause cardiovascular and respiratory depression in large doses.

Antihistamines

Promethazine is a powerful antihistamine. Like many drugs of this group, it is also a sedative and hypnotic. Promethazine may be used in children – particularly if the child cannot sleep because of an itching complaint. Promethazine, like other antihistamines, also has antiemetic properties and is useful in the prevention of travel sickness. The main objections to promethazine are the prolonged hangover of persistent drowsiness, potentiation by alcohol, respiratory depression and fits.

Barbiturates

The intermediate acting barbiturates are powerful hypnotics. Examples are amylobarbitone (Amytal), pentobarbitone (Nembutal) and quinalbarbitone (Seconal), but, current opinion is against their use except for certain specialised purposes. This is mainly because of their high addictive potential. They are therefore Controlled Drugs. Barbiturates can also produce excitement and confusion in the elderly and depress respiration. As with most hypnotic drugs, after-effects often persist for several hours after waking. These include loss of mental acuity, drowsiness or headache.

The respiratory depression caused by barbiturates made them effective and commonly used agents of suicide. In patients with emphysema or chest infections they may also precipitate respiratory failure even in normal dosage. The cerebral depressant action of barbiturates is further enhanced by taking antihistamines or alcohol at the same time. Barbiturates also have the disadvantage of causing enzyme induction in the liver and interacting with other drugs such as anticoagulants (see p. 144).

With the advent of the much safer benzodiazepines (nitrazepam and others) the barbiturates have become outmoded and are obsolete as sedatives or hypnotics.

The chief objections to the barbiturates as hypnotics are therefore:

1. Ready tendency to, and widespread addiction.
2. Respiratory depressant effect.
3. Frequent use for self-poisoning.
4. Interactions with other drugs particularly by enzyme induction in the liver.

Management of barbiturate poisoning

The main aim is to restore spontaneous respiration. There is no specific antagonist but there is no need to try to hasten recovery of consciousness.

The stomach should be washed out to remove undissolved tablets and (if possible) allow their identification. This, however, can be dangerous unless a cuffed endotracheal tube is used to prevent gastric contents from getting into the airway.

Intermittent positive-pressure ventilation is the treatment of choice once spontaneous respiration has failed.

In addition, forced diuresis can be used to help remove the drug from the body. The plasma level of the barbiturate should be assayed if possible and, if very high, dialysis may be necessary to get rid of the drug.

Analeptics (CNS and respiratory stimulants) such as doxapram may be dangerous and should not be used as the measures outlined are safer and more effective.

EPILEPSY

Epilepsy is not a single disease; it can be a sign of several disorders affecting the brain, but in many cases no cause can be found. Epilepsy is a paroxysmal dysfunction produced by abnormal electrical discharge in the brain.

There are several forms of epilepsy. The best known is major epilepsy, the most common type of which is tonic-clonic (grand mal). In the latter consciousness is lost, quickly followed by uncoordinated motor activity, typically with rigidity, then jerking and slow recovery of consciousness. Minor epilepsy includes petit mal, in which the patient, usually a child, suffers very brief lapses of consciousness ('absences') and rapidly recovers without complete loss of postural muscular control.

Drugs commonly given to control tonic-clonic epilepsy are phenobarbitone, phenytoin, primidone, carbamazepine and sodium valproate.

Phenobarbitone is an effective anticonvulsant but its use has greatly declined in recent years because of its several serious disadvantages. These are:

1. It is usually excessively sedating when therapeutic blood levels are attained.

2. On sudden cessation of the drug, rebound hyperexcitability of the motor cortex and hence severe fits result.

3. Enzyme induction.

4. Paradoxical excitement in some children.

Phenytoin and other anticonvulsants

Phenytoin is one of the drugs given for tonic-clonic epilepsy, focal fits and psychomotor epilepsy. Whenever possible the drug should be used on its own. Within the therapeutic range of plasma levels, phenytoin is not sedating but in large doses nystagmus, ataxia and other nervous system toxicity develops.

Hyperplasia of the gums can complicate phenytoin therapy. Occasionally long-term treatment may lead to folic acid deficiency and macrocytic anaemia. Phenytoin also increases the catabolism of vitamin D. This causes hypocalcaemia and histological signs of osteomalacia. The changes are usually mild and subclinical but florid rickets or osteomalacia has been described as a rare complication. Vitamin D should be given only if there is clinical evidence of bone disease. Nevertheless, phenytoin remains one of the most satisfactory drugs for the treatment of major epilepsy.

Carbamazepine rarely causes serious toxicity. It is approximately as effective as phenytoin and is the drug of choice for tonic-clonic fits.

In addition to their use for epilepsy, anticonvulsants, particularly carbamazepine, are the most effective drugs for the control of trigeminal neuralgia (see Ch. 7).

Primidone is effective in major epilepsy, but often causes sedation and cerebellar-type ataxia.

In the treatment of petit mal, ethosuximide or valproate may be used. *Ethosuximide* is the drug of choice and side-effects are not usually serious.

Benzodiazepines (particularly clonazepam) are effective in petit mal and some other forms of epilepsy, but are mainly used as intravenous injections for status epilepticus.

Sodium valproate is effective in all types of epilepsy and can give excellent control of major and many forms of minor epilepsy. Minor gastrointestinal disturbances and temporary hair loss seem to be the main side-effects but the drug is usually well tolerated. The assessment of the effectiveness of drugs in the control of epilepsy is notoriously difficult; nevertheless, sodium valproate appears to be a useful drug with the advantage that it usually seems to make patients more alert rather than drowsy. In small children, high doses of valproate occasionally cause liver failure.

Status epilepticus is a dangerous condition in which fits recur rapidly over a prolonged period. Intravenous diazepam or clonazepam is usually effective – but may have to be repeated at intervals to prevent further fits. Alternatively, intravenous chlormethiazole or intramuscular paraldehyde are effective.

PARKINSONISM AND PARKINSON'S DISEASE

Parkinson's disease mainly affects the elderly and is characterised by rigidity, akinesia (poverty of movement), tremor, a mask-like facies and excessive salivation. This neurological syndrome is a disorder of the extrapyramidal system which normally governs the quality and smoothness of voluntary movement. The lesions may be the result of arteriosclerosis or past encephalitis but in many cases no cause can be found.

Normal function of the extrapyramidal system depends on a balanced action of excitatory and inhibitory components. The excitatory transmitter is acetylcholine while the inhibitory transmitter is dopamine. In parkinsonism the inhibitory component is deficient and the concentration of dopamine in the basal ganglia may be low. Drugs can induce parkinsonism either by depleting the system of dopamine (e.g. reserpine) or by blockade of dopamine receptors (e.g. chlorpromazine).

The aim of treatment of Parkinson's disease is to restore the balance between excitation and inhibition, either by reducing cholinergic activity with an anticholinergic drug (i.e. an atropine-like agent) or by supplementing dopaminergic activity with a drug such as levodopa.

Atropine-like drugs used in the treatment of parkinsonism include benzhexol (Artane). This synthetic substance has similar actions to atropine and hyoscine, but is supposed to have less peripheral actions with equivalent central anti-parkinsonian activity. Nevertheless, dry mouth and constipation are common while urinary retention and glaucoma can also be precipitated. This type of drug is effective in reducing the rigidity but not the tremor of parkinsonism.

Levodopa produces a good response in about two-thirds of patients with Parkinson's disease. It ameliorates all the components of the syndrome. L-dopa is absorbed from the intestine, enters the brain from the circulation and is then converted to dopamine. The commonest toxic effects are nausea, vomiting and postural hypotension. Excessive doses, however, can produce involuntary movements which may be more troublesome than the parkinsonism.

Decarboxylase in the nervous system causes conversion of levodopa to dopamine. Smaller doses of levodopa are therefore effective and produce less toxicity if a decarboxylase inhibitor is given simultaneously. Such inhibitors include benserazide and carbidopa. Other drugs effective in parkinsonism are *amantadine* (which releases L-dopa from stores in the brain) and *bromocriptine* (which stimulates dopamine receptors in a similar way to L-dopa).

Amantadine is an antiviral drug which was found by chance to have anti-parkinsonian activity. It potentiates dopamine release from neuronal stores.

Bromocriptine stimulates dopamine receptors and thus has the same adverse effects as levodopa. Bromocriptine can produce nausea, postural hypotension and involuntary movements.

Selegiline is a monoamine oxidase inhibitor which is used for severe forms of Parkinson's disease.

Parkinsonism and dopamine receptor blockers

From what has been said about the pathogenesis of Parkinson's disease it may be apparent that drugs which block dopamine receptors can produce parkinsonian effects. The phenothiazine major tranquillisers (p. 93), particularly in long-term use, are the main cause of this side-effect and can cause dyskinesia (involuntary face and body movements) including parkinsonism.

Metoclopramide (p. 199), which achieves its effects partly by blocking dopamine receptors in the vomiting centre (the 'chemoreceptor trigger zone'), can cause dyskinesia and, in particular, trismus.

In the control of drug-induced parkinsonism, anticholinergic drugs are more effective than levodopa and other dopaminic agents.

NEUROSES AND PSYCHOSES

Neuroses and psychoses, particularly anxiety and depression, are some of the most common diseases dealt with in clinical practice. As a consequence, enormous quantities of psychoactive drugs, particularly anxiolytics and antidepressants, are prescribed. Although they are probably greatly overused it must be accepted that such drugs can make life tolerable for many people. Psychoactive drugs do not of course remove patients' basic problems – indeed it is not often possible to remove such problems – but treatment with suitable drugs may at least make it possible for patients to face their difficulties and, with sympathy and support from doctor or family, help them to seek some solution.

Anxiety and anxiolytic agents

Anxiety is fear. The essential difference between physiological anxiety and anxiety neurosis is the disparity between the severity of the response in relation to the cause. Suddenly meeting an angry cobra in one's bedroom would (reasonably enough) provoke some anxiety. No one could deny that this is a physiological response. By contrast, panic when confronted with a pigeon or having to leave the house to go shopping are inappropriate responses and suggest the presence of an anxiety neurosis. Such a neurosis may also manifest itself as feelings of anxiety or tension in the absence of any known external precipitating factor.

Anxiety provoked by the prospect of dental treatment is almost universal, but ranges from controllable apprehension to a phobia which makes treatment impossible. It is obviously not possible to draw a line between the normal and the neurotic response in such circumstances.

Anxiety neurosis is very common and is often difficult to treat. Psychotherapy (particularly listening patiently and sympathetically to the patient) may be helpful, but there is little objective evidence of its effectiveness and psychoanalysis is of questionable value.

The manifestations of anxiety are not only sensations of fear, but also the peripheral manifestations of excessive sympathetic activity. There may therefore be a dry mouth, rapid forceful beating of the heart (palpitations), rapid breathing, tremor and sweating.

The drugs (sedatives or anxiolytics) most used in the short-term treatment of anxiety are the benzodiazepines, especially diazepam. Anxiety may be associated with depression but tranquillisers are *not* antidepressant drugs. They may occasionally make depression worse or at least more obvious by their 'releasing' action and should not be given for the long-term treatment of anxiety.

Psychotic agitation and hyperactivity is a feature of schizophrenia. These and other symptoms of this disease need to be treated with the neuroleptics such as the phenothiazines described later.

Sedatives and 'dental sedation'

A great variety of sedatives (anxiolytics) exist, and among them, the benzodiazepines are currently the most widely used. However, the term 'dental sedation' is usually used in a fairly specific sense for brief induction of a sleep-like state for the duration of a dental operation. Since patients naturally wish to resume normal life as soon as possible after the treatment, sedating agents with the shortest possible duration of action, namely nitrous oxide and oxygen or intravenous midazolam are used. Nitrous oxide, though a powerful anxiolytic, is not of course a sedative for day-to-day use by those who find their lives uncomfortably stressful.

Benzodiazepines

With the introduction of the benzodiazepines, the barbiturates have become obsolete for the relief of anxiety. The benzodiazepines are powerful anxiolytic drugs which are much less sedative than the barbiturates, but large doses can cause drowsiness. Individual susceptibility varies widely and a satisfactory dosage regime has to be established for each patient.

Drugs in this group include diazepam (Valium), medazepam (Nobrium) and temazepam (Normison).

As mentioned earlier, benzodiazepines are anxiolytic: they are therefore effective in the symptomatic treatment of anxiety neuroses. The term 'minor' tranquilliser is misleading but is used to avoid confusion with the major tranquillisers (antipsychotic agents). The major tranquillisers (such as the phenothiazines) are effective in excited psychotic states such as delirium, hypomania and schizophrenia. Even though the minor tranquillisers are by no means minor in their actions, they are not effective in psychotic states such as these.

Benzodiazepines are effective in treating the central and peripheral manifestations of the anxiety state. Muscle tension and palpitations, as well as feelings of fear, may be suppressed. However, tolerance and dependence can develop within 6 weeks.

In dentistry this mild muscle relaxant effect, as well as the anxiolytic effect of benzodiazepines, may sometimes be useful in temporomandibular pain-dysfunction syndrome where spasm of the masticatory muscles appears to be the main cause of the symptoms.

Benzodiazepines such as lorazepam or flunitrazepam are frequently also used as premedication for general anaesthesia.

β blockers

β blocking agents, such as propranolol and oxprenolol, may be more useful than benzodiazepines for patients whose symptoms of anxiety are mainly peripheral. For example, palpitations (awareness of rapid or forceful beating of the heart) may be suppressed by blockers of β adrenergic (sympathetic) activity. Tremor is also diminished.

Other aspects of the management of anxiety

In anxiety, particular complications may require specific treatment. Difficulty in falling asleep and disturbed sleep are common and may be avoided by a slightly larger dose of diazepam in the evening. Alternatively, nitrazepam or temazepam may be given half an hour before going to bed. In general, when possible, it is preferable to resist the temptation to prescribe hypnotic drugs – fatigue is a much safer hypnotic. On the other hand, tiredness caused by lack of sleep makes emotional and other problems more unmanageable.

Acute panic attacks may punctuate the course of anxiety. These may be precipitated by a trivial stimulus or may be the result of confrontation with a 'phobic situation' – such as visiting the dentist.

Excessive anxiety in the dental chair can often be managed by giving temazepam by mouth (5 mg the night before and 5 mg 1 hour before treatment). This is often strikingly effective, but while this dosage may be inadequate for some, others are made drowsy. It may therefore be worthwhile to trying varying the dose until a satisfactory level is found. It is essential of course to warn the patient against driving a car.

The effect of oral diazepam on 'difficult' children as dental patients is more unpredictable, possibly because individual dosage needs vary widely and also because the response of children to psychoactive drugs can sometimes differ considerably from that of adults. Children may occasionally show paradoxical reactions to benzodiazepines or other sedating agents and become violent or hostile.

Where oral diazepam is unsatisfactory, intravenous diazepam or midazolam can be used, are effective and are generally safe. Their use is described in more detail in Chapter 8. Intravenous benzodiazepines should not be given to patients with chronic obstructive pulmonary disease (chronic bronchitis and emphysema) because they are mild respiratory depressants. Although this effect is usually insignificant in normal persons, rapid injection can sometimes cause apnoea.

DEPRESSION AND ANTIDEPRESSIVE AGENTS

Although all normal persons experience variations of mood, they are usually related to external events and are not socially disabling. The depressed patient, however, suffers dramatic lowering of the spirits and the mood is one of misery, hopelessness and despair quite disproportionate to the life situation. Work may become impossible and death by suicide may be felt to be preferable. What is called a 'nervous breakdown' is usually severe, disabling depression. An attack of depression may last for weeks, months or even years and then characteristically lifts. Patients usually have repeated attacks of depression but a few swing rapidly from depression to elation or mania. The phenomenon of such swings of mood is called cyclothymia and the depressive diseases are called the manic-depressive psychoses. Depression is, however, by far the most common state.

Chemical basis for the drug treatment of depression

There is substantial evidence that mood depends partly or entirely on chemical events in the brain and in particular on the levels of cerebral amine transmitters. Low cerebral levels of these amines – particularly noradrenaline – appear to be the mechanism of production of depression.

Supportive evidence is provided by the effects of the hypotensive drug reserpine for example. Reserpine depletes cerebral amines (including noradrenaline) and at the same time causes depression. Recovery of normal levels of cerebral amines after stopping the drug is accompanied by recovery of normal mood.

The only site of action of chemical transmitters in the nervous system is the receptor area on the cell membrane of the neurone.

This indicates that only noradrenaline, released into the synaptic cleft, is able to stimulate receptors and thus influence mood. The stored noradrenaline in the presynaptic neurone is pharmacologically inactive. The most important route by which released noradrenaline is removed from the synaptic cleft is by reuptake into the presynaptic nerve storage vesicles. The tricyclic antidepressant drugs block this reuptake mechanism and, by raising the concentration of noradrenaline in the synaptic cleft, enhance and prolong stimulation of the receptors. Other antidepressant drugs probably also act by raising the levels of cerebral amine transmitters.

Clearly, there must also be central mechanisms which trigger these chemical events as it is only too evident that external events, such as bereavement, can precipitate depression.

Drugs are extensively used in the treatment of depression. Psychotherapy can also be given, although its effectiveness is doubtful.

There are several types of antidepressive drug:

1. Monoamine oxidase inhibitors (familiarly known as MAOI) such as phenelzine.
2. Tricyclic antidepressants such as imipramine, amitriptyline and related drugs.
3. The 'new generation' of antidepressive drugs, with miscellaneous structures, such as mianserin, viloxazine and trazodone.

Monoamine oxidase inhibitors (MAOI)

These drugs inhibit a wide range of oxidative enzymes – including brain monoamine oxidase. If any noradrenaline leaks out of the vesicles into the cytoplasm it is normally destroyed by the enzyme monoamine oxidase. The function of this enzyme is the maintenance of low levels of noradrenaline in the neuronal cytoplasm outside the vesicles. The result of inhibiting this enzyme with MAOI drugs is that there is an increase in the quantity of noradrenaline (and other amines) stored within nerve endings. Thus, when a nerve impulse arrives more noradrenaline is available for release and the postsynaptic receptors are more strongly stimulated. This is possibly the basis of their antidepressive activity.

Uses of MAOI in depression

The MAOIs take 1-3 weeks to become effective, and it is usual to continue treatment for at least 4 weeks before deciding whether or not there will be a favourable response. The effect of these drugs persists for at least 2 weeks and during this period after stopping a MAOI there can be a serious drug or food reaction.

If adequate precautions are taken with the kinds of food eaten (especially avoidance of cheese) and against administration of interacting drugs the MAOIs appear generally to be safe and effective. However, the precise indications for the use of MAOIs in depression remain somewhat controversial and the number of foods and drugs with which they can interact remains as a serious limitation on their use.

Toxic effects

1. Interactions with foods. The main toxic effects of MAOIs result from their severe interactions with indirectly acting sympathomimetic agents, which, surprisingly, are present in many foods. Tyramine, in cheese and other foods, is one such agent.

If food containing tyramine is eaten by a normal person the tyramine is oxidised by amine oxidase enzymes in the gut wall and in the liver. In patients who are being treated with MAOI, ingested tyramine raises tyramine levels throughout the body. Tyramine acts as an indirectly acting sympathomimetic agent – it enters storage vesicles in the adrenergic nerve ending and liberates noradrenaline by displacement. The free noradrenaline diffuses across neuroeffector junctions and causes vasoconstriction. Since blood pressure depends partly on the state of arteriolar tone, the blood pressure rises. Furthermore, individuals treated with MAOIs have considerably enlarged noradrenaline stores. Thus the hypertensive action of tyramine is very great and the rise in blood pressure may be severe enough to cause a cerebral haemorrhage and even death.

Cheese is rich in tyramine. The most serious, and occasionally fatal, reactions of this type are caused by cheeses such as Camembert, Stilton, Brie or matured Cheddar in which microbial activity has converted tyrosine to tyramine. Other foods may contain vasoactive amines which can also cause hypertension in patients treated with MAOIs. For example, broad beans (the second most dangerous food on this list) contain dopamine while yeast extracts contain histamine. Ripe bananas, Chianti, beer and some other alcoholic drinks containing yeast by-products have also caused hypertensive attacks in patients taking MAOIs. In general, reactions with these substances are less severe than with cheese.

A hypertensive crisis such as that caused by interaction between an MAOI and tyramine can be treated by giving an α blocker, such as phentolamine, intravenously.

2. Interactions with sympathomimetic drugs. As indicated above, MAOIs can interact with sympathomimetic agents of the *indirectly acting type.* This has led to unjustifiable confusion and the belief that they interact with all sympathomimetic agents. However, this is not the case and MAOIs do NOT interact with the vasoconstrictors, adrenaline or noradrenaline since they are directly acting sympathomimetic agents.

If this seems inconsistent with what has been said earlier concerning the destruction of noradrenaline in the CNS by MAOI, the situation may, we hope, be clarified by saying that:

a. Noradrenaline is destroyed *within* the cytoplasm of the cells of the nervous system by MAO.

b. Noradrenaline which is injected (for example, with a local anaesthetic) is mainly removed from the circulation by uptake into the nervous system.

c. Monoamine oxidase inhibitors do *not* inhibit removal of noradrenaline from the circulation by this uptake mechanism. This means in effect that MAOI drugs, although inhibiting the destruction of noradrenaline *within* the central nervous system, play no significant role in the removal of noradrenaline from the circulation and hence on its circulatory effects.

d. Residual noradrenaline (or adrenaline) that is not taken up into the nervous system is destroyed by another enzyme, namely COMT (catechol-*O*-methyl transferase). This takes place within the cytoplasm of other cells – including smooth muscle and glands.

e. During treatment with MAOI drugs noradrenaline accumulates in greater than normal quantities in the cells (see 'a' above). Under these circumstances, *indirectly acting* sympathomimetic agents can displace excessive amounts of noradrenaline from the sympathetic terminals and in this way cause acute hypertension.

3. Interactions with opiates. Drugs which are normally metabolised by oxidation have a more intense or long-lasting effect in patients taking MAOIs. Morphine and pethidine are examples of drugs handled in this way and if administered to a patient receiving MAOIs, the interaction can cause prolonged unconsciousness with deep respiratory

Interactions with pethidine can be particularly dangerous and can result in severe respiratory depression or, alternatively, excitation, delirium, hyperpyrexia and convulsions which can have a fatal termination.

4. Interactions with other drugs. When given in combination with tricyclic antidepressants, MAOIs can give rise to excitement, confusion and hyperpyrexia. Nevertheless, MAOIs and tricyclic antidepressants are occasionally given together for the treatment of severe depression, under expert supervision.

MAOIs can interact with the hypotensive drug methyldopa to produce excitement and confusion.

Some MAOIs, particularly phenelzine, lower the blood pressure and therefore increase the effect of many hypotensive agents. In contrast, the hypotensive effect of guanethidine is reduced.

The tricyclic antidepressants

The most widely used tricyclic antidepressant drugs are imipramine, dothiepin and amitriptyline. These are similar drugs except that imipramine is mildly stimulating and can cause insomnia, while amitriptyline is mildly tranquillising and may cause drowsiness. Their antidepressant activity does not start immediately but there is a latent period of 1–3 weeks before the mood improves. Minor side-effects are common – particularly dry mouth, constipation and postural hypotension. These drugs can also potentiate the peripheral actions of noradrenaline by an inhibition of neuronal uptake.

Imipramine and amitriptyline are usually given in gradually increasing doses until the optimal response is attained. This dose is then maintained for several months; then the drug gradually withdrawn. In about half the patients so treated the attack of depression is terminated.

Amitriptyline was probably the most widely used

of the tricyclic antidepressants and is often used as a standard against which newer agents are tested. Prothiaden is another widely used tricyclic which has additional anxiolytic activity.

Side-effects of tricyclic antidepressants

1. Anticholinergic. Tricyclic antidepressants are strongly anticholinergic and dry mouth caused by amitriptyline can be so severe as occasionally to lead to ascending parotitis. Other effects are constipation, tachycardia and paralysis of accommodation.

2. Cardiotoxic. Dysrhythmias particularly in the elderly can be fatal.

3. CNS. Amitriptyline is sedating but imipramine is mildly stimulant. There can be sleep disturbances or, occasionally fits.

4. Interactions with sympathomimetic agents. Tricyclic antidepressants have been shown to enhance the effects of adrenaline, but only in some bizarre experiments in which volunteers (pre-treated with tricyclics) were given adrenaline in enormous doses by continuous *intravenous* (!) infusion for no less than 25 minutes. The main effect was then to produce a rise in systolic but a fall in diastolic blood pressure. The amount of adrenaline in local anaesthetic solutions for dental purposes is too small to produce this effect and there is *no clinical evidence of interactions between tricyclic antidepressants and adrenaline in local anaesthetic solutions.* However, this myth of dangerous interactions between dental local anaesthetics and tricyclic antidepressants is still widely believed, partly because it is perpetuated by 'experts' who presumably have never read the relevant report.

Amitriptyline remains the standard by which other antidepressants are judged. Nevertheless, its unpleasant anticholinergic effects and the risk of more dangerous toxic effects have led to the development of other, possibly safer antidepressants.

The 'new generation' antidepressants

Newer antidepressants include mianserin, viloxazine and trazodone. They are not tricyclic in structure but have similar properties in that they enhance the actions of amine transmitters in the brain. However, they have little or no anticholinergic activity and are safer in normal use and in overdose. They have less cardiovascular toxicity, but mianserin can cause postural hypotension and dizziness, and rarely, agranulocytosis.

It is particularly difficult to compare the effectiveness of antidepressant drugs, hence psychiatrists vary widely in their preferences. However, amitriptyline, the value of which has well been established over many years, is still widely used despite its disadvantages.

Adrenergic uptake blockers and adrenergic receptor blockers

As mentioned earlier, noradrenaline once released, is removed from the synaptic cleft by *uptake* into the presynaptic nerve storage vesicles. Uptake of amines such as noradrenaline is blocked by tricyclic antidepressants, particularly in the CNS. Relief of depression by such drugs is attributed to this mechanism. However, tricyclic antidepressants have relatively little effect on sympathetic activity in the rest of the body. Nevertheless, drugs such as tricyclic antidepressants may be described as 'adrenergic uptake blockers' and this may cause confusion with 'adrenergic *receptor* blockers' which are drugs which have a quite different action.

Adrenergic receptor blockers are the α and β blockers such as phentolamine and propanolol respectively. The β blockers, widely used for angina or to lower blood pressure, also have central activity but their difference from the 'adrenergic uptake blockers' is shown by the fact that they can actually *cause* depression.

Electroconvulsive therapy

Electroconvulsive therapy (ECT) is a non-drug treatment used for severe depression. The patient is anaesthetised and given a short-acting muscle relaxant such as suxamethonium. An electric current (250–500 mA at up to 150 V) is then applied across the temples for not more than 1 second and, but for the muscle relaxant, would cause violent convulsions. This procedure is repeated once or twice weekly for about 5 weeks.

ECT was for long given empirically and without objective substantiation of its benefits: some psychiatrists even believed that it was more effective when given without an anaesthetic — this probably tells us more about those psychiatrists than the alleged benefits of the treatment. However, controlled trials of ECT suggest that it increases cerebral amine levels and is one of the most effective treatments for severe depression.

Amphetamines

Amphetamines have no place in the treatment of depression. They produce elation in individuals who are not depressed, and are addictive. Depressed patients usually do not respond at all or may transiently improve then relapse into a state worse than before.*

Hypomania

Hypomania is abnormal elation. The patient is overactive mentally and physically and feels euphoric and confident. The patient therefore feels extremely well and has no complaints, but it is his anxious and often also exhausted relatives who bring, or try to bring, him to the physician.

This illness can lead to many social complications such as starting (but not finishing) too many projects, taking out hire-purchase agreements and simultaneously attempting overambitious entertainment programmes. An attack of hypomania is usually self-limiting and a more normal mood may be restored quite suddenly. Alternatively, the mood may equally suddenly plunge into depression. Quite often the mood swings rapidly and repeatedly from one extreme to the other (cyclothymia). Although hypomania is the opposite side of the coin to depression, it is very much less common.

An episode of hypomania can usually be terminated by the use of one of the major tranquillisers such as chlorpromazine (Largactil) or haloperidol (Serenace). Dosage has to be adjusted to the patients' response – too much may swing the mood to depression.

Lithium salts have the remarkable property of stabilising mood. They are particularly successful in cyclothymia and may be effective in preventing repeated attacks of hypomania or depression. The dose has to be controlled by monitoring the blood levels of lithium. Raised blood levels may lead to intestinal disturbances, involuntary movements and cardiac arrhythmias. The risk of arrhythmias is greatly increased by general anaesthetics.

Schizophrenia and the neuroleptic major tranquillisers

Schizophrenia is a truly terrible mental illness which affects nearly 1% of the population. In everyday speech it is madness and quite unlike disorders such as depression which are a recognisable, if exaggerated, disturbance of mood.

Schizophrenia predominantly affects personality, but it is incorrect to call it split personality; it is rather a disintegration of personality. The idea that in schizophrenia a person can become two quite separate individuals like Dr Jekyll and Mr Hyde, each behaving rationally but unaware of the other, is the creation of a novelist. In life the patient becomes progressively more out of touch with or completely inaccessible to others, while his responses to everyday situations become totally inappropriate. The patient may have auditory hallucinations and delusions of persecution. He may feel that others are controlling his thoughts and actions. This delusion that thoughts or actions are being controlled by outside human or physical influences is a form of paranoia. He may also feel that his thoughts are being blocked. There may be bizarre bursts of excitement, or prolonged periods of statue-like immobility.

Without treatment, few patients used to be able to live outside long-stay mental hospitals and it was mainly because of schizophrenia that strait-jackets and padded cells had to be used. In the 1950s chlorpromazine was introduced and enabled many of these patients to live at home and even resume some kind of work. Even more impressive, the early stages of the disease were completely arrested and deterioration prevented. Patients are now given neuroleptics for 1 or 2 years and these usually prevent acute episodes and relapse of the illness.

The neuroleptics include many groups of drugs, of which the most important are still the phenothiazines.

---

* Depression and suicide: the catch 22 of antidepressant treatment is that without such treatment the patient may commit suicide, but some patients are so determined upon self-destruction that they use the antidepressant drug as the agent for suicide.

The phenothiazine neuroleptics

The phenothiazines include chlorpromazine (Largactil), trifluoperazine (Stelazine) and fluphenazine (Moditen).

The central effects of these major tranquillisers include a diminished emotional responsiveness to external stimuli, sedation (in large doses), inhibition of hypothalamic activity producing hypothermia and hypotension, and depression of the vomiting centre. The major tranquillisers potentiate the action of other cerebral depressants such as alcohol or the barbiturates, but also usefully potentiate the action of analgesics and this latter effect is therapeutically valuable for severe pain.

Phenothiazines* are also weak muscle relaxants peripherally and block the actions of the catecholamines.

Phenothiazines are used for acute schizophrenia, in the long-term management of chronic schizophrenia, and in many forms of excited psychotic states including senile confusion, drug withdrawal syndromes, delirium and hypomania.

Fluphenazine enanthate is given by deep intramuscular injection at intervals up to 28 days in the long-term treatment of schizophrenia because patients cannot be relied upon to continue to take tablets.

Phenothiazines such as chlorpromazine or trifluoperazine are also used to suppress vomiting of central origin.

Other groups of neuroleptics are butyrophenones and thioxanthines, such as thiothixine.

Adverse effects. The most common toxic effects are postural hypotension and tremor of a parkinsonian type. Chlorpromazine occasionally causes a reversible type of intrahepatic obstructive jaundice.

Other side-effects of phenothiazines are involuntary facial movements, pigmentation of the oral mucosa and decreased salivation.

If the phenothiazine neuroleptics are used for many months or years a serious toxic effect develops in about one-third of patients. This is tardive

dyskinesia and presents as involuntary movements which typically involve the face. Repeated grimacing and chewing movements may be so violent that biting causes scarring and deformity of the tongue. Other parts of the body may be involved including the limbs and muscles of respiration. Other neuroleptics, such as haloperidol (a butyrophenone) and the antiemetics metoclopramide and domperidone can also cause tardive dyskinesias. This terrible complication may be irreversible and may even worsen when the drug is withdrawn.

In recent years, antipsychotic neuroleptics have been developed which appear to have a more specific effect on psychotic activity with relatively little tendency to cause extrapyramidal toxicity such as parkinsonism. These drugs include pimozide and, more recently, sulpiride.

The butyrophenones

The main example is haloperidol which has actions similar to the piperazine group of phenothiazines and thus causes less sedation than older phenothiazines. Like the phenothiazines, haloperidol causes mild hypotension. Nevertheless, haloperidol is sometimes used as a premedicating agent before surgery and in some techniques of dental sedation, but has the disadvantage of being a respiratory depressant.

---

* One of the writers was once taken to see the vast stockyards of Fort Worth, Texas, by a psychiatrist from nearby Dallas. A large advertisement hoarding extolling the virtues of a particular phenothiazine stood over the cattle pens and was a source of considerable puzzlement to both of us who were unaware that phenothiazines were originally introduced to treat worm infestations.

SUGGESTED FURTHER READING

Anon 1981a Hypnotic drugs and treatment of insomnia. Journal of the American Medical Association 245: 749

Anon 1981b ECT in Britain: a shameful state of affairs. Lancet ii: 1207

Anon 1981c Levodopa: long-term impact on Parkinson's disease. British Medical Journal 282: 417

Anon 1988 Mianserin 10 years on. Drug and Therapeutics Bulletin 26: 17

Bateman D N, Chaplin S 1988 Centrally acting drugs. British Medical Journal 296: 417

Blackwell B 1981 Adverse effects of antidepressant drugs. Drugs 21: 201

Bloom F E, Morrison J H 1986 Neurotransmitters of the human brain. Human Neurobiology 5: 1003

Braestrup C, Nielsen M 1982 Anxiety. Lancet ii: 1030

Brandon S 1982 Monoamine oxidase inhibitors in depression. British Medical Journal 285: 1594

Cassidy S, Henry J 1987 Fatal toxicity of antidepressant drugs in overdose. British Medical Journal 295: 1021

Coppen A, Abou-Saleh M T 1983 Lithium in the prophylaxis of unipolar depression: a review. Journal of the Royal Society of Medicine 76: 297

Deakin J F W 1983 Antidepressant effects of electroconvulsive therapy: current or seizure? British Medicine Journal 286: 1083

Delgado-Escueta A V, Treiman D M, Walsh G O 1983 The treatable epilepsies. I and II. New England Journal of Medicine 308: 1508, 1576

Gibberd F B 1987 Management of Parkinson's disease. British Medical Journal 294: 1393

Glassman A H, Roose S P 1982 Tricyclic drugs in the treatment of depression. Medical Clinics of North America 66: 1037

Greenblatt D J, Shader R I, Abernethy D R 1983 Current status of benzodiazepines. New England Journal of Medicine 309: 354

Greenblatt D J, Woo E, Allen M D, Orsulak P J, Shader R I 1978 Rapid recovery from massive diazepam overdose. Journal of the American Medical Association 240: 1872

Hamilton M. The clinical distinction between anxiety and depression. British Journal of Clinical Pharmacology 15: 165S

Hassell T M, White II G C, Jewson L G, Peele III L C 1979 Valproic acid: a new antiepileptic drug with potential side effects of dental concern. Journal of the American Dental Association 99: 983

Heel R C, Brogden R N, Speight T M, Avery G S 1981 Temazepam: a review of its pharmacological properties and therapeutic efficacy as an hypnotic. Drugs 21: 321

Higgitt A C, Lader M H, Fonagy P 1985 Clinical management of benzodiazepine dependence. British Medical Journal 291: 688

Hockings N, Ballinger B R 1983 Hypnotics and anxiolytics. British Medical Journal 286: 1949

Hollister L E 1981 Current antidepressant drugs: their clinical use. Drugs 22: 129

Hollister L E, Conley F K, Britt R H, Shuer L 1981 Long-term use of diazepam. Journal of the American Medical Association 246: 1568

Lader M 1982 Some newer antidepressants. Hospital Update, 8: 895

Lader M L 1987 Clinical pharmacology of benzodiazepines. Annual Preview of Medicine 38: 19

Parke J D 1981 Adverse effects of antiparkinsonian drugs. Drugs 21: 341

Paykel E S 1983 The classification of depression. British Journal of Clinical Pharmacology 15: 155S

Perucca E, Richens A 1981 Drug interactions with phenytoin. Drugs 21: 120

Petursson H, Lader M 1983 Rational use of anxiolytic/sedative drugs. Drugs 25: 514

Pollitt J 1983 New drugs in psychiatry. British Journal of Hospital Medicine 29: 340

Rickels K, Case G, Downing R W, Winokur A 1983 Long-term diazepam therapy and clinical outcome. Journal of American Medical Association 250: 767

Rosenbaum J F 1982 Current concepts in psychiatry. New England Journal of Medicine 306: 401

Skegg K, Skeff D C G, Richards S M. Incidence of self poisoning in patients prescribed pyschotropic drugs. British Medical Journal 286: 841

Spero L 1982 Epilepsy. Lancet ii: 1319

Study R E, Barker J L 1982 Cellular mechanisms of benzodiazepine action. Journal of the American Medical Association 247: 2147

W H O Review Group 1983 Use and abuse of benzodiazepines. Bulletin of the World Health Organization 61: 551

7. The nervous system
III. Analgesics and drug dependence

ANTI-INFLAMMATORY AND OTHER NON-NARCOTIC ANALGESICS

These drugs are often referred to as 'minor' analgesics. This implies that they are useful only for the management of mild pain, but this understates their effectiveness. They are effective in very painful conditions such as rheumatoid arthritis, other forms of skeletal disease and cancer, and are likely to be particularly useful for dental pain since the latter is typically inflammatory in origin. They are less potent analgesics than the opioids such as morphine but many of the 'minor' analgesics are in fact at least as effective as some of the narcotic analgesics that are given by mouth.

Representative and commonly used drugs in this group are:

1. Aspirin and other salicylates.
2. Paracetamol.
3. Pyrazolones.
4. Mefenamates.
5. Indomethacin and related drugs.
6. Propionic acid derivatives and related drugs.

Aspirin

Aspirin is acetylsalicylic acid. It is mainly absorbed from the small intestine, but some is absorbed from the stomach. The main site of aspirin's action is in the peripheral tissues, where it has an anti-inflammatory effect. This is the main analgesic action of aspirin; it may also have some central (thalamic) inhibitory action, but this is controversial.

Aspirin is the archetype (and still one of the most useful) of the now almost innumerable Non-Steroidal Anti-Inflammatory Agents (NSAIAs) of which all the above (except paracetamol) are examples.

One of the important chemical mediators of pain and inflammation in injured or diseased tissues is a group of lipid substances called the prostaglandins. Aspirin and some of the other minor analgesics prevent the synthesis of prostaglandin E_2, and hence diminish peripheral manifestations of tissue injury (see Fig. 7.1). Thus pain, some of the swelling and impaired function of inflamed tissues are lessened.

Aspirin is antipyretic by its action on the hypothalamus This may also be due to inhibition of prostaglandin synthesis, which is a mediator of the febrile response to infections.

Side-effects

1. Gastric irritation. A common and important side-effect of the non-steroidal anti-inflammatory agents in general is irritation of the gastrointestinal mucosa. The particles of these drugs are particularly damaging and may cause acute ulceration or aggravate chronic ulceration in the stomach. These lesions frequently bleed – sometimes torrentially. Even in the absence of any clinical evidence of gastric irritation, about 70% of people taking aspirin regularly lose up to 10 ml of blood a day and this is detectable in the faeces. Bleeding is aggravated by taking alcohol and diminished by simultaneous administration of alkalis, or using buffered aspirin. Other anti-inflammatory agents are also gastric irritants.

2. Effects on haemostasis. Aspirin-induced gastric bleeding is so frequent that it is one of the most common single causes of emergency admissions for acute haematemesis. In most cases, bleeding is subclinical but aspirin should not be given to a

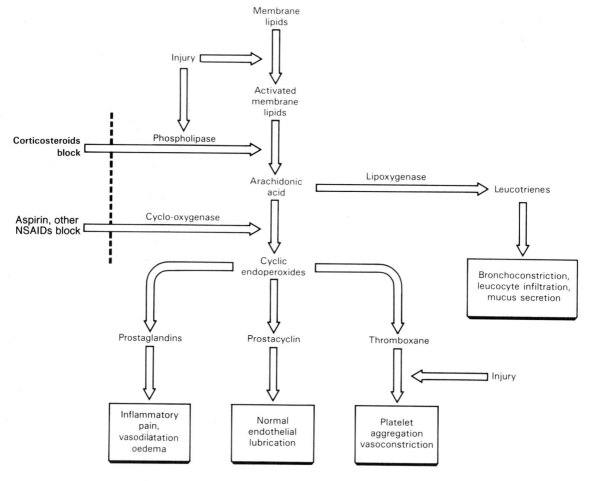

Fig. 7.1 Sites of action of aspirin and of other agents blocking the synthesis of mediators of inflammation.

patient with a known haemorrhagic tendency (such as haemophilia or as a result of anticoagulant therapy) or with a history suggestive of peptic ulceration ('indigestion' or epigastric pain).

In addition to provoking gastric bleeding, aspirin itself impairs haemostasis mainly by interference with platelet aggregation and even in normal doses prolongs the bleeding time. Since the initiation of thrombus formation in arteries is dependent on platelet adhesion and aggregation, it is interesting that some evidence has been found to suggest that chronic aspirin takers have a lower than average mortality from myocardial infarction, but more recently this has been disputed.

Large doses of aspirin are said to cause hypoprothrombinaemia, but the evidence is scanty.

However, the effect of aspirin on platelet function means that it potentiates haemorrhagic disorders of any sort, particularly those where the clotting process is defective. Aspirin has recently been shown also to have fibrinolytic activity. The clinical importance of this effect is not yet known. Aspirin on its own, however, is rarely a significant cause of abnormal bleeding except from the stomach where other mechanisms are acting.

3. Allergy. Aspirin may occasionally cause allergic reactions – including bronchospasm and urticaria. Aspirin should preferably not be given to patients with a history of bronchial asthma. Rashes (petechial or erythematous but sometimes mimicking measles or scarlet fever) are another type of side-effect.

4. Reye's syndrome. Reye's syndrome is a rare combination of liver and brain damage which usually presents as deepening drowsiness and can be fatal. It particularly affects young children. Its pathogenesis is unknown but it can follow viral infections such as chickenpox and there is an association with the administration of apirin. Aspirin is therefore contraindicated for children under 12 and particularly if they are febrile.*

5. Overdose. Large doses of aspirin cause tinnitus and temporary deafness. Moderate overdose stimulates the respiratory centre, causing increased rate and depth of respiration and ultimately respiratory alkalosis, due to rapid excretion of carbon dioxide via the lungs. Dangerous aspirin overdose produces an intracellular acidosis that can be fatal. Aspirin is a common means of self-poisoning because the tablets are so easily obtainable. Aspirin accounts for about 200 suicides a year in Britain.

All this suggests that aspirin is a dangerous drug. In fact, it is estimated that at least 2000 *tons* (6000 million tablets) are taken each year in Britain and many patients (such as those with arthritis) are taking considerable quantities of aspirin every day for years on end. The frequency of toxic reactions is remarkably low considering the scale of use.

With reasonable care aspirin is a safe and effective drug and remains, for example, the single most generally useful drug in the long-term management of rheumatoid arthritis. After three-quarters of a century aspirin has not been superseded as a general purpose analgesic.

The *main effects* of aspirin can be summarised as:

1. Analgesic. Mainly peripheral action and due to its anti-inflammatory action by inhibiting prostaglandin synthesis.
2. Antipyretic.

Adverse effects:

1. Gastric bleeding.
2. Interference with platelet function causing a prolonged bleeding time.
3. Tinnitus, deafness.

---

* Reye was an Australian pathologist of German parentage. For those who care about such matters, the correct pronunciation is probably therefore 'Rye' rather than 'Ray'.

4. Hypersensitivity.
5. Poisonous in overdosage by its metabolic effects.
6. Reye's syndrome in childhood.

Paracetamol

Paracetamol is a widely used analgesic derived from a much older drug, phenacetin. Phenacetin is obsolete in Britain because it can cause renal papillary necrosis if large doses are given over a long period. Although paracetamol is the active derivative of phenacetin produced in the body, it does not appear to be significantly nephrotoxic. Phenacetin and paracetamol are antipyretic and analgesic but have no anti-inflammatory or anti-rheumatic effect. The mode of action of paracetamol appears to be essentially similar to that of other NSAIDs, namely, inhibition of prostaglandin synthesis. However, this action appears to be mainly central; there is no significant anti-inflammatory effect peripherally and the associated gastric irritant effect is also therefore absent.

The main toxic effect of paracetamol is that it can cause hepatic damage and even liver failure in mild overdose. This can be particularly dangerous because overdose of paracetamol is not followed by immediate coma. If an overdose has been taken therefore, the patient may think it has had no effect as the symptoms of liver damage may not appear for several days. In addition, the liver damage, which is difficult to treat effectively, is more likely to be fatal than the effects of aspirin poisoning.

Paracetamol taken in normal doses for occasional use seems otherwise to be safe and it is a useful alternative to aspirin for patients with gastric ulceration or who react to aspirin in other ways.

In view of the risk of Reye's syndrome with aspirin, paracetamol is the analgesic of choice for children under 12.

Mefenamic acid

Mefenamic acid is structurally unrelated to other anti-inflammatory analgesics but has properties and effectiveness generally similar to those of aspirin. Mefenamic acid occasionally causes rashes or diarrhoea, in which case it should be stopped. Anaemia, thrombocytopenia, leucopenia or renal damage are rare side-effects which have been reported after prolonged use.

Other anti-inflammatory analgesics

These drugs have a potent anti-inflammatory action and are useful only for pain due to inflammation. These drugs are therefore mainly used for the rheumatic disorders and not as general purpose analgesics. In spite of these potent anti-inflammatory actions, aspirin still remains one of the most useful and effective drugs in the treatment of rheumatoid arthritis, although it may be necessary to give very large doses. Even these, however, are usually less likely to cause side-effects than the

potent anti-inflammatory drugs. There are now very many of these agents and they include the drugs in Table 7.1.

Phenylbutazone and oxyphenbutazone

These are potent anti-inflammatory analgesics. Phenylbutazone and its analogues are pyrazolone derivatives of which the forerunner was amidopyrine (aminopyrine). Amidopyrine is an effective analgesic but is prone to cause leucopenia and agranulocytosis. These toxic effects on the marrow have caused amidopyrine to be discarded, but its derivatives share its toxicity to the marrow and other organs.

Table 7.1   Non-steroidal anti-inflammatory drugs (NSAIDs)

Approved name	Trade name	Tolerability	Clinical usefulness
Aspirin Soluble aspirin Aloxiprin Benorylate Sustained release aspirins	Disprin Solprin Palaprim Benoral Levius	Excellent in acute illness. Large doses cause gastric irritation in prolonged use. Better tolerated than plain aspirin in prolonged use	Very useful. Effective antipyretic, analgesic and anti-inflammatory. Contraindicated in childhood.
Diflunisal	Dolobid	Less irritant to stomach	Similar to aspirin
Pyrazalones Phenylbutazone Oxyphenbutazone Azapropazone	Butazolidin Butacote Tanderil Tandacote Rheumox	Rashes and gastro-intestinal disturbances common Agranulocytosis*	Effective but because of toxicity use reserved mainly for ankylosing spondylitis. Highly effective anti-inflammatory agents. Effective analgesic and anti-inflammatory agent
Fenamates Mefenamic acid	Ponstan	Diarrhoea common.	Analgesic, but weak anti-inflammatory properties
Indomethacin group Indomethacin Sulindac	Indocid Mobilan Imbrilon Clinoral	Headache common Gastrointestinal disturbances fairly common	Highly effective anti-inflammatory agents
Propionic acid derivatives and similar drugs Ibuprofen Ketoprofen Naproxen Flurbiprofen Fenoprofen Diclofenac Fenbufen Piroxicam Tolmetin	Brufen Orudis Naprosyn Synflex Froben Fenopron Progesic Voltarol Lederfen Feldene Tolectin	Little gastric irritation Moderate–mild gastric irritant	Mild analgesic, and anti-inflammatory Moderate–powerful analgesic and anti-inflammatory agent

* Phenylbutazone was the most common cause of drug-related marrow depression in the UK

The main metabolite of phenylbutazone is oxyphenbutazone which is also an anti-inflammatory analgesic and is used in eye ointments. Both are gastric irritants and can precipitate severe gastric haemorrhage. These drugs also produce sodium and water retention. This may aggravate hypertension and congestive cardiac failure.

Phenylbutazone and oxyphenbutazone were widely used in the treatment of osteoarthritis, rheumatoid arthritis, phlebitis, gout and ankylosing spondylitis.

Phenylbutazone and oxyphenbutazone are important causes of fatal aplastic anaemia however.

It has been estimated that these drugs have caused more than 1000 deaths in Britain. Since phenylbutazone and oxyphenbutazone have no major advantages over other non-steroidal anti-inflammatory drugs to compensate for their dangers, they have been withdrawn from general use.

Indomethacin

Indomethacin is a stronger anti-inflammatory analgesic which is mainly used in the treatment of inflammatory joint disease. A common side-effect of this drug is headache. Like many other anti-inflammatory drugs, indomethacin can cause gastric irritation, ulceration and haemorrhage.

Indomethacin can rarely cause agranulocytosis.

Ibuprofen, ketoprofen, fenoprofen, naproxen, flurbiprofen, fenbufen

These are anti-inflammatory agents widely used in the management of rheumatoid arthritis. They are as effective as aspirin but usually cause less gastric irritation and are therefore particularly useful when aspirin cannot be tolerated. Nevertheless, there is very wide individual variation in susceptibility to gastric irritation from different drugs in this group. Their success in rheumatic diseases appears to be solely due to their anti-inflammatory action, as they have no central analgesic activity.

The widespread use of the anti-inflammatory analgesics for rheumatoid arthritis mentioned on several occasions earlier is simply due to the fact that this is the most common disease needing treatment of this sort.

Since most dental pain is inflammatory, aspirin and these propionic acid derivatives, such as ibu-

profen, are usually the drugs of choice and are likely to be the most effective.

Ibuprofen is the NSAID least likely to cause toxic effects and is frequently therefore the first choice despite the fact that it is a weaker anti-inflammatory analgesic than others in this group.

Other minor analgesics

These include propoxyphene, which is related to methadone, and codeine. These drugs are therefore discussed with the narcotic analgesics to which they are related.

Analgesic combinations

The problem of dose-dependent toxicity in the treatment of pain can sometimes be overcome by using several drugs together in small doses. Thus, in treating mild to moderate pain, aspirin, paracetamol and codeine, or paracetamol and dihydrocodeine may have stronger analgesic effects. It is, however, difficult to assess in an objective way the potency of analgesic agents and it is possible that the effectiveness of analgesic mixtures is due to the high total amount of analgesic used.

TREATMENT OF DENTAL PAIN

Aspirin and similar drugs alone or in combination are the most widely used analgesics for dental as for most other pain and are usually effective. It has to be admitted, however, that acute pulpitis and periapical periodontitis can cause intense pain which responds poorly to any of the commonly available drugs. It is hardly feasible to give an injection of one of the narcotic analgesics on such occasions and a need remains for a remedy for this problem. At the moment the best answer is immediate elimination of the cause of the pain by appropriate dental treatment.

MANAGEMENT OF SPECIAL TYPES OF PAIN

1. Pain due to inflammation

When the inflammatory reaction can be suppressed without risk of spreading infection, as in rheumatoid arthritis, anti-inflammatory drugs may be helpful. Many non-narcotic analgesics such as aspirin and pyrazolone derivatives (phenylbutazone and its analogues) are anti-inflammatory and, as a consequence, analgesic. Others such as indomethacin and naproxen have a stronger anti-inflammatory effect.

As mentioned earlier, aspirin in adequate doses or one of the propionic acid derivatives ('profens') are the most appropriate choice for this type of dental pain and are most likely to be effective.

The mode of action of anti-inflammatory analgesics is such that they are most effective in preventing the onset of inflammatory pain, rather than countering the effects of prostaglandins already formed. Whenever possible therefore these drugs should be given when pain is anticipated. Thus, after a difficult third molar extraction, aspirin or other NSAID should be given before the local anaesthetic starts to wear off.

Corticosteroids are also widely used for their anti-inflammatory action as in rheumatoid arthritis when other means have failed. The side-effects are such that systemic corticosteroids should be given only when no other treatment is effective.

Anti-inflammatory agents may also be useful for reducing the pain and swelling that otherwise follows oral surgery.

Corticosteroids (e.g. triamcinolone) have been used topically to relieve the pain of acute pulpitis. A tetracycline is also included in the preparation with the aim of overcoming the local infection. Acute pulpitis is difficult to relieve with drugs and this preparation applied as a paste to the surface of the exposed pulp is effective. Unfortunately this preparation usually causes death of the pulp later on.

Herpes zoster which affects the posterior horn cells causes intense aching pain. When the second and third divisions of the trigeminal nerve are affected patients are often quite unable to distinguish this pain from toothache. Analgesics are helpful but use of an antiviral agent is also necessary. *Acyclovir* by mouth, or in severe cases by intravenous injection, should be given as it has been shown to be highly effective against this infection in immunodeficient patients. *Idoxuridine* can be applied as a 5% or 40% solution in dimethyl sulphoxide to enhance its absorption through the skin, but is too toxic for systemic administration. In either case administration must start at the earliest possible moment.

2. Trigeminal neuralgia

Trigeminal neuralgia is an acute paroxysmal pain often of unbearable severity and is typically precipitated by the touching or chilling of a trigger zone on the face or in the mouth. There is no peripheral cause. The most effective drugs available are *anticonvulsants*. Phenytoin is moderately effective but *carbamazepine* (Tegretol) is better. This is chemically related to the tricyclic antidepressant imipramine. Carbamazepine reduces the frequency and severity of attacks in many cases; in others, phenytoin may have to be given as well. Carbamazepine is not an analgesic and does not relieve other forms of pain. Side-effects may include nausea, rashes, drowsiness and ataxia.

The anticonvulsant benzodiazepine, clonazepam, is sometimes also effective in controlling trigeminal neuralgia and can be used if carbamazepine causes too severe side-effects, but it is more sedating.

The effectiveness of anticonvulsants in trigeminal neuralgia may be related to the fact that the latter may be a sensory counterpart to epilepsy. Sudden electrical discharges in the brain can trigger violent muscular activity (epilepsy) or pain (trigeminal neuralgia). Anticonvulsants probably act mainly by reducing the spread of excitation and responsiveness of neurones in the brain and may therefore affect sensory as well as motor cortical cells.

Anticonvulsants are not (of course) analgesics and have no effect on an attack once it has started. These drugs are only effective therefore if given on a long-term basis and will usually then control the frequency and severity of attacks. It is not uncommon, however, to find that in a patient with trigeminal neuralgia, carbamazepine has been given without benefit simply because it has been used as an analgesic when an attack has started. Carbamazepine and other anticonvulsants are also ineffective at controlling pain other than that of trigeminal neuralgia and are of no value in the treatment of post-herpetic neuralgia.

3. Migraine and migrainous neuralgia

Classical migraine is characterised by a sequence of events which typically starts with an aura (or warning) often consisting of an hallucination of a zigzag pattern of flickering light (a 'fortification spectrum'). This is followed by photophobia, nausea and intense headache of one side of the head (hemicrania) which may persist for several hours. The headache appears to be due to dilatation and stretching of vessels at or near the base of the brain. This in turn appears to be the result of the vasoactive effect of certain amines. These have not yet been identified with certainty but appear to have an action like serotonin (5HT).

Mild migraine can be managed by use of simple analgesics and 70% of attacks are controlled by aspirin or paracetamol. If nausea is severe, the absorption of analgesics is improved by giving metoclopramide. Resistant migraine is treated with *ergotamine*. This has to be given early to be effective. Oral absorption is variable and severe migraine can often only be controlled by ergotamine given by subcutaneous injection. An alternative is to inhale ergotamine powder from an aerosol inhaler (Medihaler); this is much more reliable than oral administration. Ergotamine has a wide variety of actions including peripheral vasoconstriction, but the way in which it relieves migraine is not entirely clear.

Prophylaxis of migraine

Pizotifen is an antihistamine chemically related to the tricyclic antidepressants and having antiserotinergic activity. It is effective, but can cause weight gain and drowsiness.

NSAIDs can also be effective prophylactics for migraine, but the side-effects may be unacceptable.

Beta-blockers are effective. Their use is limited mainly by their contraindications, particularly asthma or heart failure and their interaction with ergotamine.

Clonidine appears to be less effective than was previously believed. It may aggravate depression or cause insomnia.

Methysergide has dangerous side-effects, namely retroperitoneal, endocardial and pleural fibrosis, so that it is restricted to specialist use in hospital.

Migrainous neuralgia. This variant of migraine can be mistaken for pain of dental origin, since it is localised to the maxilla deep to and around the eye on one side. Young adults are mainly affected and, apart from the site, migrainous neuralgia differs from classical migraine in that the attacks may come on regularly at the same time, day after day, for weeks. One typical feature is that the attacks are often at night. Then there may be a complete remission for one to several months and the disease usually improves or ceases altogether in later middle age. Another characteristic feature of migrainous neuralgia is visible vascular changes such as reddening of the conjunctiva of the affected side, sometimes with oedematous swelling of the face which may be sufficient to close the eye. There is no aura or nausea but the condition is managed as for classical migraine with ergotamine. It is an uncommon cause of facial pain and in a rare variant of this disorder the pain is felt in the jaws or even in the mandible and is known as 'lower half headache'.

4. Spasm of voluntary muscle

Muscle spasm (tension headache) is a common cause of headache, particularly of the occipital region. Muscle spasm is probably also the main cause of the pain of so-called pain-dysfunction syndrome. Anxiety and tension seem to play a large part and anxiolytic drugs, particularly diazepam which also has a muscle relaxant action, may be helpful to some patients.

5. Ischaemic muscle pain – myocardial infarction

Myocardial infarction is one of the most severe kinds of pain that can be experienced. It occasionally presents problems of diagnosis or management in the dental surgery particularly when the pain is felt in the lower jaw. The pain of myocardial infarction can only be managed by giving strong analgesics such as morphine by injection, or nitrous oxide and oxygen (see Ch. 10).

6. Pain as a symptom of depression

A minority of depressed patients have physical rather than psychic symptoms. One of these is atypical facial pain often affecting the upper jaw. It is frequently described as severe or unbearable, aching in character, is unremitting and of very long duration. The pain may sometimes be dramatically relieved by giving an antidepressant in adequa dosage. Inevitably, however, it is difficult to exclua an organic cause with absolute certainty and a psychiatrist's opinion should be sought.

THE NARCOTIC ANALGESICS AND DRUG DEPENDENCE

The terms narcotic analgesic, major analgesic and opioid are used interchangeably, but opioid is the term more generally used. The group includes morphine, codeine and their derivatives, and synthetic morphine-like drugs. These drugs are powerful analgesics (particularly when given by injection), cough and respiratory depressants, and inhibitors of intestinal motility. Tolerance develops with all these drugs. After repeated administration the dose has to be increased to maintain the same level of effect and dependence can result.

The narcotic analgesics are most effective against severe pain, particularly of visceral or skeletal origin such as myocardial infarction, deep bone pain or postoperative pain, and the pain of advanced cancer. The accompanying emotional reaction to pain is also lessened or abolished. The tendency to cause dependence, however, restricts the use of these drugs to the relief of pain which is either nonrecurrent or caused by terminal cancer.

Dependence on the opiods readily develops and most of them therefore are Controlled Drugs.

Enkephatins and endorphins

Although the effects of morphine and other opiates have been known for thousands of years, their mechanism of action has not been understood until very recently.

Natural peptides (enkephalins and endorphins) are present in the brain and have properties mimicking those of morphine. The enkephalins react with specific opiate receptors in the brain and these receptors are also the targets for opiate drugs. The enkephalins are possibly released during pain or other stressful events and by stimulating their receptors raise the pain threshold and help the individual to adapt. Stimulation of these receptors by drugs raises the pain threshold and also induces feelings of relaxation or alternatively, of dysphoria according to which receptors are stimulated (Table 7.2). Narcotic antagonists also bind to these same opiate receptors and prevent access of analgesics, thus stopping their actions.

Narcotic analgesics

The main types are:

1. Morphine and derivatives such as heroin.
2. Codeine and derivatives such as dihydrocodeine.
3. Pethidine.
4. Propylamines – such as methadone and propoxyphene.
5. Benzomorphans – such as pentazocine and phenazocine.

Morphine

Morphine is a natural opioid readily obtained (together with other opioids such as codeine) from the juice of the unripe seed pods of the oriental poppy (*Papaver somniferum*).

Administration of morphine is usually by injection. It is also absorbed through the intestinal, nasal and respiratory epithelia, but less completely.

Shortly after an injection there may be a brief phase of excitement. In the normal (non-addicted)

Table 7.2 Opioid receptor types

Receptor type	Effect of receptor stimulation	Examples of agonists
μ	Mediates brain analgesia; respiratory depression; euphoria and dependence	Morphine; (buprenorphine is a partial agonist)
κ	Mediates spinal analgesia; sedation	Morphine; pentazocine
δ	Dysphoria; hallucinations	Pentazocine

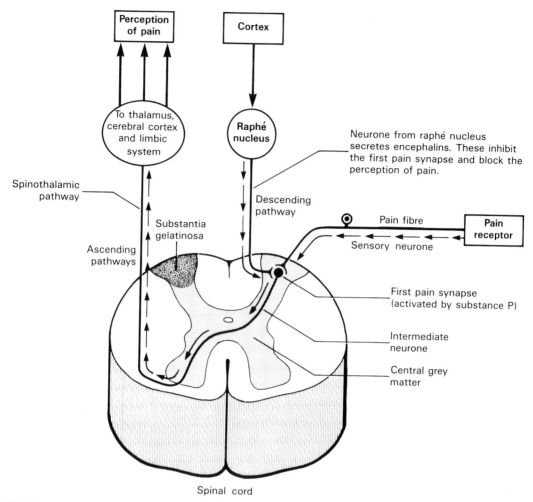

Fig. 7.2 First pain synapse in substantia gelatinosa of the spinal cord. Synapse is stimulated by pain fibres (via substance P). Synapse is blocked by encephalins secreted by descending neurones.

person this is followed by sedation and sleepiness. If the subject was previously in pain, then the relief will bring euphoria. Morphine has a strong tranquillising effect and in addicts particularly, produces euphoria and feelings of self-confidence and relaxation.

After morphine has been given, a variety of unpleasant stimuli such as pain become less effective in eliciting withdrawal reflexes and feelings of apprehension. In other words both the sensation of pain is diminished and the emotional response to pain is also suppressed.

Toxic effects. Morphine is a depressant of the brain but it also has some central stimulant effects which are, occasionally, the dominant response.

Morphine depresses the rate and depth of respiration by decreasing the sensitivity of the respiratory centre to carbon dioxide. Because of this respiratory effect, narcotic analgesics are particularly dangerous in patients suffering from lung diseases such as chronic bronchitis, asthma and pneumonia.

An added hazard to patients with asthma is that morphine releases histamine from the tissues. This produces bronchoconstriction and mucosal oedema, which aggravate the respiratory difficulties of patients with asthma.

The central sedative (and possibly the analgesic) actions of morphine are potentiated by major tranquillisers such as chlorpromazine.

Although morphine is predominantly a depressant of the brain – particularly of the respiratory centre and the thalamic areas concerned with the appreciation of pain – it also causes some stimulation. Morphine stimulates the brainstem chemoreceptor trigger zone, which activates the vomiting centre, but individual susceptibility to this side-effect varies widely. In a few susceptible individuals the motor system is stimulated and this may lead to convulsions. The pupils are also constricted by stimulation of the midbrain. Eye signs are important in the assessment of head injuries and a fixed dilated pupil is indicative of raised intraocular pressure. Morphine can disguise this change and, since it is also a respiratory depressant, is strictly contraindicated after head injuries.

Peripherally, morphine increases the tone of smooth muscle in the ureters, gall bladder and intestine. This may (theoretically) aggravate colic but prolonged use certainly causes constipation by inhibiting peristalsis in the colon. Morphine in very low concentrations is therefore used in mixtures to stop diarrhoea.

Dependence and abuse

Dependence is the state which develops when drugs (such as the opiates) are given repeatedly. If the drugs are then stopped, physical or psychological illness results.

Drug abuse refers to the use of drugs for non-medicinal purposes and frequently results in dependence.

Morphine can produce both physical and psychological dependence, particularly if given for periods of 3–4 weeks or more, and an addict can develop serious physical and mental withdrawal reactions when the drug is stopped.

Withdrawal symptoms begin with a craving for the drug, anxiety and agitation. There is restlessness and increased salivary, nasal and lacrimal secretion. In the early stages the patient becomes depressed and drowsy and may fall into a restless sleep. Later goose-flesh, nausea and loss of appetite may be prominent. The symptoms become worse and 2 days after the last dose of morphine there are abdominal pains, diarrhoea, repeated vomiting, muscle spasms, sweating, shivering and severe shock. The patient may die at this stage.

Actions of morphine – summary:

1. Potent analgesia by a central action.
2. Sedation ranging from tranquillisation to sleep or euphoria.
3. Cough suppression.

Adverse effects:

1. Respiratory depression.
2. Nausea and vomiting.
3. Contraction of smooth muscle of the gastro-intestinal tract. Sphincters close and gut movement is depressed.
4. Histamine release, e.g. constriction of bronchiolar muscle.
5. Addiction (dependence).

These effects are generally undesirable but may occasionally be exploited. It may be helpful, for example, to damp down the excessive respiratory activity and consequent load on the heart in left ventricular failure. Depression of gut movement can be helpful in diarrhoea when there is no serious infection.

Diamorphine (heroin)

Heroin is diacetylmorphine; *diamorphine* is the approved name. It is regarded in Britain (perhaps because it was first synthesised here) as being more powerfully analgesic than morphine on a weight for weight basis, but objective evidence for a clinically significant difference is hard to establish. Diamorphine is therefore regarded in the USA as having no significant advantages and is said to be more highly addictive; certainly the diamorphine withdrawal syndrome is the most severe of any of the narcotics.

Diamorphine is said to be less sedative than morphine. In Britain its use is mainly restricted to relieving very severe pain, particularly in the terminal stages of cancer and in myocardial infarction.

Codeine

Codeine (methylmorphine) is a natural opioid. Although it shows all the general pharmacological actions of morphine, it is a very much weaker analgesic. When given subcutaneously the estimated potency of codeine is only a twelfth of that of morphine (weight for weight). It is not feasible, however, to try to get the same analgesic response as to morphine, as large doses of codeine cause unpleasant side-effects. In practice, codeine cannot therefore be given in such amounts, but is usually given in doses of up to 20 mg orally with other analgesics such as aspirin. Codeine is used for the treatment of moderate pain, for the symptomatic treatment of diarrhoea and particularly for the suppression of cough. In these doses, codeine produces little or no sedation or euphoria. It is not significantly addictive but drug abuse is not unknown.

Dihydrocodeine is said to have approximately twice the analgesic effect of codeine. It possesses all the main characteristics of morphine, but its effectiveness is midway between that of morphine and codeine. In practice, it may be effective in the treatment of moderately severe pain which is not relieved by codeine. Drug dependence is rare and when it does develop withdrawal symptoms are not severe. The main side-effects with normal doses are dizziness and constipation.

Dihydrocodeine has also, incidentally, been reported to *increase* the perception of dental pain and to be less effective than aspirin. An anti-inflammatory analgesic such as aspirin is certainly an appropriate choice for most dental pain, but the measurement of pain perception is notoriously difficult, as discussed later.

Pethidine

Pethidine is a synthetic major analgesic which has many of the actions of morphine, but also has some atropine-like properties in that it relaxes the smooth muscle of the ureters. However, some constipation is common because of spasm of intestinal muscle.

The size of the pupils is not affected. The drug is a powerful analgesic (100 mg of pethidine produces the same effect as 10 mg of morphine) and, unlike codeine, pethidine can be given in doses of several hundred milligrams to get an adequate response. Respiration and cough are depressed. The drug is more likely than morphine to produce dizziness and vomiting. Euphoria, sedation and addictive potential are similar to those of morphine. As mentioned elsewhere in this text, monoamine oxidase inhibitors may give rise to a particularly

severe interaction with pethidine. In some cases, as with morphine, central depression is enhanced and the patient goes into coma, but in other cases there is hyperpyrexia and hyperexcitability which sometimes proves fatal.

Methadone

Methadone is a synthetic analgesic which has very similar potency and pharmacological properties to morphine. It is effective by mouth. Like morphine, it causes smooth muscle spasm. There is, however, an important difference: methadone has less addictive potential than morphine and pethidine. Nevertheless, dependence can develop.

Dextropropoxyphene (propoxyphene)

Dextropropoxyphene is a methadone derivative, but is not a potent analgesic. The side-effects of the drug are similar to those of codeine. Thus in high doses drowsiness, constipation, abdominal pain and anorexia are common.

Dextropropoxyphene is much less effective when taken by mouth than after subcutaneous injection. Although it is a popular analgesic, some trials have found that propoxyphene has little or no detectable analgesic effect when taken by mouth. In proprietary preparations propoxyphene is often combined with another analgesic such as paracetamol (as in Distalgesic) and its enormous popularity is almost certainly not due to its potency as an analgesic, but rather because of the effect of the narcotic component (propoxyphene) on mood (see also p. 112). The abuse potential of dextropropoxyphene is less than that of pethidine, because high doses and parenteral administration can cause unpleasant psychotic reactions. Nevertheless, Distalgesic has become increasingly widely used as a drug of addiction.

Dangers of propoxyphene. Dependence on propoxyphene has become common and withdrawal signs have been described even in an infant born to a woman regularly treated with this drug during pregnancy.

Another danger is that of self-poisoning. Partly as a result of its ready availability acute overdosage of propoxyphene is now common. This leads to rapid fluctuation between coma and convulsions together with cardiac and respiratory depression. Distalgesic, a popular proprietary analgesic, is also widely used for self-poisoning. It is hepatotoxic as a consequence of the paracetamol content in addition to its effects on the nervous system caused by the propoxyphene content. Sudden cardiac or respiratory arrest is a danger even when the patient's condition seems satisfactory. Acute cardiorespiratory depression and pulmonary oedema are important causes of death but if these hazards are survived acute liver failure often develops.

For some time Distalgesic was the most common cause of death in cases of drug overdosage referred to a forensic laboratory. The amount of overdose is estimated to be within the range of 20 to 30 tablets, but in nearly 50% of cases alcohol had been taken in addition.

The many deaths from Distalgesic poisoning may in part result from the fact that many self-poisonings may be intended as no more than dramatic gestures rather than irreversible self-destruction. For those who make such attempts in the expectation of awakening amidst a gratifying flurry of attention, Distalgesic may prove more potent than they would presumably have desired.

Quite apart from these dangers, extensive surveys have not produced convincing evidence of greater effectiveness or any other advantages of propoxyphene when compared with other analgesics.

The use of Distalgesic has therefore been discouraged and this proprietary compound is no longer prescribable in the National Health Service. However, *co-proxamol*, which has the same composition, is available.

Pentazocine

Pentazocine is a potent analgesic when given by injection. Weight for weight pentazocine is about a third as effective as morphine. The actions of pentazocine are qualitatively similar to morphine, but in doses which produce equal degrees of analgesia and respiratory depression it causes less sedation – indeed, unpleasant hallucinations and anxiety (the dysphoric syndrome) can be produced. This considerably lessens but does not abolish the risk of drug dependence.

This dysphoric effect is one of the features of pentazocine which makes it an unsatisfactory analgesic for the primary management of myocardial infarction (p. 216).

For long, pentazocine was not a controlled drug, but though it could be readily prescribed it is by no means a completely safe analgesic. It has most of the toxic effects of morphine and in particular also causes respiratory depression. The fact that it was not a controlled drug was mainly because it is less prone to dependence, but dependence is nevertheless a hazard and pentazocine has been widely abused.

Because pentazocine is a partial antagonist it is contraindicated in narcotic addicts in whom it may produce withdrawal syndromes.

Pentazocine was also used in dentistry to enhance the sedative effect of intravenous diazepam. In this application pentazocine had the sole advantage that it was not a controlled drug. Pentazocine is not significantly safer and is less sedating than other narcotics. In combination with diazepam, pentazocine can cause severe respiratory depression which has sometimes been fatal.

Phenazocine is a more potent analgesic and is about three times as active as morphine. It is otherwise similar to pentazocine. Drug dependence develops slowly, but the withdrawal syndrome is prolonged.

Nalbuphine

Nalbuphine is an opioid which is given by injection and, in adequate dosage, appears to be as effective as morphine for pain control but with fewer side-effects, and, it is thought, less potential for abuse. Like morphine, it may be given by intravenous injection for the primary management of myocardial infarction. Nalbuphine has the advantage that, although it causes respiratory depression, the latter does not progress beyond a certain level with increasing dosage ('ceiling effect'). Nalbuphine also appears to be less prone to cause nausea than morphine. It is therefore useful for perioperative analgesia.

Nalbupine may also be used to potentiate intravenous sedation with diazepam or midazolam where its limited potential for depression of respiration is an important advantage over pentazocine.

Other potent analgesics

A great variety of analgesics, some of which are not opiate in nature, is now available. Their main features are shown in Table 7.3.

Buprenorphine, for example, is an exceedingly potent analgesic, which is usually administered sublingually but can also be given by injection. One of its advantages is that it has little potential for dependence and is not, as yet, a controlled drug.

The main adverse effects are nausea, drowsiness and dizziness. Respiratory depression is rare but when it happens, is resistant to reversal by naloxone.

Despite their apparent advantages, none of these newer agents appear to have any applications in dentistry, apart perhaps, from the management of severe postoperative pain.

Uses of narcotic analgesics in dentistry

The narcotic analgesics are widely used in medicine for purposes such as those described. Their main application in dentistry is for severe postoperative pain unresponsive to the anti-inflammatory analgesics. The problem of addiction is negligible here, as this is a short course of treatment which is not likely to be repeated at frequent intervals. Pethidine is often chosen.

Morphine remains the drug of choice in the initial care of a patient who has had a myocardial infarct because of the valuable sedating as well as analgesic effect that morphine has. By contrast, pentazocine is unsatisfactory because of the dysphoria and sensations of increased anxiety that it may produce.

Analgesic potency

Analgesic potency is in some ways a misleading term. All that it means is that, weight for weight and given by the same route, drugs differ in their ability to reduce the sensation of pain. This difference is of little clinical importance. For example, if morphine is believed to possess five times the potency of pethidine, then 100 mg of pethidine can be given to achieve the same degree of analgesia as that produced by 20 mg of morphine. Of much greater practical importance is the acceptable

ceiling effect of analgesics. This refers to the greatest degree of analgesia which can be obtained with the highest dose which can be comfortably tolerated. Thus, although morphine is about 12 times more active than codeine, 240 mg of codeine cannot be used instead of 20 mg of morphine because approximately 80 to 120 mg of codeine produce unacceptable sedation, nausea, abdominal pain and vomiting in most patients.

The narcotic analgesics share many important qualities and particularly when given by injection are unrivalled for the relief of severe pain. Several of the narcotic analgesics, such as codeine, dextropropoxyphene and pentazocine when given by mouth may not be significantly more effective than the minor (anti-inflammatory) analgesics and in some situations are less so.

Pain is a subjective phenomenon and is difficult to measure in a precise manner for research purposes. Because of this it is impossible to be dogmatic about the potency of analgesic drugs. Some work, for instance, has claimed to demonstrate that even morphine does not influence pain threshold but merely reduces the emotional response to pain. In practice one must be directed by the patient's description of how much the drug has lessened his discomfort.

Narcotic antagonists

Respiratory depression is the cause of death after overdosage of morphine or its derivatives. Respiratory depression from this cause can often be treated effectively with naloxone.

Naloxone

Naloxone is a narcotic antagonist which differs from older agents such as levallorphan in having no agonist activity and is also effective against pentazocine overdose, which the other antagonists are not. Naloxone is now the antagonist of choice in most cases of narcotic overdose. It should be noted, however, that naloxone has little effect in cases of overdose with buprenorphine.

Naloxone, like other narcotic antagonists, has no beneficial effect on overdose of other depressants such as barbiturates or general anaesthetics and in

Table 7.3 Properties of other major analgesics

Approved name	Proprietary name	Analgesic potency	Dependence liability	Special features
Dextromoramide	Palfium	Equivalent to morphine	Similar to morphine	Duration of action 4h. Useful drug for severe pain
Codeine (methyl ester of morphine)	in Codis, Pharmidone, Pardale, Panadeine, Sonalgin, Solpadeine, Veganin	One-tenth analgesia of morphine (converted to morphine in brain; some morphine also present in plasma)	Rare	For mild pain and symptomatic treatment of cough and diarrhoea
Dihydrocodeine	DF 118	Equivalent to codeine	Rare	Mild to moderate pain only. Also cough suppression
Diphenoxylate	Combined with atropine in Lomotil		Possible but risk negligible with short-term use	Can cause euphoria. Use limited to treatment of diarrhoea
Dipipanone	Diconal (10 mg with cyclizine 30 mg)	25 mg equivalent to 10 mg morphine	Similar to morphine	Frequently abused powerful analgesic which can be given orally
Ethoheptazine	Combined with aspirin and meprobamate in Equagesic	Equivalent of codeine	None	For mild to moderate pain
Levorphanol	Dromoran	3–4 times that of morphine	Similar to morphine	Only clinically available member of the morphinan series. No advantages over morphine. Less nausea
Nalbuphine	Nubain		Less potential for abuse	Has some atropine-like activity
Pethidine	Pamergan	Half that of morphine	Similar to morphine	For moderate to severe pain. Well absorbed orally
Phenazocine	Prinadol Narphen	3–4 times that of morphine	Similar to morphine	
Other potent analgesics				
Pentazocine	Fortral	About half as effective as morphine	Low. Produces dysphoria	Opiate antagonist with strong agonist properties. Well absorbed from intestine or s.c. or i.m. injection. Can precipitate withdrawal syndrome in opiate addicts
Buprenorphine	Temgesic	15 times as effective as morphine	Appears to be low	Powerful and equal opiate antagonist and agonist properties. Overdose responds poorly to naloxone
Nefopam	Acupan	Somewhat less potent than morphine	Not yet demonstrated	No response to naloxone
Meptazinol	Meptid	Similar potency to pethidine	Not yet demonstrated	Less sedating and less respiratory depression than morphine. Given by injection

large doses will itself cause dangerous respiratory depression. Accurate diagnosis of the cause of respiratory depression is therefore essential before naloxone is given.

Naloxone precipitates withdrawal symptoms when given to an addict and is itself a drug of addiction.

Some of the newer narcotic analgesics such as pentazocine and buprenorphine are opiate antagonists but are also partial opiate agonists, i.e. they have both agonist and antagonist properties. Thus these drugs antagonise the action of morphine and can, for example, precipitate withdrawal symptoms in opiate addicts; nevertheless, they are potent analgesics.

As mentioned earlier, naloxone is relatively ineffective for buprenorphine poisoning.

DRUG DEPENDENCE

Drug dependence is the term used to describe a condition in which an individual who has repeatedly taken a drug finds himself compelled to go on taking it to maintain his physical and mental wellbeing. This means that the sudden withdrawal of the drug produces craving for it and may also cause dangerous physical changes. In everyday speech this condition is called addiction.

Although many individuals are dependent on or habituated to nicotine (in cigarettes) and caffeine (in tea and coffee), this does not lead to deterioration in their personal relationships and ability to work. On the other hand, dependence on drugs such as heroin, barbiturates and alcohol is almost invariably severely socially disruptive.

Alcohol

Alcohol is the most common cause of serious drug dependence in the UK. Its incidence may be 5% of the population.

There is no precise definition of alcoholism – certainly not every heavy drinker is an alcoholic. The term alcoholic means that an individual is dependent on alcohol and this implies that he has lost control of his drinking. The compulsion to become intoxicated leads to psychological and social disability (disruption of family life and of work) or physical illness.

The causes of alcoholism are not understood, but the availability of the drug, social and emotional deprivation, and possibly genetic traits are important predisposing factors.

The delightful taste of many alcoholic drinks also does little to discourage its habitual use or abuse.

The psychological causes of many forms of drug dependence are desire for pleasure and escape. Either of these desires can lead to powerful emotional dependence on a drug. Alcohol is mainly a depressant of brain function and is a powerful anxiolytic agent. It is particularly its ability to allow individuals to escape from anxiety and tension which makes alcohol liable to abuse.

In the early stages of alcohol dependence it is the wish to repeat the calming and tranquillising experience which provides the stimulus to continue drinking. Later the anxiolytic properties of alcohol become less, but attempts to stop the habit cause deep anxiety and distress. Drunkenness during the day or drinking before the day's work starts and the wish to drink alone are early signs of the process of social alienation.

Tolerance to the tranquillising actions of alcohol soon develops and leads to a progressive increase in the amount drunk. Severe bouts of drinking may terminate in coma.

Sudden cessation of drinking may precipitate tremor, anxiety and convulsions. Delirium tremens is one form of withdrawal state in which delirium, panic and hallucinations are prominent. These hallucinations are of a peculiar character; the stories of pink elephants and green rats are not inaccurate (although insects are seen more often than elephants), but do not emphasise adequately the element of terror that is always present. Sedative anxiolytic drugs such as diazepam are used to treat this reaction. Chlormethiazole is also effective.

Alcohol should be withdrawn gradually and tranquillisers are used during this process. In the attempt to prevent relapse, disulphiram (Antabuse) is sometimes given. If alcohol is taken whilst on the drug, flushing, headache, nausea and vomiting will result. This treatment is deliberately unpleasant but rarely effective. Metronidazole has a similar effect and has been used for the same purpose.

Toxic effects of alcohol abuse. The main toxic effects of alcohol abuse are as follows:

1. *Gastrointestinal*: gastritis, hepatitis, cirrhosis and pancreatitis.

2. *Cardiac*: arrhythmias and cardiomyopathy.

3. *Nervous system*: cerebral damage.

4. *Bone marrow*: depression of erythropoiesis.

Causes of death among alcoholics:

1. Accidents.

2. Suicide.

3. Overdose (respiratory depression or inhalation of vomit).

4. Bleeding (from oesophageal varices or haemorrhagic gastritis).

5. Liver failure.

6. Heart failure.

Alcohol also has teratogenic effects and pregnant women taking large quantities of alcohol can produce infants with a characteristic facies, varying degrees of mental defect and other abnormalities.

Narcotic analgesics

The narcotic analgesics vary in their addictive potential. Amongst the ones most likely to lead to dependence are diamorphine, morphine and pethidine. These drugs produce sedation in normal individuals but are euphoriant in dependent subjects. Withdrawal should be gradual – by replacement with less powerfully addictive narcotics such as methadone. The withdrawal reaction begins as craving for the drug several hours after the last dose. The most severe illness is about 48 hours later and may lead to coma and death. At the height of the illness there are severe abdominal pains, diarrhoea, vomiting, shivering and shock.

The many other complications of narcotic abuse or of the way in which injections are used are discussed on page 114.

Pentazocine, in spite of its tendency to produce dysphoria, has become increasingly widely abused, and in the US pentazocine in combination with an antihistamine (tripellenamine) is a popular street drug. The pentazocine and tripellenamine tablets are crushed and added to water for injection and this combination has been widely used as a cheaper and more easily obtainable substitute for heroin.

The benzodiazepines

Dependence on the benzodiazepines frequently results from taking these drugs for prolonged periods. In benzodiazepine-dependent patients, stopping the drug can cause anxiety or panic attacks, insomnia and gastrointestinal disturbances. Fits may be another effect: they start several days after drug withdrawal and can be continuous and severe or, occasionally, fatal.

The withdrawal state can persist for many weeks and be accompanied by muscular pains, photophobia, hyperacusis and hypersensitivity to touch. Depression is common.

The barbiturates

Addiction is common and can cause severe psychological and physical withdrawal illnesses. The features of the withdrawal state include anxiety, insomnia, twitching and convulsions. Status epilepticus can lead to death. Other hypnotics – including glutethimide, nitrazepam and methaqualone – can produce the same picture.

Cannabis

Cannabis is the generic name for a group of drugs which includes hashish and marihuana. For many years it was considered that cannabis produced no harmful effects other than intoxication. Recent evidence suggests that chromosomal damage, interference with sex hormone function, bronchial irritation, personality changes and irreversible brain damage may be caused by these substances. A striking change is loss of ambition and indifference to external events (apathy syndrome).

It must be emphasized that opiates and other depressants of the nervous system have been used and abused for many centuries. In the USA for example the term 'narcotic' has for long been used as a catchall term for all drugs of abuse. Nevertheless, drugs of abuse fall into two main groups, namely:

1. Opiates and other nervous system depressants.

2. Stimulants of the nervous system such as cocaine.

Although these two groups of drugs have opposing central effects they both produce pleasurable changes in mood, which is the reason for their being abused.

Cocaine

Sigmund Freud is credited with having created the first cocaine addict – he used it to wean a colleague off morphine.

Unlike the previously mentioned drugs, cocaine is a stimulant and euphoriant drug. It readily produces psychological dependence. A physical withdrawal state does not develop, yet the drug is notorious for its deleterious effects on the patient's personality.

Cocaine is absorbed by any route but is commonly inhaled and absorbed through the nasal mucosa to prolong its duration of action to 1–1.5 hours. However, cocaine is a potent vasoconstrictor and can eventually cause ischaemic necrosis of the nasal septum. It can also be smoked as it is heat stable.

Cocaine was at one time so expensive that it was fashionable as a drug of abuse for the wealthy. It is now exported on so vast a scale from South America that the price has fallen and its abuse has become widespread.

A particularly dangerous form of cocaine is when it is prepared as a free base, by heating in an alkaline solution such as sodium bicarbonate (baking soda). The cocaine crystals thus extracted, are known as 'crack' as they crackle when they are heated. Smoking free base cocaine allows respiratory absorption and provides central stimulation almost as rapidly as intravenous injection. In the USA, intravenous injection of a mixture of heroin and cocaine ('speedball') has become increasingly popular, probably because it is less sedating than heroin alone.

The toxic effects of cocaine, particularly after intravenous injection, are arrhythmias which can terminate in ventricular fibrillation or myocardial infarction. Alternatively, central stimulation may lead to fatal convulsions.

A peculiar effect of cocaine abuse is the sensation of insects running over the skin – a symptom termed formication (*please* note the spelling). As discussed earlier, cocaine is strongly sympathomimetic and this is illustrated by its effects on the addict who becomes what has been colourfully described as a 'sexed-up extrovert with dilated pupils'.

Note: A cause of acute fatal cocaine poisoning is what is termed, bizarrely but appropriately, the 'body packer' syndrome. This refers to the carriage of ingested packets of cocaine by smugglers. Rupture of such a packet in the gut releases a massive dose of cocaine. Among those few who have been detected, the mortality has been 56%. In view of the value of smuggled cocaine, one would have thought it worthwhile to invest a few pence in better quality plastic bags.

Amphetamine

Amphetamine is another stimulant drug with sympathomimetic activity and; in particular, a strong central euphoriant effect like that of cocaine. It is however taken by mouth and its effects then last several hours. Like cocaine it produces psychological but not physical dependence. Large doses may precipitate a schizophrenia-like psychosis with hallucinatory and paranoid features. This psychotic reaction may persist for many days after the last dose of the drug.

Anaesthetic agents

Many anaesthetic agents have been used as drugs of abuse – a practice which dates back to within a year or two of their introduction.

Naturally, dependence on these drugs is more common among medical or paramedical personnel who have easier access to them and is, therefore, an occupational hazard of anaesthetists and dentists.

Nitrous oxide in particular has a strong potential for abuse as it appears to have direct interactions with the endogenous opiate system. There is some evidence that it acts at the mu, kappa and sigma opioid receptors and that it may be a partial agonist.

In view of its low toxicity, nitrous oxide might seem to be an 'ideal' drug of dependence but for the effect of prolonged intake on vitamin B12 metabolism (see Ch. 8). As a result, the majority of patients (including dentists) dependent on nitrous oxide have developed neurological damage.

In practical terms, the chief factor that limits nitrous oxide abuse, is the inconvenience of having to hump around the heavy steel cylinders. Nevertheless, such is human determination that medical and dental students in the USA have been known to steal the large hospital cylinders of nitrous oxide for their own nefarious purposes.

Other abused substances

The term 'substance abuse' is now widely used because many other compounds, such as solvents in glue or other materials, are increasingly abused.

An additional problem is the home production of drugs such as amphetamine, but worse is the production of 'designer drugs'. These are compounds which are chemically related to opiates or other drugs of dependence and with similar potential for abuse, but since they are not officially 'drugs' are difficult to control.

The situation is however continually changing. This is partly a consequence of political events, whereby it becomes important for countries to produce opium or cocaine on an enormous scale for profit (often to buy weapons) with the result that such drugs flood the market and become so cheap as to displace alternatives.

Complications of drug abuse

The pharmacological actions of the drugs of dependence account for only a part of their effects on addicts. An equally important factor is the mode of life of many addicts, who may be unlikely to be careful and methodical in their habits. Even minimal cleanliness in relation to injections is often neglected. Overdosage is common. Irregular or inadequate meals and insanitary living conditions also contribute to morbidity.

The most common complications of injected drugs are hepatitis B, AIDS and other generalised infections such as infective endocarditis, local infections and venous thrombosis. Fungal septicaemia is a recognised but less common hazard. Malnutrition is frequent and may predispose to respiratory infections, particularly tuberculosis and pneumonia.

An additional problem may be caused by mixed drug taking, especially among heroin addicts who may take cocaine to counteract the hypnotic effect of the opiate. Overdosage of cocaine can cause sudden death by its effects on the heart and nervous system.

At the other extreme, many (so-called) heroin addicts can unknowingly be taking at least as much barbiturate (or other diluent) as of opiate, since the narcotic drugs are progressively diluted as they are passed along the chain of drug traders who each take their profits at every stage of the process. A parcel of heroin which has been cut in half (i.e. diluted by 50%) five times between producer and addict contains only about 3% of its original opiate content.

Since the total number of addicts and the precise nature of their drug intake is unknown, reports of morbidity and mortality are of little statistical significance. Many addicts are not recognised as such, until they die as a direct or indirect result of their habits. Those cases which are liable to reach the headlines are adolescents who die within a matter of months. A few addicts can, however, lead relatively normal lives with little or no apparent impairment of health. Overall, however, it is clear that the life expectation of addicts is very much shorter than that of the remainder of the population.

The management of the physical aspects of dependence on drugs is relatively straightforward in expert hands. The main difficulty is prevention of relapse and the treatment of the underlying social and psychological problems of the patient. Even the most energetic, persistent and enthusiastic psychotherapy may not be successful.

Although the availability of the drug and intolerable personal and social stresses from which the individual wants to escape are factors which contribute to drug dependence, people vary in their susceptibility to dependence on drugs. There appears, nevertheless, to be no specific personality type identifiable as a potential addict and it is safer not to succumb to the temptation to resort to drugs for entertainment or escape. Insight into the actions of drugs does not protect against dependence. The addiction rate in dentists, doctors and nurses, who have relatively easy access to drugs of addiction, is higher than that of the rest of the population.

The hazards of drug abuse to the addict can be summarised as follows:

1. Infections (hepatitis, infective endocarditis, tetanus, septicaemia, AIDS).
2. Overdose.
3. Malnutrition and its consequences.

The hazards to the community are considerably more important than the risks to the addicts. They include the following:

1. Thefts (to obtain money for drugs.)
2. Crimes of violence, either to further theft or as a result of the effects of drugs (especially alcohol and the hallucinogens).
3. Road traffic accidents.

SUGGESTED FURTHER READING

Amin M M, Laskin D M 1983 Prophylactic use of indomethacin for prevention of postsurgical complications after removal of impacted third molars. Oral Surgery 55: 448

Anderson W H, Kuehnle J C 1981 Diagnosis and early management of acute psychosis. New England Journal of Medicine 305: 1128

Anon (LA) 1987 Dying for a drink? Lancet ii: 1249

Anon (LA) 1987 The chemoreceptor trigger zone revisited. Lancet i: 144

Anon (LA) 1987 Screening for drugs of abuse. Lancet i: 365

Blau J N 1982 A plain man's guide to the management of migraine. British Medical Journal 284: 1095

Bullingham R E S 1981 Synthetic opiate analgesics. British Journal of Hospital Medicine 25: 59

Cesselin F 1986 Endomorphins and nociception (review). Revue Neurologique (Paris) 142: 649

Coles L S Fries J F, Kraines R G, Roth S H 1983 Side effects of nonsteroidal anti-inflammatory drugs. American Journal of Medicine 74: 820

Council on scientific affairs 1981 Marijuana: its health hazards and therapeutic potentials. Journal of the Amercian Medical Association 246: 1823

Cregler L L, Mark H 1986 Medical complications of cocaine abuse. New England Journal of Medicine 315: 1495

Crossley H A, Wynn R L, Bergman S A 1983 Nonsteroidal anti-inflammatory agents in relieving dental pain: a review. Journal of Amercian Dental Association 106: 61

Day R O 1988 Mode of action of non-steroidal anti-inflammatory drugs. Medical Journal of Australia 148: 195

Dingfelder J R 1982 Prostaglandin inhibitors. New England Journal Medicine 307: 746

Editorial 1981 Aspirin or paracetamol? Lancet ii: 287

Editorial 1981 Prostacyclin in therapeutics. Lancet i: 643

Editorial 1982 Classification of headache. Lancet ii: 1318

Editorial 1982 Endogenous opiates and their actions. Lancet iii: 305

Editorial 1982 Solvent abuse. Lancet ii: 1139

Editorial 1982 Treatment of migraine. Lancet i: 1338

Editorial 1983 Meptazinol Lancet ii 384

Gawin F H, Ellinwood E H 1988 Cocaine and other stimulants. New England Journal of Medicine 318: 1173

Ghodse A H 1983 Treatment of drug addiction in London. Lancet i: 636

Ghodse A H, Edwards G, Stapleton J et al. 1981 Drug-related problems in London accident and emergency departments. Lancet ii: 859

Gilbert D G, Hagen R L, D'Agostino J A 1986 The effects of cigarette smoking on human sexual potency. Addictive Behaviours ii: 431

Gillman M A 1986 Nitrous oxide, an opioid addictive agent. American Journal of Medicine 81: 97

Gravenstein J S, Kory W P, Marks R G 1983 Drug abuse by anesthesia personnel. Anesthesia and Analgesia 62: 467

Greenbaum R A, Kaye G, Mason P D. 1987 Experience with nalbuphine, a new opioid analgesic, in acute myocardial infarction. Journal of the Royal Society of Medicine 80: 418

Hall S M 1986 Reye's syndrome and aspirin: a review. Journal of the Royal Society of Medicine 79: 596

Hill R G 1981 Endogenous opioids and pain: a review. Journal of the Royal Society of Medicine 74: 448

Hull C J 1988, Control of pain in the perioperative period. British Medical Bulletin 4: 341

Johnson R P, Connelly J C 1981 Addicted physicians. Journal of the American Medical Association 245: 253

Langman M J S, Coggon D, Spiegelhalter D 1983 Analgesic intake and the risk of acute upper gastrointestinal bleeding. American Journal of Medicine 74: 79

Lorenzen I B 1983 Treatment of severe rheumatoid arthritis. Annals of Chemical Research 15: 80

Manschreck T C 1981 Schizophrenic disorders. New England Journal of Medicine 305: 1628

McCarron M. M., Wood J. D. 1983 The cocaine 'body packer' syndrome. Journal of the American Medical Association 250: 1417

Neuberger J, Davis M, Williams R 1980 Long-term ingestion of paracetamol and liver disease. Journal of the Royal Society of Medicine 73: 701

Peatfield R 1983 Migraine: current concepts of pathogenesis and treatment. Drugs 26: 364

Persson J, Magnusson P-H 1987 Prevalence of problem drinkers among patients attending somatic outpatient clinics: a study of alcohol related medical care. British Medical Journal 295: 467

Prescott L F 1982 Analgesic nephropathy. Drugs 23: 75

Rees W D W, Turnberg L A 1980 Reappraisal of the effects of aspirin on the stomach. Lancet ii: 410

Relman A S 1982 Marijuana and health. New England Journal of Medicine 306: 603

Seymour R A, Blair G S, Wyatt F A R 1983 Post-operative dental pain and analgesic efficacy – part II. British Journal of Oral Surgery 21: 298

Simpson G M, Pi E H, Sramek Jr J J 1981 Adverse effects of antipsychotic agents. Drugs 21: 138

Spector R G, Rogers H J, Roy D 1984 Psychiatry. Common drug treatments. Martin Dunitz, London

Thompson T L, Moran M G, Nies A S 1983 Psychotropic drug use in the elderly (II). New England Journal of Medicine 308: 194

Wall R, Linford S M J, Akthter M I 1980 Addiction to Distalgesic (dextropropoxyphene). British Medical Journal 280: 1213

Wetli C V, Wright R K 1979 Death caused by recreational cocaine use. Journal of the American Medical Association 241: 2519

Woods J H, Katz J L, Winger G 1988 Abuse liability of benzodiazepines (1214 refs). Pharmacological Reviews 39: 254

Young R J, Lawson A A H 1980 Distalgesic poisoning – cause for concern. British Medical Journal 280: 1045

8. General anaesthesia and sedation

The introduction of general anaesthesia has been one of the greatest advances in medicine in that it has made possible the enormous range of complex surgical operations that are now taken for granted.

Although Humphrey Davy noticed the analgesic effects of nitrous oxide in 1800 and even suggested its use for surgical anaesthesia, it was not put to any such practical use until nearly half a century later. This was mainly due to two American dentists, Horace Wells who showed the effects of nitrous oxide in 1844, and William Morton who introduced ether in 1846.

Dentists have undoubtedly therefore made one major contribution to reducing suffering and to the physical welfare of the world.

The anaesthetic state

General anaesthesia is a state of unconsciousness from which the patient cannot be aroused by external stimuli. The depth of anaesthesia must be such as to abolish pain but still be controllable and reversible by the anaesthetist.

All nervous system depressants, in overdose, produce unconsciousness, but this is not controllable and may not be readily reversible. Anaesthetic agents, by contrast, induce unconsciousness rapidly and, ideally, without depression of respiratory or cardiovascular function. Most surgical operations also require abolition of reflex movements and often, complete muscular relaxation. These can all be achieved by use of a potent anaesthetic agent in sufficiently high dosage as to cause deep anaesthesia but at the cost of increased risks, a prolonged recovery period and, usually, unpleasant after-effects.

The appreciation that the many requirements of the surgeon could be met by use of different drugs each having a specific effect, for example muscle relaxation, has led, when necessary, to the use of a combination of drugs – a technique termed 'balanced anaesthesia'.

Mechanism of action of anaesthetic agents

In spite of the great advances in the techniques of anaesthesia, the mode of action of anaesthetic agents is by no means fully understood and there is no known single property possessed by all agents.

Lipid-solubility hypothesis

Many anaesthetic agents (but not all) are lipid soluble. There is some correlation between fat solubility and potency, but there are many exceptions. One such exception is chloral hydrate which is hypnotic but poorly lipid soluble. However, in the body chloral is converted into a highly lipid-soluble metabolite (trichloroethanol). Other exceptions therefore may perhaps be more apparent than real.

The lipid solubility of an anaesthetic suggests that the mechanism of action is by way of an effect on cell membranes within the brain.

In spite of the limitations of this hypothesis in explaining a highly complex process, part at least can be substantiated and it appears that:

a. chemically inert agents which are to some degree lipid soluble have an anaesthetic effect, and

b. the potency of anaesthetic action is related to the degree of affinity for lipid in the presence of body fluid.

The concentration ratio (partition coefficient) in favour of a lipid such as olive oil compared with water has, however, been shown to have poorer correlation with anaesthetic potency than the partition coefficient between octanol and water. Newer evidence also suggests that the action of anaesthetics is by binding to specific proteins or to synapses rather than to lipids in the nervous system.

In addition, there is circumstantial evidence to suggest that the analgesic effect of general anaesthetics such as nitrous oxide may be mediated by inducing enkephalin release.

Essential properties of general anaesthetic agents

The three main objectives of general anaesthesia are:

1. Abolition of consciousness.
2. Analgesia.
3. Muscular relaxation.

These can all be achieved by an anaesthetic agent in high dosage but is more safely done, as mentioned earlier, by using a combination of drugs each having a specific effect. No single general anaesthetic agent has all the properties required to meet the diverse needs of modern surgery.

Desirable properties of an anaesthetic agent are that it should:

1. Produce a controllable and rapidly reversible level of unconsciousness.
2. Have a wide margin of dosage between that inducing unconsciousness and that causing medullary paralysis.
3. Give a rapid, smooth and pleasant induction.
4. Have no adverse effects on the cardiovascular system causing either significant disturbances of cardiac rhythm or depression of blood pressure.
5. Have no toxic effects on other organs such as the liver.
6. Have no irritant effect on the respiratory tract (if an inhalational agent).
7. Cause no local irritant effect at the site of injection (if an intravenous agent).
8. Be non-inflammable. (Inflammable agents with oxygen produce a powerful explosive mixture that can be ignited even by an invisible spark of static electricity.)
9. Have no undesirable interactions with other drugs likely to be given before or during anaesthesia.

10. Be quickly metabolised and/or excreted.
11. Allow pleasant and (preferably) rapid recovery.

Analgesic properties of general anaesthetic agents

Since the patient is deeply unconscious during anaesthesia, there would seem to be little value in the agents having an analgesic action. Analgesic properties in general anaesthetic agents are, however, valuable in that they allow surgery to be carried out at a very light level of anaesthesia, provided that muscular relaxation is not required. If needed, the latter can be produced by muscle relaxants.

In dentistry particularly, anaesthesia should always be light in the interests of safety. Nitrous oxide is therefore valuable as it is a potent analgesic, although it may have to be supplemented with halothane. Methohexitone, by contrast, is not analgesic and may be anti-analgesic. As a result, during light anaesthesia the patient is restless when painful stimuli are applied and there may be a temptation to deepen the level of anaesthesia.

General considerations

The management of a general anaesthetic is, to a large degree, acute applied pharmacology. The pharmacological effects are exceptionally rapid and the patients' reactions almost immediate, as are the many complications that can arise. Generally speaking too, the level of dosage needed to produce deep unconsciousness is close to that which depresses the respiratory or cardiovascular centres.

General anaesthetic agents vary widely in their toxicity but anaesthesia is a craft where the skill of the anaesthetist is generally more important than the nature of the drugs used. Naturally, however, the expert anaesthetist chooses agents whose potentialities he knows and is also prepared for and skilled in the management of emergencies.

Special risks are associated with anaesthesia irrespective of the agents used, particularly because of the loss of reflexes which normally protect the airway. Acute respiratory obstruction is a special danger. This is an even greater hazard in dentistry than in other types of surgery because the operating site is at the upper end of the respiratory tract and because material can only too easily fall into the unprotected airway. In other cases respiratory exchange may be inadequate and cause gradual (often barely perceptible) but none the less dangerous hypoxia.

The techniques of general anaesthesia can only be learnt by adequate practical instruction and experience. Some of the precautions that must be taken whenever an anaesthetic is given are nevertheless so important that they must be regarded as an essential part of the procedure however brief the anaesthetic or however trifling the operation.

Precautions

1. Before administration of the anaesthetic. A general anaesthetic should only be given when:
   a. The patient is fit enough to withstand it and has no history of adverse reactions to anaesthesia.
   b. There are no serious problems relating to any drugs the patient is taking (*see later*).
   c. The patient has had nothing to eat or drink for 4 hours previously.
   d. The patient or a parent is able to give informed consent, which should be obtained in writing.

In the case of outpatient anaesthesia, it is a good idea to make sure that the patient's bladder has been emptied.

Another person should also be available to accompany the patient home afterwards.

2. Factors affecting the administration of the anaesthetic:
   a. An anaesthetist and a nurse should be present.
   b. The anaesthetic equipment must be in full working order.
   c. Plenty of oxygen must be available (both in the anaesthetic apparatus and in reserve) together with means for positive pressure inflation of the lungs.
   d. Effective throat packs must be used to protect the airway.
   e. Efficient suction apparatus must be handy to keep the airway clear.
   f. Resuscitative equipment including facilities for endotracheal intubation or tracheostomy and appropriate drugs must be ready.

3. After the operation the patient must be:
   a. Put in a position where blood or saliva do not drain back into the pharynx.
   b. Kept under supervision until conscious.
   c. Allowed home when conscious provided that it is reasonably certain that the accompanying adult can be responsible for the patient.
   d. Forbidden to drive a car or operate unguarded machinery until the following day at the earliest.

Fitness for anaesthesia

Fitness for anaesthesia is a relative term. Complex surgical procedures may have to be undertaken on desperately ill patients kept alive by multiple drug therapy. Anaesthesia in such patients, however, is feasible only in the hands of skilled anaesthetists with all the facilities of a modern hospital at their disposal and in situations where the risks of anaesthesia have deliberately to be balanced against the chances of the patient's survival without surgery. General anaesthesia for dentistry in general practice represents the complete antithesis of this situation, that is, no risk to the patient's life or health is acceptable.

The following should be regarded as relative or absolute contraindications to general anaesthesia for dental outpatients where limited facilities are available:

1. Cardiovascular disease especially severe hypertension and ischaemic heart disease.
2. Respiratory disease especially asthma and chronic bronchitis with emphysema.
3. Gastrointestinal disease where there is an increased risk of vomiting.
4. Anaemia, including sickle cell disease or trait.
5. Haemophilia or other comparably severe haemorrhagic disease.
6. Liver disease (especially if barbiturates or halothane are to be used).
7. Corticosteroid, antidepressant and antihypertensive therapy. These and other drugs which may complicate general anaesthesia are discussed later.

Drugs used in anaesthesia

In addition to the anaesthetic agents themselves it is usual in hospital practice, to give drugs before the operation (premedication) and sometimes also afterwards, to assist recovery or to make it more pleasant.

Premedication

Premedication is given before anything more than a minor operation. Premedication is not usually given in dental practice partly because it is rarely necessary and partly because it tends to delay recovery.

The purposes of premedication are:

1. To allay anxiety.
2. To make induction more pleasant.
3. To minimise oral and bronchial secretions.
4. To reduce the amount of anaesthetic agent needed.
5. To protect against some of the possible adverse effects of the anaesthetic agents.

Sedation. Sedation helps to protect the patient against anxiety about the anaesthetic or the operation. Since anxiety increases production of adrenaline or noradrenaline, sedation may also protect the patient against their cardiovascular effects. This is particularly important with agents such as halothane which sensitise the heart to catecholamines.

Sedation, particularly with morphine or its derivatives, potentiates the anaesthetic. This may be useful when a weak agent such as nitrous oxide is used. On the other hand, sedatives increase the hazards of potent agents especially the intravenous barbiturates.

For general surgery, morphine (or its derivatives) is often used. These are sedative and analgesic, and are valuable if the patient is already in pain. Analgesic drugs also diminish reflex movements during light anaesthesia and reduce postoperative restlessness due to pain. The disadvantages of opiates is that they are respiratory and (to a lesser extent) cardiac depressants. They also increase the likelihood of postoperative nausea and vomiting.

For anxiety alone, a benzodiazepine is useful. Diazepam, 5 or 10 mg, can be given orally on the night before the operation and repeated an hour before operation. This is often satisfactory for dental operations and many other surgical procedures.

An antihistamine such as promethazine (which is also a phenothiazine) is another alternative popular for children since it has a strong and prolonged sedative effect, but tends to cause postoperative restlessness.

Inhibition of secretions. Atropine is given to reduce salivary, pharyngeal, bronchial and gastric secretions. This reduces aspiration of saliva, mucus and gastric contents and lessens the chance of postoperative pulmonary collapse and aspiration pneumonia. Hyoscine has the same peripheral actions as atropine, but in addition is sedative and depresses the vomiting centre.

Anticholinergic drugs, such as atropine and hyoscine, may also reduce the chance of sudden death during induction of anaesthesia, particularly, in the past, with chloroform, which can cause excessive vagal slowing of the heart.

When halothane is used (as it often is) a β blocker may be given for cardiac arrhythmias if conditions precipitate them.

Generally a sedative analgesic and anticholinergic drug are given together. A common combination is hyoscine and pethidine, but a benzodiazepine is probably, overall, the most satisfactory choice; many anaesthetists use no other premedication, unless the patient is in pain.

Inhibition of bronchial secretions is less necessary now that irritant agents such as ether are no longer used. Excessive drying can also cause postoperative discomfort. There is no consensus about the most useful premedicant regimen at the moment.

Stages of anaesthesia

Anaesthesia is divided into four stages which, during the slow induction with open ether, could easily be identified. Nowadays, particularly when powerful intravenous agents are used, the stages often merge so smoothly and quickly as to be barely identifiable.

Stage 1: Analgesia. Analgesia is not complete (although it varies with the drug used) in the first stage. Consciousness is progressively lost, but at first hearing is enhanced to the extent that the quiet routine of the operating theatre may sound to the patient like a mounting roar of violent activity.

Some anaesthetic agents such as the barbiturates have no analgesic action.

Stage 2: Excitement. The patient is unconscious, reflexes are intact and there may be automatic movements. In extreme cases the patient shouts, struggles violently and has to be restrained to prevent injuries. These unpleasant effects can be avoided by quick, skilful induction or by use of a powerful intravenous agent such as thiopentone.

This stage is sometimes the most dangerous in that very occasionally the patient may suddenly die. The cause of such deaths is not always clear but there may be vagal overactivity slowing the heart excessively, or alternatively, release of endogenous adrenaline may precipitate ventricular fibrillation, especially when the heart is sensitised to catecholamines by the anaesthetic agent. The danger of vagal inhibition of the heart may be reduced by premedication with atropine.

Stage 3: Surgical anaesthesia. This is usually divided arbitrarily into four planes of increasing depth. Reflex activity and muscle tone are progressively lost until in the fourth stage there is complete muscular relaxation. The depth of anaesthesia can be recognised by testing reflex responses at various sites and by movements of the eyeballs, the state of the pupils and the rate, depth and rhythm of respiration.

Stage 4: Medullary paralysis. This is the stage which must *not* be reached. It is the result of overdose or may be a complication of hypoxia or both. Immediate resuscitative measures must be started.

ANAESTHETIC AGENTS

Anaesthetic agents fall into the following categories:

I. Inhalational agents
  1. Gases
    Nitrous oxide
    Cyclopropane
  2. Volatile liquids
    Ether
    Halogenated hydrocarbons and ethers
    Chloroform
    Trichloroethylene
    Halothane
    Enflurane
    Isoflurane
II. Intravenous agents
  1. Barbiturates
    Thiopentone
    Methohexitone
  2. Non-barbiturate
    Ketamine
    Etomidate
    Propofol

The anaesthetic gases are a heterogeneous collection of agents varying widely in their chemical structure, actions and potency. Several have passed out of use but nitrous oxide remains outstandingly important as a very safe – though weak – agent with a strong analgesic action.

The ethers have the common properties of being generally safe, giving a reasonable degree of muscular relaxation and, when properly used, have minimal adverse effects on the heart and liver. In spite of being intensely irritant, inflammable and difficult to administer, ether itself remained the standard anaesthetic agent for more than a century. It has been supplanted by halothane, enflurane or isoflurane and is virtually obsolete.

The halogenated hydrocarbons have the common properties of being (a) potent, (b) non-irritant, (c) non-inflammable and (d) easy to administer. They have however adverse effects on the heart (causing disturbances of rhythm in particular) and on the liver. Chloroform is the most dangerous member of this group and is obsolete. Halothane is one of the safest. It has for long been the standard inhalational anaesthetic agent for general and dental surgery but enflurane and isoflurane are increasingly being used.

The intravenous agents such as the barbiturates have the common properties of being pleasant for the patient but are somewhat dangerous in unskilled hands because they are (a) highly potent and (b) strong depressants of respiration.

An overdose is only too easy to give but difficult to manage.

The non-barbiturate intravenous agents are heterogeneous and vary widely in their chemical nature and effects.

INHALATIONAL AGENTS

The most widely used anaesthetic mixture is halothane, enflurane or isoflurane with nitrous oxide and oxygen.

Nitrous oxide

Nitrous oxide is a colourless, non-irritant gas with a faint odour. It is neither inflammable nor explosive but will support combustion.

Nitrous oxide was the first anaesthetic agent to be introduced and has remained in use for nearly 150 years. It is one of the safest agents available, but this is partly because it is so weak an anaesthetic that in the highest acceptable concentrations (80% with 20% oxygen) it is unable to depress the medulla. It also has no adverse effects on the heart, respiratory tract, liver or kidneys.

In addition to its weak anaesthetic properties, nitrous oxide is a potent analgesic and anxiolytic even in subanaesthetic doses.

Induction with nitrous oxide is rapid and pleasant. Recovery is also rapid as the gas is excreted unchanged from the lungs.

Adverse effects

1. Hypoxia. This is not an effect of nitrous oxide itself but merely a consequence of the temptation to deepen anaesthesia by decreasing the oxygen concentration below 20%. In the past it was common in 'dental gas' sessions to induce many patients with 100% nitrous oxide for a short period, with cyanosis as an inevitable consequence. Even so, adequate anaesthesia was not always achieved. However undesirable such manoeuvres may be, some millions of 'dental gases' have been given in this way without fatalities.

The low anaesthetic potency is overcome by giving an adjuvant such as halothane.

2. Vomiting. Nitrous oxide occasionally causes nausea or vomiting if it is given too rapidly in high concentration. The mechanisms are unknown but it may be a central effect like that of the opiates, with which nitrous oxide has many properties in common.

3. Depression of vitamin B12 metabolism. Nitrous oxide inactivates vitamin B12 in the form of methyl cobalamin and can therefore, on prolonged exposure, cause depletion of methionine and have similar effects to pernicious anaemia, namely megaloblastic anaemia, leukopenia and neurological damage.

This effect is not normally significant in fit patients, as megaloblastic marrow changes are not detectable until after 5–6 hours' exposure to 50% nitrous oxide. Moreover in some of the earlier reports of this effect, patients had been exposed to nitrous oxide continuously for many days or intermittently, in some cases, for months – itself a remarkable tribute to the safety of this drug in other respects.

This toxic effect of nitrous oxide is a cause for concern for surgical and dental staff (especially women who are or likely to be pregnant) exposed to traces of nitrous oxide in the atmosphere. Although there is little firm evidence of significant adverse effects, effective scavenging is desirable.

The dyshaemopoietic effect of nitrous oxide can be prevented, when necessary, or reversed by giving folinic acid.

Paradoxically, in long-term abusers of nitrous oxide, neurological complications are the main effect but megaloblastic anaemia is rare. Some compensatory mechanism seems therefore able to develop and overcome the effect of nitrous oxide on the bone marrow.

Entonox is pre-mixed, 50 : 50 nitrous oxide and oxygen. It is used as an analgesic and sedative for such purposes as the immediate management of myocardial infarction or obstetric analgesia. Cylinders of Entonox are standard equipment in many ambulances and it is given by ambulance personnel for patients in transit to intensive care units.

Entonox has also been used for dental sedation.

The analgesic power of nitrous oxide is difficult to estimate. At concentrations between 50% and 80% it seems to be comparable to morphine, and has at least as great a sedative effect. It has the great advantage that it causes no respiratory depression and its effects can be instantly reversed when necessary.

Cyclopropane

Cyclopropane is an inflammable and explosive gas. It is only slightly irritant to the bronchial mucosa.

Induction is rapid due to its high potency. The cardiac rate is usually normal but if high concentrations of the gas are used or if there is CO_2 accumulation, then ventricular arrhythmias can develop. Blood pressure is unaltered and there is no hepatotoxicity. Recovery is rapid but nausea and vomiting are common.

The mortality associated with the use of cyclopropane, even when all other factors have been taken into account, is higher than with any other agent. Its highly explosive nature has also limited its use.

Ether (diethyl ether)

Ether is a volatile liquid with a pungent vapour that is inflammable and forms a highly explosive mixture with oxygen. Ether is so intensely irritating to the bronchial mucosa that even in skilled hands induction is slow and unpleasant. Nevertheless, nitrous oxide, oxygen and ether was a standard anaesthetic mixture used for countless surgical operations with an excellent record of safety since its introduction in 1846, for about a century.

Ether is important as a 'classical' anaesthetic agent and the defined stages of anaesthesia describe the sequence seen when open ether is used but are not easily seen with modern anaesthetic techniques.

The irritant nature of ether allows only low concentrations to be used at first and the slow induction may be followed by a long excitement stage. Muscular relaxation is produced in deep anaesthesia so that ether was satisfactory for abdominal surgery.

Ether does not cause cardiac arrhythmias or increased myocardial excitability and the depth of anaesthesia can be reliably gauged by the levels of reflex activity, eye signs (movement or position of the eyeballs and degree of dilatation of the pupils), and depth and rhythm of respiration. Overdose, with toxic effects (medullary paralysis), is therefore readily avoidable with normal skill and care.

Recovery is slow and unpleasant; postoperative vomiting and lung complications are common.

The unpleasant induction period was mitigated by premedication with morphine and hyoscine, or overcome by use of an intravenous agent (thiopentone) for induction. Ether (with nitrous oxide and oxygen) was then used to maintain more prolonged anaesthesia. This was common practice.

Ether has been little used for dental anaesthesia because of its unpleasantness and the difficulties of administration.

Chloroform

Chloroform was the forerunner of modern inhalational agents which reproduce its desirable properties but with greatly reduced toxic effects.

Chloroform is a sweet-smelling, volatile liquid which induces anaesthesia quickly and relatively pleasantly. There is good analgesia in subanaesthetic doses and it is not inflammable.

Not surprisingly, chloroform was thought, in comparison with ether, to be the ideal anaesthetic agent and its use was greatly encouraged by Queen Victoria's acceptance of it during labour. In fact, chloroform is considerably more toxic and dangerous than ether.

Chloroform causes cardiovascular and respiratory depression even in relatively low concentrations but, even worse, was prone to cause sudden cardiac malfunction, such as ventricular fibrillation or arrest, during induction. The introduction of atropine in premedication was partly with the aim of reducing vagal inhibition, which was responsible for some of these cardiac complications.

Chloroform is also a potent cause of postoperative liver damage.

In spite of these dangers, the ease and convenience of administration of chloroform with minimal equipment were such that it continued to be used for domiciliary midwifery until comparatively recently. However, it should now be regarded as obsolete.

Halothane

Halothane has been the standard inhalational anaesthetic agent for several decades and is widely used in dentistry.

Halothane is non-inflammable and non-explosive. It is given with nitrous oxide and oxygen, at a concentration of 2–3% for induction, then continued at 0.5–2%. For this purpose a calibrated vaporiser has to be used to ensure accurate regulation of the concentration.

Induction is smooth and more pleasant than with newer agents. There is minimal excitement and surgical anaesthesia can be induced in 2 to 3 minutes. Muscle relaxation is usually good but muscle relaxants can be given if necessary.

Overdose causes depression of the respiratory centre, but depression of the vasomotor centre follows less quickly than with chloroform. There is therefore time to start resuscitative measures. Recovery is usually rapid but depends on the total dose given. Nausea and vomiting are rare but there may be shivering during recovery.

Adverse effects

Overall, halothane has a remarkable record of safety but (like chloroform) it can cause liver damage and sensitises the heart to catecholamines to cause dysrhythmias.

*1. **Hepatotoxic reactions to halothane.*** Liver damage can follow administration of halothane. Reactions range from abnormalities of liver function detectable only by laboratory tests, to fatal massive hepatic necrosis. The latter is so uncommon however, that surveys on an immense scale have had to be carried out to confirm whether there was a cause-and-effect relationship or whether the reaction was merely coincidental and due, for example, to viral hepatitis. It is remarkable, in fact, that generally accepted figures for the incidence of hepatic reactions to halothane are considerably lower than the incidence of unexpected abnormalities of liver function found in patients before undergoing surgery.

It is now clear that a minority of patients can have hepatotoxic reactions to halothane, particularly after repeated exposure. However, after years of intensive study, the mechanism of the hepatotoxic effects remains unclear and controversial. One of the difficulties is that it does not appear possible to reproduce this reaction in animals in the same form as it affects humans and many of the animal findings are at variance with the clinical findings in humans.

In rats in particular, a change from oxidative to reductive metabolism as a result of hypoxia or depression of the circulation appears to make halothane hepatotoxic. Unlike humans however, halothane hepatoxicity tends to be dose related, but repeated exposure is not otherwise particularly dangerous. In other animals, halothane hepatoxicity does not appear to result from metabolic products.

Overall, because repeated exposure presents the greatest risk and because only a minority of individuals appear to be susceptible, it appears most probable that halothane-induced liver damage is immunologically mediated. This may in turn, result from metabolic production of an antigen or hapten, but if so neither it nor any immunological mechanism have been identified with certainty.

In summary:

1. Halothane can rarely cause fulminant and occasionally fatal hepatitis.

2. This risk is greater with halothane than with enflurane or isoflurane.

3. Only certain individuals appear to be at risk from halothane hepatitis, but can only be identified after the event.

4. On general grounds, and because of the findings in animals, it appears to be particularly important to avoid hypoxia or anything that might cause depression of the circulation when halothane is given.

5. Most important, halothane should not be given again to anyone who has had a reaction to it.

6. Even in patients who have had no reaction to halothane, this agent should not be given again within an interval of less than 6 months.

Although there is no doubt about the potential hepatotoxicity of halothane, it has been used and investigated on so vast a scale over the years that no other anaesthetic agent is known with certainty (with the precautions indicated above) to be safer.

*2. **Dysrhythmias.*** Like most anaesthetics, halothane causes dose-related depression of the blood pressure. In addition, halothane sensitises the heart to catecholamines such as adrenaline. The latter (given in oral surgery to produce a bloodless field) and hypoxia or excessive accumulation of CO_2 increase the tendency to dysrhythmias. Beta blockers are effective but rarely used, as a brief period of controlled ventilation is usually sufficient to stop them.

Overall, halothane remains a useful and generally safe general anaesthetic agent as indicated by the fact that it remains in use decades after its introduction and has not been rendered obsolete by newer agents.

Enflurane

Enflurane is a halogenated ether which gives a relatively pleasant induction (although less pleasant than halothane) and has a very rapid onset of action.

Only about 2.5% of enflurane is metabolised and systemic effects seem to be minimal. Cardiac rhythm is more stable than with halothane and there is less sensitivity to injected adrenaline. There is no firm evidence that enflurane can cause hepatitis, but occasional cases of hepatitis following administration of enflurane have been reported.

The chief disadvantages of enflurane are that it depresses respiration more than halothane and also has epileptogenic potential.

Enflurane has been used satisfactorily for brief dental operations. Its advantages in this application are the low risk of arrhythmias, the rapid induction, which is complete in about a minute and a half, and the more rapid recovery than with halothane.

Isoflurane

Isoflurane is an isomer of enflurane and has similar properties in terms of rapidity of induction. Its advantages are that (a) it causes less respiratory depression than enflurane (but nevertheless more than halothane), (b) adverse cardiac effects are minimal and it is a coronary vasodilator, (c) it is not epileptogenic and (d) it does not appear to have any potential for liver damage.

The disadvantages of isoflurane are that it is pungent and causes undesirable degrees of salivation, coughing and laryngospasm. Induction is therefore considerably less pleasant than with halothane and recovery is slower. Many therefore feel that isoflurane does not have any significant advantages over halothane, especially for dental anaesthesia for children, to compensate for its much greater cost. However, isoflurane is valuable as an anaesthetic agent for anyone who has had a hepatic reaction to halothane.

Trichloroethylene (Trilene)

Trilene is a relatively weak anaesthetic but a potent analgesic. It is non-irritant and induction is rela-

tively rapid and pleasant. It causes little cardiovascular disturbance although it is probably inadvisable to give adrenaline. There is no significant muscle relaxation and Trilene is most suitable for use as a supplement to nitrous oxide and oxygen to abolish pain during dental treatment or minor surgical procedures. Trilene was widely used in this way before the introduction of halothane and is still available. However, slow recovery and a tendency to postoperative vomiting are probable reasons why it is less used now and regarded by many as obsolete.

Closed circuit anaesthesia is contraindicated as breakdown products of Trilene when drawn over sodalime (for rebreathing) have a specific toxic action on the trigeminal nerve.

INTRAVENOUS ANAESTHETICS: BARBITURATES

Many patients fear anaesthetics given via a mask over the face and in the past, inhalational agents, particularly ether, were irritant and nauseating. As a consequence, intravenous barbiturates and in particular thiopentone are almost universally used in general surgical practice to give rapid and pleasant induction of anaesthesia which can then be continued with the more readily controllable inhalational agents.

Short operations can be carried out with these agents alone and methohexitone was widely used and became notorious in dental practice where it was popular with patients who disliked inhalational anaesthesia. However, these agents have caused several deaths in dental patients and, relatively speaking, have caused more fatalities than inhalational agents.

The dangers of intravenous barbiturates include the following:

1. They are very powerful anaesthetics. Overdose is easy to give and once injected their action is not reversed until they have been metabolised.

2. They are potent respiratory depressants and severe hypoxia can result if there is any respiratory obstruction. The latter is a major hazard in operations, such as dental surgery, at the upper end of the airway.

3. They also depress cardiac output and this can aggravate the effects of hypoxia.

4. Intravenous barbiturates can occasionally cause severe hypersensitivity reactions which may not be recognised as such.

It may be worth emphasising that respiratory obstruction, even if mild, can interfere with the giving of inhalational agents. By contrast, intravenous agents can be injected, irrespective of the state of the airway.

Thiopentone

Thiopentone has remained the standard induction agent in general surgical practice since its introduction in the 1930s. It is usually given as a 2.5% solution and induces unconsciousness smoothly and pleasantly in little more than the arm to brain circulation time. An increasing dose can then be given slowly until the required level of unconsciousness is reached.

There is no analgesia in moderate dosage so that surgical stimulation causes reflex movements. Increased doses however cause respiratory and circulatory depression and intravenous barbiturates should never be used unless the airway can be maintained with absolute certainty. This entails the ability to carry out endotracheal intubation.

The circulatory effects of thiopentone also make it dangerous for patients with poor cardiac function or in shock. Thiopentone is reputed to have caused more deaths among American troops injured during the bombing of Pearl Harbour than did the enemy.

Waking after a moderate dose of thiopentone is rapid, but largely due to redistribution of the drug. Metabolism is slower, so that variable degrees of sedation persist for up to 24 hours and is further delayed if liver function is impaired.

Adverse effects

1. Laryngeal spasm. This is common during induction and is probably due to overactive laryngeal reflexes. The spasm is usually short lived but administration should stop until it relaxes. If it persists a muscle relaxant and artificial ventilation may need to be given.

2. Extravascular injection. Thiopentone is irritant, so that extravascular injection can cause pain,

swelling and local tissue necrosis. Local infiltration of the area with procaine and hyaluronidase may help to relieve symptoms and disperse the drug.

3. Intra-arterial injection. The irritant effect of thiopentone on arterial walls is such that accidental intra-arterial injection can cause intense arterial spasm. The risk is mainly with strong (5%) solutions and typical symptoms are sudden pain in the arm and if the spasm leads to thrombosis, blanching of the fingers. In extreme cases this has terminated in gangrene necessitating amputation. An attempt to relieve the spasm should be made by giving an alpha-blocking agent and anticoagulants.

4. Overdose. Respiratory depression is the first and most important effect. Immediate positive pressure mechanical ventilation must be given as there is no specific antagonist. Respiratory stimulants are of little value.

5. Hypersensitivity reactions. Thiopentone can cause histamine release or, rarely, hypersensitivity reactions of various types. In a typical, severe reaction, there is bronchospasm, flushing, oedema and vasodilatation, and a sharp fall in blood pressure. Occasionally, such reactions have been fatal. The treatment is essentially the same as that for similar reactions to penicillin as described earlier.

In spite of these hazards, thiopentone has over many years proved, in expert hands, to be a safe and useful drug which has not been displaced by newer agents. Its principal use is as an induction agent or in short operations. However, it must be emphasized that its safety record, despite its low therapeutic index, is largely a reflection of anaesthetists' skill.

Methohexitone

Methohexitone is in most respects similar to thiopentone, as described above. The chief differences are as follows:

1. It is 2.5 times as potent as thiopentone.
2. Recovery is more rapid, mainly because of more rapid redistribution but also, to some extent, more rapid metabolism than thiopentone.
3. It causes excitatory activity (involuntary movements and hiccup).
4. It has epileptogenic potential.
5. It is less prone than thiopentone to cause laryngeal spasm.

6. It is much less irritant when an accidental intravascular injection is given.

Methohexitone has never become so widely used as thiopentone as an induction agent in general surgical practice, probably because of the involuntary movements it causes and lack of any significant advantages. In dental practice, however, methohexitone had a widespread vogue, and is still used by some, because it is popular with patients (if they are unaware of the hazards), and because of the apparently rapid recovery and the lesser dangers from extravenous injection than with thiopentone.

Hazards with methohexitone in dental practice

The use of methohexitone in dental practice has resulted in several deaths, and its use, especially by the 'operator-anaesthetist' is rightly condemned. A variety of difficulties and complications can develop in these circumstances.

1. Light anaesthesia with methohexitone produces a restless patient who responds to surgical stimuli by involuntary movements – a state hardly conducive to good dentistry.
2. Restlessness of the patient is a temptation to increase the dose of methohexitone and deepen the anaesthesia.
3. Mild hypoventilation and some depression of cardiac output seem to be common effects of methohexitone.
4. The airway is difficult to protect, especially when the patient is supine. No throat pack gives 100% protection and blood and mucus readily leak back towards the larynx: if you care to try eating a sandwich, lying on your back without a pillow, don't blame us if you choke. Respiratory efficiency is also somewhat less in the supine position.

In a fit young patient these items, individually, may be of little consequence, but their cumulative effect combined with the respiratory depression caused by methohexitone can be disastrous.

If the dentist is trying both to administer methohexitone and to supervise the patient's condition as well as carry out a dental procedure, then the patient may not survive. To act as operator-anaesthetist is therefore an invitation to disciplinary action when anything goes wrong – as it will, sooner or later. When this happens the dentist is likely to get a distinctly chilly response from the coroner.

Now that simple and safer techniques of intravenous or inhalational dental sedation are available there is no justification for the use of methohexitone for this purpose.

Non-barbiturate intravenous agents

Two intravenous anaesthetic agents, Althesin and, particularly, propanidid, gave a rapid recovery and were used in dentistry. However, they caused hypersensitivity reactions so much more frequently than the barbiturates that they have been withdrawn.

Ketamine

Ketamine differs from other anaesthetic agents in that it produces a state of so-called dissociative anaesthesia, in which, apart from loss of consciousness and analgesia, bodily responses are quite different from those to conventional anaesthetics.

Ketamine can be given by intramuscular but more usually by intravenous injection which is quickly followed by loss of consciousness. Reflexes however typically remain intact so that there is increased muscle tone instead of relaxation. There is also cardiovascular stimulation so that both the blood pressure and pulse rate can increase. Ketamine is therefore contraindicated in hypertensive patients.

Analgesia is intense but the main limitation of ketamine is that it is prone to cause vivid and terrifying nightmares or hallucinations during recovery, particularly in adults. These effects can be reduced or abolished by premedication with, for example, diazepam.

Ketamine is useful for anaesthesia in children and particularly if it has to be given repeatedly, but recovery is slow. It also has the advantage that it can be given by intramuscular injection, which is valuable for an otherwise uncontrollable child.

Etomidate is an induction agent which causes less hypotension than comparable agents. Recovery is rapid, but injection is painful, involuntary movements are common and there have been reports that repeated doses may cause adrenocortical suppression.

Propofol is a newer induction or maintenance agent which is also followed by rapid recovery without after-effects and little involuntary movement. It is being increasingly widely used and has the advantage that it seems to have anti-emetic properties, but injection can be mildly painful.

INTRAVENOUS AND INHALATIONAL SEDATION IN DENTISTRY.

As mentioned earlier, the term 'dental sedation' refers to rapid abolition of anxiety for the relatively brief period of a dental procedure. Only a few agents have suitable properties, as most of the commonly used sedatives taken by mouth are not sufficiently rapid in onset and usually, are too long acting to be useful for this purpose.

Diazepam

The use of oral diazepam as an anxiolytic has been discussed earlier. For a more rapid effect and associated hypnosis, diazepam or the related agent, midazolam, can be given intravenously. Full anaesthesia is not achieved, reflexes are little depressed and there is usually complete amnesia afterwards.

The usual procedure is to prepare the patients essentially as for a brief anaesthetic but they do not need to be starved. Diazepam is injected very slowly, with the patient in the supine or near-supine position. The usual dose is 10–15 mg but is determined by the response. If quiet conversation is maintained during administration, it will be noticed that the patient's responses suddenly weaken or stop. There may be obvious ptosis with drooping of the eyelid half across the pupil (Verrill's sign) or the patient may suddenly and obviously fall asleep. Nevertheless, the patient should remain responsive to verbal contact. A sponge or similar pack is inserted to protect the airway. A local anaesthetic is given as there is no analgesia. If this is not done or is ineffective the patient will respond to pain with unconscious facial or other movements, or will cry out.

With normal doses, the patient remains sedated for about half an hour but remains drowsy and co-operative for a longer period when such procedures as cavity lining or filling can be completed.

Once recovery is complete, there are no after-effects and there is usually complete amnesia for the period after the start of the injection or even for the period when the patient was apparently still awake, or for any of the rare episodes of moaning or shouting during sedation. Amnesia can occasionally be prolonged and there are stories – some of which may even be true – of episodes of bizarre behaviour long afterwards.

Adverse effects

Diazepam like other benzodiazepines is remarkably safe and most of the hazards of its use by the intravenous route in healthy patients are little more than theoretical. However, they include the following:

1. Respiratory depression. Diazepam causes slight but measurable respiratory depression. It should not therefore be given to hypoxic patients, particularly those with chronic bronchitis and emphysema. Rapid injection in normal patients can also cause temporary apnoea.

Respiratory depression is however greatly enhanced if diazepam is given with an opiate adjuvant, such as pentazocine, to deepen the sedation. Some deaths have resulted as a consequence.

2. Hypotension. There can be mild postural hypotension and, in patients whose blood pressure has been raised by anxiety, there may be a sharper fall, but the effect is unlikely to be dangerous.

3. Delayed recovery. The slow recovery from diazepam sedation is one of its major disadvantages and is the result of two factors, namely:

a. Formation of active metabolites – the half-life of diazepam is up to 50 hours while that of one of its metabolites, desmethyldiazepam, is up to 200 hours. In the case of gross overdose in suicide attempts, metabolites may continue to be excreted for weeks afterwards.

b. Enterohepatic recirculation – as a result, patients may be awake about an hour after treatment but not in full posession of their faculties until some hours afterwards. Worse perhaps is the so-called *second peak effect* (mainly due to enterohepatic recirculation), when the patient suddenly becomes drowsy and can fall asleep after apparent recovery.

It is essential therefore that patients should not drive a motor vehicle for at least 12 hours after intravenous diazepam, but should be taken home by a responsible adult. In view of car drivers' proclivities for ignoring instructions of this sort, it would be interesting to know how many road accidents have resulted from intravenous diazepam. It is undoubtedly safe for patients but may be lethal for pedestrians.

4. Vascular damage. Diazepam is insoluble in water and the standard solute is propylene glycol which is irritant to endothelium. This can lead to thrombophlebitis or, in the case of accidental intra-arterial injection, spasm and tissue damage. In rare cases this has resulted in gangrene of the fingers.

This problem may be overcome by withdrawing blood to dilute the diazepam after entering the vein but before making the injection. An alternative is to use *Diazemuls* (diazepam in a lipid emulsion) but this is viscous and is less potent. A better alternative is midazolam.

Midazolam

Midazolam has the following advantages over diazepam:

1. It is water soluble and non-irritant to vessel walls.
2. It is metabolised considerably more rapidly than diazepam. It has no persistent active metabolites and does not undergo enterohepatic recirculation. There is therefore no second peak effect, but the period of initial recovery is no more rapid.
3. It appears to give even more complete amnesia than diazepam.

Midazolam is more potent than diazepam and if not used in the more dilute formulation, the passage through the conventional stages of sedation can be so rapid that too large a dose may be given.

Overall, the advantages of midazolam over diazepam are so great that it has largely replaced the latter for intravenous sedation and many regard intravenous diazepam as obsolete.

Benzodiazepine antagonists

Benzodiazepine receptors have been described in the CNS, and antagonists which bind to these receptors have been developed. One of them, *flumazenil*, reverses all the actions of benzodiazepines, as discussed earlier. It can be used for rapid

arousal after midazolam-induced sedation and for treatment of benzodiazepine overdose. The action of flumazenil is brief however, so that to reverse the action of diazepam, repeated doses of this antagonist have to be given.

In dentistry, flumazenil may also be useful for waking a patient sedated with midazolam, immediately after the more traumatic procedures have been completed, so that subsequent procedures can be carried out with full patient co-operation.

Nitrous oxide-oxygen sedation

The technique of sedation known as 'Relative Analgesia' depends on the analgesic and anxiolytic properties of nitrous oxide in concentrations too low to induce anaesthesia. Reduction of anxiety raises the threshold of pain perception so that otherwise intolerable procedures may be accepted calmly.

The aim of the technique is to keep the patient conscious and co-operative but in a state of complete tranquillity. Ideally, the patient should have sensations of warmth, confidence and a pleasant degree of dissociation from the realities of his situation – the feelings, in fact, of mild inebriation. The level of analgesia is variable, but local anaesthesia is usually necessary for cavity preparation. The injection can be easily and painlessly given.

It should be made clear to patients that they are not having an anaesthetic and the concentration of nitrous oxide is adjusted to provide the degree of tranquillisation required. Individual patients' levels of anxiety and response to nitrous oxide vary widely but an effective concentration may be as low as 20%.

To retain the co-operation and confidence of the patient, the operator needs to keep up a flow of gentle, encouraging conversation. This also ensures that descent of the patient into unconsciousness is immediately apparent and the concentration of nitrous oxide reduced accordingly.

Administration of nitrous oxide should stop shortly before treatment has been completed and washed out with pure oxygen to hasten recovery.

Advantages of nitrous oxide sedation

1. The patient remains conscious and co-operative. Reflexes are retained.

2. There is no respiratory depression or undesirable cardiovascular effects.

3. Recovery is almost immediate. However, it is desirable to give patients about 15 minutes to make sure that they have fully recovered their faculties.

It must be emphasised, however, that nitrous oxide should only be given from apparatus with a fail-safe device that makes it impossible to administer it with less than 30% oxygen.

RESPIRATORY STIMULANTS (ANALEPTICS)

Analeptics can produce widespread central arousal (amphetamines and cocaine) or act on the brainstem (doxapram, ethamivan or nikethamide). The potential use for such drugs in anaesthesia is for respiratory depression as a result, for example, of overdose of a barbiturate or of hypoxia.

However, barbiturate overdose is better managed conservatively mainly by intubation and maintained mechanical ventilation. In the case of hypoxia, or overdose of an anaesthetic, the respiratory centre responds poorly to respiratory stimulants. The latter also have a low therapeutic ratio, so that increasing the dose can cause convulsions. Doxapram is somewhat safer than other analeptics but has a brief duration of action and has to be given as a continuous intravenous infusion.

For opiate overdose a specific antagonist, naloxone, is available and rapidly reverses the narcosis and respiratory depression. Naloxone should *not* however be given for barbiturate overdose as it has partial agonist activity and may deepen barbiturate-induced respiratory depression.

SUGGESTED FURTHER READING

Alagesan K, Nunn J F, Feeley T W, Henegan C P H 1987 Comparison of the respiratory depressant effects of halothane and isoflurane in routine surgery. British Journal of Anaesthesia 59: 1070

Alexander C M, Gross J B 1988 Sedative doses of midazolam depress hypoxic ventilatory responses in humans. Anesthesia and Analgesia 67: 377

Atkinson R S Adams A P (eds) 1985 Anaesthesia and analgesia. In Jones R M (ed) 1. Isoflurane. Churchill Livingstone, Edinburgh, pp 1–11

Brogden R N, Goa K L 1988 Flumazenil. Drugs 35: 448

Cattermole R W, Verghese C, Blair I J, Jones C J H, Flynn P J, Sebel P S 1986 Isoflurane and halothane for outpatient dental anaesthesia in children. British Journal of Anaesthesia 58: 385

Eger E I II, Smuckler E A, Ferrell L D, Goldsmith C H, Johnson B H 1986 Is enflurane hepatoxic? Anesthesia and Analgesia 65: 21

Franks N P, Lieb W R 1987 Anaesthetics on the mind. Nature 328: 113

Galletly D, Forrest P, Purdie G 1988 Comparison of the recovery characteristics of diazepam and midazolam. British Journal of Anaesthesia 60: 520

Gelman S, Van Dyke R 1988 Anesthesiology 68 (no 4): 479

Halsey M J 1987 Drug interactions in anaesthesia. British Journal of Anaesthesia 59: 112

Hook P C G, Lavery K M 1988 New intravenous sedative combinations in oral surgery: a comparative study of nalbuphine or pentazocine with midazolam. British Journal of Oral and Maxillofacial Surgery 26: 95

Langley M S, Heel R C 1988 Propofol: a review. Drugs 35: 334

McAteer P M, Carter J A, Cooper G M, Prys-Roberts C 1986 Comparison of isoflurane and halothane in outpatient paediatric dental anaesthesia. British Journal of Anaesthesia 58: 390

McCollum J S C, Dundee J W 1986 Comparison of induction characteristics of four intravenous anaesthetic agents. Anaesthesia 41: 995

McLaughlin W, Broomhead L, Hill C M 1987 A 25-year review of general anaesthesia at the Leeds Dental Hospital. British Dental Journal 163: 317

Milligan K R, Howe J P, Dundee J W 1988 Halothane and isoflurane in outpatient anaesthesia. Anaesthesia 43:

Sear J W 1987 Toxicity of IV Anaesthetics. British Journal of Anaesthesia 59: 24

Sharer N M, Nunn J F, Royston J P, Chanarin I 1983 Effects of chronic exposure to nitrous oxide on methionine synthase activity. British Journal of Anaesthesia 55: 693

Skelly A M, Nelson I A 1986 Clinical assessment of a new dilution of midazolam hydrochloride for dental sedation. British Dental Journal 162: 99

Spence A A 1988 Antibody to halothane-induced liver antigen. British Journal of Anaesthesia 60: 1202

Stoelting R K 1983 Allergic reactions during anaesthesia. Anesthesia and Analgesia 62: 341

Thornton J A 1982 The problem of histamine in anaesthesia. British Journal of Anaesthesia 54: 1

White P F 1986 Pharmacologic and clinical aspects of preoperative medication. Anesthesia and Analgesia 65: 963

Whitwam J G 1987 Benzodiazepines. Anaesthesia 42: 1255

Wood N, Sheikh A 1986 Midazolam and diazepam for minor oral surgery. British Dental Journal 160: 9

9. Local analgesia

The term 'analgesia' is preferred since, to some, anaesthesia implies unconsciousness. This may or may not be pedantic but the term 'local anaesthetic agent' still persists and both 'local anaesthesia' and 'local analgesia' are currently used and equivalent terms.

Mechanism of conduction of the nerve impulse

A nerve impulse (irrespective of whether it is afferent from a sense organ or efferent to a neuro-muscular junction) is in effect a wave of electrical activity passing along the fibre. This electrical activity is the result of exchange of cations (sodium and potassium) across the nerve cell membrane.

In the resting state the nerve cell membrane is permeable to potassium ions but relatively impermeable to sodium ions, so that there is a minute potential difference between the inside and the outside of the cell. In this resting state sodium ions are forced outwards (by the so-called sodium pump) and the intracellular concentration of sodium kept at a low level – the concentration of sodium ions outside the cell is approximately 10 times higher than inside.

When a nerve impulse is initiated the permeability of a short length of an axon is momentarily but greatly increased. Sodium ions diffuse rapidly into the cell, overwhelming the sodium pump and suddenly reversing the polarity of the interior of the fibre relative to the exterior. The inrush of sodium ions is then balanced by escape of potassium ions. This membrane change, with resulting reversal in polarity of the interior relative to the exterior of the cell, is referred to as a *wave of depolarisation*. Its rapid movement along the fibre constitutes the nerve impulse (Fig. 9.1).

Immediately in the wake of the wave of depolarisation the membrane starts to recover. Sodium ions are ejected by the sodium pump and potassium ions move in. The relative concentration of these two ions inside and outside the cell is quickly restored to the levels characteristic of the resting state.

Mode of action of local anaesthetic agents

The mode of action of local anaesthetic agents is complex but in essence they can be regarded as reversibly blocking sodium channels and thus, the rapid inflow of sodium ions on which neural transmission depends.

The fact that local anaesthetics appear to act selectively on sensory fibres is due to the greater diffusion barriers around A fibres (motor and other functions) than around C fibres. Motor fibres are thickly myelinated. An unusual local analgesic, etidocaine, is highly lipid soluble; therefore it rapidly causes both motor and sensory blockade. Most other local anaesthetics are poorly soluble in lipids and rapidly enter C fibres, but penetration of the diffusion barriers around motor fibres is so slow that, normally, no significant block develops.

Toxic effects of local anaesthetics

Most local anaesthetics if absorbed in sufficient quantity into the circulation have toxic effects on the CNS (typically, stimulation followed by depression) and on the heart. With the exception of cocaine which increases myocardial activity and excitability, most local anaesthetic agents have a depressant action on the heart. This may sometimes be sufficient to cause a significant fall in cardiac

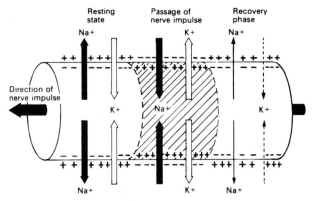

1. Resting state. The intracellular concentration of potassium ions greatly exceeds the extracellular concentration. The opposite is true for sodium which is actively 'pumped' out

2. Passage of impulse. There is a transient inrush of sodium ions and outflow of potassium ions and the polarity of the interior of the cell relative to the exterior is reversed (depolarisation).

3. Recovery phase. Sodium ions are ejected and replaced by potassium ions until the relative concentration of these two ions inside and outside the cell is restored to that of the resting state.

Fig. 9.1 Conduction of a nerve impulse

output; lignocaine by contrast can be used therapeutically to stabilise irregular heart rhythm particularly after a myocardial infarct.

Bupivicaine (see below) is an exception in that it can cause life-threatening cardiac arrhythmias which have caused over 50 deaths in a short period in the USA, mostly as a consequence of extradural blocks for obstetrics.

The action of lignocaine on the nervous system seems somewhat paradoxical in that overdoses in bolus injections can cause fits, but smaller doses of intravenous lignocaine can be used as an anticonvulsant for status epilepticus.

The toxic effects of local anaesthetics cannot be predicted in any simple way for reasons connected with the practical aspects of local anaesthetic techniques.

Local anaesthetics generally used in dentistry are given with a vasoconstrictor (such as adrenaline) to prevent rapid absorption and to give a prolonged effect. Any toxic effect of a local anaesthetic agent is therefore the combined action of both substances. If some or all of the local anaesthetic mixture gets into a blood vessel, the adrenaline – small though the amount is – may have a significant cardiovascular effect, namely palpitations and possibly cardiac irregularities, outweighing any toxic action of the local anaesthetic itself. Catecholamine vasoconstrictors have a slight but detectable systemic effect even when they are localised to the site of injection by their own vasoconstrictor effect.

Generally speaking, modern local anaesthetic preparations are nevertheless remarkably safe and effective; toxic effects are exceedingly uncommon but most of them are due to the vasoconstrictor component.

Effectiveness of local anaesthetic agents

The effectiveness of a local anaesthetic agent under clinical conditions is affected by several variables including:

1. The analgesic potency of the agent itself.

2. The proximity of the point of injection to the appropriate nerves, i.e. the skill of the operator.

3. The persistence of the agent at the site of injection. This mainly depends on the concentration and effectiveness of the added vasoconstrictor.

4. The rate at which the agent is metabolised at the site of injection.

5. The extent of spread of anaesthesia.

In addition to the operator's skill, anatomical variations may result in the local anaesthetic being injected further from the nerve trunk than expected when a regional block is being carried out. Some spread of the anaesthetic effect is therefore desirable to cover such contingencies and also to provide an adequate field of analgesia without having to give too many local infiltrations. Modern agents, particularly lignocaine and its successors, give a very good spread of anaesthesia but none of the more recently introduced agents seems to be so effective in this respect as 2% lignocaine (with 1 : 80 000 adrenaline) which as a consequence has retained a well-deserved popularity.

To try to get an effective inferior dental nerve block using procaine is a salutary experience which makes the advances in local anaesthetic agents only too apparent.

Local anaesthetic agents

The composition of a typical local anaesthetic solution is as follows:

Lignocaine hydrochloride (usually 2%) or other local anaesthetic agent.
Adrenaline (usually 1:80 000 = 12.5 μg/ml) or other vasoconstrictor.
Antioxidant (such as sodium metabisulphate).
Preservative (such as a parabens or sodium benzoate).
Modified Ringer's solution.

Cocaine

Cocaine was the first effective local anaesthetic agent. Its properties were the subject of early research by Sigmund Freud.* Freud, however, after a relatively short time handed these investigations over to an ophthalmologist colleague, Koller, and went on to what he regarded as more interest-ing and important matters. After Koller's introduction of cocaine as an effective local anaesthetic for ophthalmology, Freud (with tiresome facetiousness) used to refer to his friend as 'Coca Koller'.

Cocaine remains an outstandingly effective surface anaesthetic agent but is too toxic for use by injection.

Cocaine is also a drug of addiction but differs fundamentally from morphine and similar drugs in that it is a cardiac and cerebral stimulant. It has a strong amphetamine-like, sympathomimetic action and induces a sense of excessively lively well-being and abolishes fatigue and hunger. Overdose causes restlessness, excitement and convulsions.

Since cocaine has both direct and indirect sympathomimetic actions it is unique as a local anaesthetic agent in being a strong vasoconstrictor. Hence cocaine produces not merely a localised and persistent effect but protects the patient against its own systemic actions to some degree.

The toxic effects of cocaine are mainly those of sympathetic overactivity and central stimulation. In addition to the effects on the central nervous system mentioned above, heart and respiration rates accelerate. Increased myocardial excitability leads to progressively more severe disturbance of rhythm. Ventricular fibrillation or convulsions may be fatal.

Applications. Cocaine should only be used as a surface anaesthetic but is so effective for this purpose that an ointment containing 20% of cocaine on cotton wool placed against the antral wall allows the underlying bone to be painlessly opened with a trocar. Topical cocaine has therefore remained in use for this purpose in ENT departments and is still sometimes used in ophthalmology.

In dentistry cocaine is occasionally used topically in the depths of an apicectomy cavity when an orthodox local anaesthetic has failed.

The cerebral stimulant effect of cocaine makes it liable to addiction but though it resembles the amphetamines in this respect addiction has much more serious effects. Cocaine is, therefore, a Controlled Drug and a Class A Poison.

Patients are not incidentally very likely to become addicted to cocaine used for dental purposes. If that were so, all our parents or grandparents in the cocaine era would have become addicts. It is the

---

* Freud himself was not apparently averse to taking cocaine from time to time, (and who can blame him), but the suggestion by a recent biographer that the whole of Freudian sexual and psychoanalytic theory is no more than the vapourings of a cocaine addict, seems a somewhat extreme view.

dentist who has access to the drug who is more likely to become dependent

Procaine

Procaine consists of a para-amino benzoic acid residue linked to an ester group. The linking group is readily hydrolysed by cholinesterase and this contributes to the short duration of action of procaine when given by local infiltration. In addition, procaine is a weak vasodilator and is rapidly absorbed. Thus the much lower toxicity of procaine when compared with cocaine is counterbalanced by the rapid absorption of procaine into the circulation. As a consequence, procaine must be given with a vasoconstrictor to ensure adequate duration of action and to minimise systemic toxic effects.

Procaine has no surface anaesthetic action.

Toxic effects. The main effect is cerebral stimulation or excitement and restlessness going on to depression and ultimately, coma.

The cardiovascular effects are depression of myocardial excitability and of cardiac output. In addition there may be peripheral vasodilatation with the overall result that the blood pressure falls severely.

Hypersensitivity to procaine can develop particularly among those who use it frequently.

For dental and most other purposes procaine is obsolete.

Lignocaine

Lignocaine differs from procaine in that an amide group links the two parts of the molecule. As a result it is not affected by cholinesterase and it is less rapidly metabolised than procaine. Lignocaine has no vasoconstrictor effect; as a result a vasoconstrictor (usually adrenaline at a concentration of 1 : 100 000 or 1 : 80 000) is needed to give lignocaine adequate duration and reliability of action.

The combination of 2% lignocaine with 1 : 100 000 or 1 : 80 000 adrenaline in 2 ml cartridges provides a highly effective, reliable and generally safe local anaesthetic for dental purposes.

Lignocaine without adrenaline can be given when thought necessary, but its action is unreliable and brief. If the analgesia is inadequate, pain will cause endogenous catecholamine secretion. If, therefore, the patient is thought to be at risk from cardiovascular disease omission of adrenaline has no practical advantages. Theoretically prilocaine, with or without felypressin, may be safer, but its advantages in such situations are unproven and it may provide no more than a false sense of security.

Lignocaine has some surface anaesthetic activity (although this is weak in comparison with cocaine and some other agents) and is widely used for this purpose. Preparations are usually in the form of an ointment and hyaluronidase may be added with the idea of improving absorption. To be effective and to obliterate the pain of an injection, such preparations must be in contact with the oral mucosa for an adequate time (at least a minute) and protected from dilution by saliva.

Toxic effects

*1. **Cerebral.*** Lignocaine in overdose usually causes cerebral depression without preliminary excitement. Moderate doses of lignocaine as mentioned earlier are anticonvulsant.

*2. **Cardiovascular.*** In gross overdose lignocaine causes cardiac depression, but depresses cardiac excitability before it significantly reduces the force of contraction. Lignocaine, as a consequence, is the treatment of choice for the control of dangerous arrhythmias after myocardial infarction. For this purpose it is given intravenously as a bolus of 100 mg.

*3. **'Lignocaine allergy'.*** Although isolated cases of 'lignocaine allergy' have been very occasionally reported, it is doubtful whether there have ever been any full authenticated and immunologically confirmed cases of hypersensitivity reactions to lignocaine. This is particularly surprising in that local anaesthetics are often given repeatedly to the same individuals (some of whom inevitably are susceptible to such reactions) for successive sessions of treatment. These conditions are ideal for the induction of hypersensitivity.

In most cases of so-called allergy to lignocaine it has usually been unclear which component of the solution has caused the trouble. In particular, most local anaesthetic solutions contain a benzoic acid derivative (a parabens) as a preservative. Parabens are however well-recognised sensitizing agents. As a consequence, parabens-free local anaesthetics have been introduced.

Despite the persistence of the belief in lignocaine allergy in some circles, the vast scale of use of this agent for well over a quarter of a century in the UK, USA and other countries, but at the same time the rarity of reports of adverse reactions, indicates that hypersensitivity to this drug is unlikely to be a significant possibility.

Although lignocaine and adrenaline have been proved to be remarkably safe in practice, they should not and do not need to be given in unlimited quantities. If a couple of cartridges in any given area fail to produce the desired effect, then there is something wrong with the solution, the patient, or (most often) the operator, and the attempt should be abandoned until the problem has been investigated.

The maximum dose of lignocaine (local anaesthetic solution) that should be given to a healthy adult is 5 (2 ml) cartridges over the space of an hour.

Prilocaine

Prilocaine is chemically similar to lignocaine and has very similar properties. Prilocaine has a weak but significant vasoconstrictor activity which enables it to be used effectively (as a 4% solution) without an added vasoconstrictor. Under such circumstances it provides more reliable analgesia than lignocaine alone and this can be used for brief procedures.

Prilocaine is rapidly redistributed around the body and metabolised after absorption; it has as a result a lower nominal toxicity than lignocaine. Prilocaine is therefore used in a higher concentration (3%) than lignocaine; this also makes use of the weak vasoconstrictor action and only a very low concentration of adrenaline (1 : 300 000) has to be added.

Three per cent prilocaine with 1 : 300 000 adrenaline appears to be nearly as effective as 2% lignocaine with 1 : 80 000 adrenaline. Another alternative available (as described later) is 3% prilocaine with felypressin, a synthetic (non-catecholamine) vasoconstrictor. Only prilocaine is

available with felypressin since they are both produced by the same manufacturer. The main toxic effect reported of prilocaine is cyanosis due to methaemoglobinaemia.

Allergy to prilocaine has also been reported. The claim that prilocaine, with or without felypressin, is safer than lignocaine with adrenaline for patients with heart disease is unsupported by the morbidity and mortality data on local anaesthetics.

Mepivacaine

Mepivacaine is also similar to lignocaine in chemical constitution and properties. It can be used as a 3% solution without a vasoconstrictor when it provides adequate local analgesia of short duration. It is not clear whether this preparation has any advantages over 4% prilocaine used in the same way.

Two per cent mepivacaine with 1 : 200 000 adrenaline is available and has the theoretical advantage of a lower vasoconstrictor content.

Allergy to mepivacaine has also been reported.

Bupivacaine

Bupivacaine is an ultralong-acting local anaesthetic. Complete analgesia of the related area after an inferior block may last for 8–12 hours. This is only useful in dentistry for some forms of otherwise intractable pain.

As mentioned earlier, bupivacaine is considerably more cardiotoxic than other currently used local anaesthetic agents, but probably only in the larger doses required for extradural regional analgesia.

Vasoconstrictors for use with local anaesthetic agents

The purpose of adding a vasoconstrictor to local anaesthetic agents is to reduce the local circulation at the site of injection sufficiently to prevent the agent from diffusing away too rapidly.

The much reduced rate of absorption is often said to minimise any toxic effects the local anaesthetic might cause when it reaches the general circulation. Such statements seem, however, to betray a certain confusion of thought, in that the most toxic component of anaesthetic solutions is the vasoconstrictor itself. On the other hand the vasoconstrictor effect of catecholamines (such as adrenaline or noradrenaline) is protective since vasoconstriction slows their own absorption. If, however, the injection accidentally gets into a blood vessel the vasoconstrictor (if a catecholamine) may have more serious effects than the local anaesthetic agent.

Another effect of the vasoconstrictor with local anaesthetic is that when given as a local infiltration, it provides a relatively bloodless field of operation.

The main agents that have been used are adrenaline, noradrenaline and felypressin.

Adrenaline

Adrenaline is an effective vasoconstrictor and in the usual concentration of 1 : 80 000 in a healthy patient causes no more than transient palpitations on injection. The chief objections to adrenaline result from its adrenergic activity and in particular the increased myocardial excitability. In overdose this can lead to disturbance of cardiac rhythm and even ventricular fibrillation.

Adrenaline can raise the systolic pressure transiently but tends to lower the diastolic pressure.

In spite of these drawbacks clinical evidence of serious adverse reactions to adrenaline-containing local anaesthetics is very hard to find.

The main systemic effect of adrenaline in local anaesthetics is to cause, in some patients, tachycardia (palpitations) but these are of no significance.

Drug interactions (theoretical or real). As discussed in Chapter 6, interactions with antidepressants have been postulated but not substantiated.

There is no evidence that either adrenaline or noradrenaline is potentiated by monoamine oxidase inhibitors since they are broken down by another enzyme, catechol O-methyl transferase (COMT) (see Ch. 6).

As discussed earlier, interactions between adrenaline and tricyclic antidepressants have been demonstrated only by giving volunteers tricyclic antidepressants and then infusing them with *intravenous* adrenaline at the rate of 18 μg/min for *25 minutes*. One can only wonder both at the heroism of the volunteers, and also that the consequences were so slight.

There is *no clinical evidence* that adrenaline in the amounts used in dental local anaesthetics (as mentioned in Ch. 6) has any significant interaction with tricyclic antidepressants.

Interactions with beta blocking drugs. Adrenaline, if given in sufficiently large doses, can interact with drugs such as propranolol to raise the blood pressure. This results from the fact that adrenaline causes constriction of skin and visceral vessels (α effect) but dilatation of muscle arterioles (β effect). Since the muscles contain the larger vascular bed, the net effect is that peripheral resistance is slightly lowered and, typically, the diastolic pressure falls.

When however adrenaline is administered to a person receiving propranolol (for example) its beta effect of dilating muscle vessels is blocked but the alpha effect on skin and visceral vessels is unopposed. The consequent constriction of both muscle and skin vessels raises the peripheral resistance and blood pressure.

Clinically, occasional cases of hypertensive interactions between adrenaline and propranolol have been, as yet, reported only in patients receiving relatively large amounts of adrenaline in local anaesthetics for plastic surgery.

Noradrenaline

Noradrenaline has no direct effects on the heart but since it is alpha adrenergic it can cause a rise in blood pressure by widespread vasoconstriction. Some cases of acute hypertension, including several deaths, have resulted from use of *high* concentrations (1 : 20 000) of noradrenaline or from the use of four or more cartridges containing 1 : 80 000 noradrenaline.

A few of the patients suffering these severe reactions were also taking tricyclic antidepressant agents which may have potentiated the effect of the noradrenaline, but those patients who had the most severe reactions apparently received only noradrenaline.

Noradrenaline can therefore cause severe complications, particularly when used in excessive amounts. Noradrenaline has no advantages as a vasoconstrictor and unlike adrenaline (in spite of the latter's *theoretical* disadvantages) has been shown to cause serious clinical complications.

There is, therefore, no indication for the use of noradrenaline as a vasoconstrictor in local anaesthetic preparations for dentistry.

Felypressin (Octapressin)

Felypressin is a synthetic analogue of the pituitary hormone vasopressin. It is an effective vasoconstrictor although less powerful than adrenaline. Felypressin appears to have no adverse systemic effects in concentrations normally used; it does not appear to have any untoward effects on the heart and does not seem to increase myocardial excitability. As far as is known, felypressin does not seem to have any adverse interactions with other drugs, but its advantages appear to be no more than theoretical.

Felypressin is available commercially only with prilocaine (3%) but has *theoretical* advantages over adrenaline. When a bloodless field is needed for oral surgery under anaesthesia, felypressin is so much less effective that adrenaline is still preferred.

The periodontal ligament injection

A recent modification to local anaesthetic technique has been the introduction of special syringes to facilitate the injection of a local anaesthetic into the periodontal ligament. Only a minute amount of solution is injected but great pressure and a fine bore (30 gauge) short needle have to be used. A conventional syringe can be used but is more difficult.

Before giving an intraligamentary injection, it may be desirable incidentally to irrigate the gingival sulcus with an antiseptic such as chlorhexidine in alcohol, to avoid propelling bacteria into the bloodstream. There is however no evidence as yet that intraligamentary injections are a cause of infective endocarditis.

The mechanisms of anaesthesia produced by intraligamentary injection are unknown but experiments have shown that with this technique sterile normal saline or adrenaline alone is as effective as 2% lignocaine with 1:50 000 adrenaline. The pressure used seems to be the determining factor and is so high with an intraligamentary injection that the solution may either interrupt the blood supply to

the pulp or simply compress the sensory nerve fibres.

Intraligamentary injection for local anaesthesia has the following advantages:

1. It can produce effective pulpal anaesthesia or analgesia for extractions when conventional injections have failed.
2. Single tooth anaesthesia is possible and enables individual teeth in different quadrants to be treated without the widespread numbness that results from conventional injections.
3. The onset of analgesia can be very rapid, even immediate or within 30 seconds. The duration is typically up to an hour.
4. The injection can be painless.
5. Using the special syringes available the amount of local anaesthetic solution injected is small, usually about 0.2 ml, although this is usually no more than of theoretical benefit.

The disadvantages are:

1. Postoperative pain may persist for several days but the frequency with which such pain develops is controversial.
2. The amount of damage caused to the periodontal membrane is unknown but extrusion of a tooth has been reported.
3. If a conventional syringe is used the pressure necessary for the injection can burst the cartridge.
4. Accurate placement of the needle may be difficult.
5. Overall, it is less reliable than conventional injections for local analgesia. Some experiments suggest that the failure rate may be as high as 30%. Even so, it may sometimes be effective when conventional injections fail.

Intraligamentary injection has both its enthusiasts and its opponents. Its main applications are those where the advantages listed above are important considerations and in particular when a conventional injection has failed to produce adequate pulpal anaesthesia.

Surface anaesthetic agents

The usefulness of surface anaesthetics is limited. Painful conditions of the mouth should not be treated symptomatically and untreatable disease such as hopelessly advanced cancer needs to be managed by generous use of narcotic analgesics.

A 'sensitive palate' (a tendency to retch during dental treatment) is probably mainly caused by anxiety so that a sedative such as diazepam by mouth is usually more effective than a surface anaesthetic. Benzocaine lozenges are available for this problem or for painful oral lesions unresponsive to other treatment.

Surface anaesthetics are also used as ointments or sprays to lessen the pain of injection of local anaesthetics.

Cocaine is a highly effective surface anaesthetic but the nuisance involved in carrying out the regulations necessary to obtain and use it far outweighs its advantages.

Amethocaine is an effective surface anaesthetic but is too toxic for injection and is a potent sensitiser. If used as an ointment the operator can develop contact dermatitis of the fingers. Amethocaine is sometimes included in proprietary surface anaesthetic sprays.

Lignocaine has some surface anaesthetic action but unlike cocaine the action is relatively superficial. Once the needle is through the surface the discomfort from the injection is much as usual. In proprietary preparations hyaluronidase is sometimes added. Hyaluronidase depolymerises hyaluronic acid which forms part of the connective tissue ground substance and should allow the local anaesthetic to spread. This improves the effectiveness to some degree but even so, enough time – preferably 1 or 2 minutes – must be allowed for a lignocaine-based surface anaesthetic to act. During this time the paste should be protected from being washed away by saliva.

In fact, most of the discomfort from a local anaesthetic seems to come during the injection itself when the tissues are being torn apart by the injected fluid. A surface anaesthetic such as lignocaine has little effect at this level and the main precaution is to make the injection very slowly. This is particularly important when injections are made into the palate where the tissues are tightly bound down to bone.

Lignocaine gel is useful for painful oral lesions such as major aphthae, for which no satisfactory or specific treatment is available, and allows eating and swallowing in relative comfort.

Obtundents

Obtundents were used to dull the sensitivity of dentine in the days when local anaesthetics were less reliable and effective. Alcohol 70–100%, phenol, clove and other essential oils, thymol and many others have been used with the object of precipitating or dehydrating the contents of the dentinal tubules. Local anaesthetics themselves are ineffective when applied to dentine.

Obtundent dressings such as zinc oxide and clove oil are also used (with other measures) to relieve the pain of an infected ('dry') socket.

SUGGESTED FURTHER READING

Anon 1983 Use of local anaesthetic drugs in hospital practice. British Medical Journal 286: 1784

Cawson R A, Curson I, Whittington D R 1983 The hazards of dental local anaesthetics. British Dental Journal 154: 253

Chandler M J, Grammer L C, Patterson R 1987 Provocative challenge with local anaesthetics in patients with a prior history of reaction. Journal of Allergy and Clinical Immunology 79: 883

Council on dental materials, instruments and equipment 1983 Status report: the periodontal ligament injection. Journal of the American Dental Association 106: 222

Covino B G 1986 Pharmacology of local anaesthetic agents. British Journal of Anaesthesia 58: 701

Handler L E, Albers D D 1987 The effects of the vasoconstrictor epinephrine on the duration of pulpal anesthesia using the intraligamentary injection. Journal of the American Dental Association 114: 807

Incaudo G, Schatz M, Patterson R, Rosenberg M, Yamaoto F, Hamburger R 1978 Administration of local anaesthetics to patients with a history of prior adverse reaction. Journal of Allergy and Clinical Immunology 61: 339

Johnson W T, DeStigter T 1983 Hypersensitivity to procaine, tetracaine, mepivacaine, and methylparaben: report of a case. Journal of the American Dental Association 106: 53

Kreutz R W, Kinni M E 1983 Life-threatening toxic methemoglobinemia induced by prilocaine. Oral Surgery 56: 480

Miller A G 1983 A clinical evaluation of the Ligmaject periodontal ligament injection syringe. Dental Update 10: 639

Rosenberg H, Orkin F K, Springstead J 1979 Abuse of nitrous oxide. Anaesthesia and Analgesia 58: 104

Schorr W F 1968 Paraben allergy. Journal of the American Medical Association 204: 107

Scott D B 1986 Toxic effects of local anesthetic agents on the central nervous system. British Journal of Anaesthesia 58: 732

Strichartz G R 1987 Local anaesthetics. Handbook of experimental pharmacology, vol. 81. Springer, Berlin

Tucker G T 1986 Pharmacokinetics of local anaesthetics. British Journal of Anaesthesia 58: 717

Wildsmith J A W 1986 Peripheral nerve and local anaesthetic drugs. British Journal of Anaesthesia 58: 692

10. The cardiovascular system

Hypertension

Hypertension is an abnormally and persistently raised blood pressure. In a minority of patients this may be secondary to kidney or endocrine disease. In over three-quarters of patients the primary cause of the raised blood pressure is not known and the disease is called essential hypertension.

It is important to lower a raised blood pressure to avoid complications such as ischaemic heart disease, left ventricular failure, secondary renal damage, cerebral vascular disease and retinal changes. Hypertension and ischaemic heart disease are now the most common causes of death in the Western world.

Although there is no evidence that overactivity of the sympathetic nervous system is the major cause of essential hypertension, many drugs which lower a raised blood pressure block the sympathetic outflow to the arteriolar smooth muscle (Fig. 10.1).

The action of drugs in reducing blood pressure is complex and is often the result of action at several sites. Antihypertensive agents fall into the following broad categories:

1. Diuretics.
2. Calcium channel blockers.
3. Beta adrenergic blockers.
4. Alpha adrenergic blockers.
5. Vasodilators.
6. Angiotensin-converting enzyme inhibitors.
7. Others.

1. Diuretics

The thiazides such as *bendrofluazide* and *cyclopenthiazide* (Navidrex) lower blood pressure by several actions, namely:

a. Vasodilatation.
b. Inducing sodium loss.
c. Reducing circulating blood volume.

The first two of these actions are the most important.

Thiazides are the first choice for the treatment of mild hypertension, especially in the elderly.

2. Calcium channel blockers (calcium antagonists)

This group of drugs includes *verapamil, nifedipine* and *diltiazem*. They act by inhibiting the flow of calcium through membranes in cells. Nifedipine acts mainly on peripheral arterioles causing vasodilatation and hence reducing peripheral resistance and lowering the blood pressure. Verapamil is also a useful antihypertensive drug but, in addition, reduces the excitability of the atria of the heart and so is used in supraventricular tachycardia. Verapamil, nifedipine and diltiazem dilate coronary arteries and are effective in angina pectoris.

3. β blockers

β blockers (such as *propranolol, oxprenolol, metoprolol* and *atenolol*) are very useful in treating hypertension of all grades of severity. They act by several mechanisms. These include:

1. Reduced cardiac output.
2. Reduced renin release from the kidneys.
3. Reduced sympathetic outflow from the CNS.
4. Reduced release of noradrenaline from peripheral sympathetic nerves.

They are unusual amongst hypotensive drugs in that they do not cause postural hypotension. At present the β blockers are extensively used in the

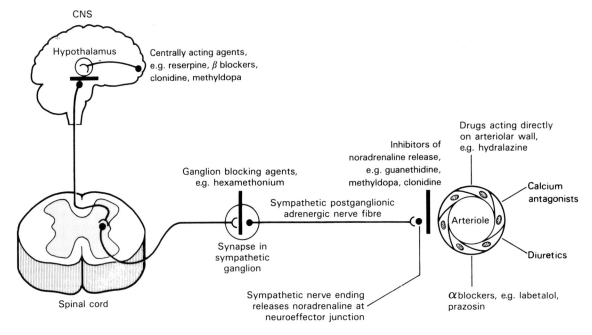

Fig. 10.1   Main sites of action of important drugs used to lower the blood pressure.

treatment of hypertension but often cause lassitude and sometimes depression. The β blocker *labetalol* also has some α blocker activity and is a valuable antihypertensive agent.

β blockers also appear to give better protection than other antihypertensive drugs against recurrences or complications of, and hence have significantly lowered the mortality from myocardial infarction.

4. Alpha adrenergic blockers

Prazosin acts on α 1 receptors in the arteriolar walls and has a vasodilator action. It is a powerful antihypertensive with relatively little toxicity. It is widely used for hypertension of all degrees of severity. *Indoramin* is similar.

Other α adrenergic blockers such as *phenoxybenzamine* or *phentolamine* are less effective and have many side-effects.

5. Vasodilator drugs

Vasodilator drugs include the following:

a. **Hydralazine** is useful in the treatment of severe hypertension due to kidney disease because,

unlike many other hypotensive drugs, renal blood flow is not reduced.

A disadvantage of hydralazine is that it can produce serious autoimmune reactions resembling systemic lupus erythematosus in patients who metabolise the drug slowly. These complications can be prevented by limiting the maximum dose to 200 mg daily.

b. **Diazoxide** is particularly used in severe hypertension when a rapid fall in blood pressure is wanted.

c. **Diuretics** such as the thiazides and also frusemide have, as mentioned earlier, a vasodilator action separate from their diuretic effect and this contributes to their ability to lower blood pressure.

d. **Minoxidil** is a powerful vasodilator used in the specialist treatment of severe hypertension refractory to other drugs. Minoxidil can, however, induce diabetes mellitus and cause hypertrichosis. Application of minoxidil to the scalp is therefore used as a cure for baldness.

6. Angiotensin-converting enzyme (ACE) inhibitors

Captopril and *enalapril* are examples of these drugs. Angiotension II is an endogenous vasoconstrictor; it

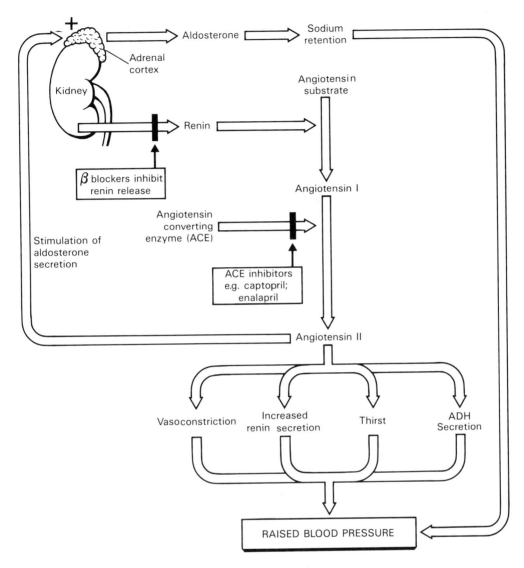

Fig. 10.2 Effects of antihypertensive agents on the renin angiotensin pathway.

can also stimulate aldosterone release from the renal cortex and thus cause sodium retention. These drugs prevent the formation of angiotension II and therefore lower the blood pressure. Captopril and enalapril are used for moderate and severe refractory hypertension.

7. Others

a. Methyldopa. Centrally acting and powerful stimulator of α 2 (prejunctional) receptors inhibiting noradrenaline release. Effective but causes

sedation and depression. (Clonidine has a similar action.)

b. Clonidine and reserpine. Centrally acting. Effective but virtually obsolete because of side-effects, particularly depression.

c. Adrenergic neurone blocking agents (e.g. guanethidine and debrisoquine.) These agents' main action is to block the release of noradrenaline from sympathetic junctional nerve endings. Effective but cause postural hypotension and failure of ejaculation.

d. Ganglion-blocking agents. Obsolete because

parasympathetic ganglia are also blocked with severe side-effects such as dry mouth.

General management of essential hypertension

If no primary cause (such as chronic renal disease) can be found, the usual principles of management are as follows:

1. Body weight. If the patient is overweight, attempts must be made to bring this back to a reasonable level.

2. Smoking. Cigarette smoking should be stopped as it is an important risk factor for athero-sclerosis.

These measures alone may sometimes be sufficient to control mild hypertension.

3. Diuretics. Regular use of one of the thiazides is often the first type of treatment to be considered. This alone can control mild hypertension, or in moderately severe cases will usefully potentiate other hypotensive agents.

4. Antihypertensives. These are needed for moderate and severe hypertension. For moderate hypertension (diastolic pressure above 110 mmHg) β blockers are most favoured because of their effectiveness and relatively few side-effects unless these drugs are contraindicated because of asthma. For more severe hypertension a vasodilator such as hydralazine is given in addition to a β blocker.

5. Relaxation exercises and meditation.

6. Reducing alcohol intake. More than 4–8 units of alcohol (2–4 pints of beer) each day may contribute to raising the blood pressure.

7. Regular 'aerobic' exercise (such as jogging for 20 minutes at least three times weekly) may contribute to blood pressure lowering.

8. A great reduction in dietary salt intake may lower blood pressure.

9. There is some evidence that changing to a vegetarian diet (in particular a reduction in animal fats) lowers the blood pressure.

It has to be emphasised that these are only general principles. New drugs are constantly being introduced and views change about older drugs as experience accumulates. There are therefore no hard and fast rules about the treatment of this common and serious disease.

Ischaemic heart disease

The coronary arteries supply the myocardium with oxygenated blood. Ischaemic heart disease is caused by atherosclerotic narrowing of the coronary arteries. The reduced blood supply causes both atrophy of cardiac muscle with fibrous replacement and, in addition, damages the conducting tissues causing unstable cardiac rhythm. Myocardial ischaemia can lead to either angina pectoris or myocardial infarction.

Angina pectoris and myocardial infarction

Angina pectoris is a pain in the chest, often substernal and radiating down the left arm. It is brought on by exercise, cold or emotion. Angina due to effort is relieved by rest within a few minutes. The pain appears to be caused by transient oxygen deficiency in the myocardium, but is not severe enough to produce permanent structural damage.

Myocardial infarction produces prolonged severe chest pain which is not relieved by rest. The underlying myocardial oxygen lack is so severe that an irreversible necrotic injury is inflicted on the heart.

Management of angina. The mainstay of treatment is glyceryl trinitrate. In addition, any predisposing causes such as obesity, hypertension or anaemia should be treated. Violent effort and exposure to cold should also be avoided.

1. Glyceryl trinitrate is a short-acting anti-anginal drug which is absorbed from a tablet put under the tongue. This allows rapid absorption of the drug into the systemic circulation without passage through the liver, where it would be metabolised.

Glyceryl trinitrate relaxes and dilates venulae – but obstructed and rigid coronary arteries are not affected. Nevertheless, this drug is one of the most effective in treating anginal attacks because venous return and peripheral resistance are lessened and the work done by the heart is reduced. The tension in the ventricular wall in diastole is also lessened and this contributes to the reduced oxygen needs of the heart.

The long-acting nitrates and nitrites (such as pentaerythritol tetranitrate) are clinically very much less effective than short-acting drugs such as glyceryl trinitrate and amyl nitrite. Isosorbide dinitrate orally or sublingually is as effective as glyceryl trinitrate.

2. β blocking drugs. Activation of the sympathetic nervous system by anger, fear, anxiety or effort may bring on an attack of angina. Blockade of the effects of the sympathetic nerves on the heart by β blockers such as propranolol and oxprenolol is often very effective in reducing the frequency and severity of anginal attacks. Whereas glyceryl trinitrate is taken when the anginal pain appears (or just before it is anticipated), β blockers are taken regularly several times a day.

Although β blockers are often effective in the treatment of severe angina a few patients are made worse. Bronchospasm may also be a problem.

3. Drugs which block the flow of calcium into the heart (such as nifedipine and verapamil) are of great benefit in angina and are increasingly widely used.

Nifedipine is, in addition, an effective antihypertensive agent and verapamil is an antidysrhythmic agent.

Angina is not always persistent. In some, attacks stop completely after a time: in such cases drugs need only to be kept in reserve against the possibility of recurrence.

Myocardial infarction. This is usually characterised by agonisingly severe chest pain – often radiating into the neck or down the left arm.

The pain persists for several hours and is not relieved by rest or by glyceryl trinitrate. *Myocardial infarction and angina can occasionally cause pain felt only in the left jaw. Rare though this, is the importance of accurate diagnosis and the avoidance of operative treatment for the pain will be obvious.* Characteristic electrocardiographic changes follow and indicate that part of the ventricular wall has suffered irreversible damage. There is no curative treatment but several measures may lower the mortality.

The underlying cause is severe reduction in the oxygen supply to the myocardium. This was thought at one time to follow occlusion of a major coronary artery by thrombus but this is rarely the case. Although atherosclerosis is virtually invariably associated with myocardial infarction, the precipitating event seems to be the development of a severe dysrhythmia. Infarction does not develop until a little while after the acute attack. Patients who die suddenly during a so-called myocardial infarct show no necrosis of the myocardium at post-mortem.

If patients are monitored during the acute attack, electrocardiograms always show arrhythmias. They increase the oxygen demands of the heart and also decrease the output. This in turn further lowers the heart's blood supply. If this situation persists the patient either dies or an infarct develops.

The main treatment, therefore, to reduce the mortality and effects of the acute attack is to do everything possible to stop the development of cardiac arrhythmias. Survival from the acute attack almost invariably leaves the patient with an area of myocardial necrosis. The size of this infarct is an important factor affecting the prognosis.

A controlled trial in over 3000 patients has shown that the administration of a β blocking agent reduced the mortality of myocardial infarction to a significant degree. In this trial the reduction in mortality was 38% and it was recommended that long-term β blockade should be continued after uncomplicated myocardial infarction.

Summary of management:

a. Pain and anxiety may be greatly reduced by giving a narcotic analgesic. Morphine is still widely used. Nitrous oxide and oxygen are also highly effective and safe.

b. If left ventricular failure follows it should be vigorously treated with oxygen and frusemide (a diuretic) and then with a vasodilator in resistant cases (see p. 146).

c. A frequent cause of death soon after the onset of infarction is ventricular fibrillation. Ventricular arrhythmias may be treated or prevented with a β blocking drug, lignocaine or procaineamide, but ventricular fibrillation cannot be controlled with drugs and is managed by electrical defibrillation.

Myocardial infarction is the chief cause of sudden death but even this may sometimes be preventable if immediate cardiopulmonary resuscitation is given. Obviously this is not always successful but the more quickly this is started and the more efficiently it is done the better the results.

Prevention of atherosclerosis and coronary heart disease

These two diseases go hand in hand and any measures which reduce the severity of atherosclerosis are likely also to reduce the risk of coronary heart disease.

The main risk factors for atherosclerosis are as follows:

1. Age.
2. Hypertension.
3. Cigarette smoking.
4. High blood cholesterol levels.
5. Insufficient exercise.
6. Diabetes mellitus.

Substitution of animal fats by polyunsaturated vegetable fats in the diet lowers blood cholesterol levels. There is however controversy as to whether there is any significant clinical benefit, as the effect is small.

In the USA the mortality from coronary heart disease (CHD) between 1950 and 1963 increased by 19%, but between 1964 and 1975 there has been a significant decrease in CHD mortality. Since that time the consumption of tobacco and of dairy products has fallen in the USA. The consumption of butter, for instance, fell by nearly 32% and of animal fats and oils fell by more than 56% between 1963 and 1975. By contrast, the consumption of vegetable fats and oils increased by over 44%.

These associations may be merely coincidental. Nevertheless, similar findings have been reported from other countries.

Contributory factors to this decline in CHD mortality may be the better management of the acute emergency and the introduction of such drugs as β blockers which help prevent the lethal effects of severe arrhythmias after myocardial infarction.

Clinical trials have also shown that treatment of hypertension reduces CHD mortality.

While the epidemiological evidence for the beneficial effects of polyunsaturated fatty acids may look impressive it has still to be accepted that their actual role remains unproven. Reducing total fat intake is probably, and stopping smoking is certainly more important. Equally, improvements in the treatment of hypertension may also make a further impact on CHD statistics.

Management of thrombotic diseases

Thrombosis is a complex process involving both platelets and the clotting mechanism. On the venous side deposition of fibrin predominates, but in the fast-moving arterial blood, thrombi consist mainly of platelets with little fibrin. The nature of so-called coronary thrombosis is more obscure but platelet thrombi play a part in the production of most cases of myocardial infarction.

Drugs used in the management of thrombotic disease, therefore, comprise two main groups, namely:

1. Anticoagulants.
2. Antiplatelet drugs.

Anticoagulants

The aim of treatment with anticoagulants is to prevent thrombosis. Clinically, however, anticoagulants have not lived up to their expectations. The problems are:

a. Thrombosis in arteries is initiated primarily by platelet activity. Fibrin is deposited on the platelet thrombus but anticoagulants can do little more than prevent extension of fibrin deposition.

b. Laboratory control of anticoagulant dosage has to be constantly maintained. Without such control the dangers of haemorrhage, especially in older patients, are considerable. Some anticoagulants have other side-effects and, in addition, anticoagulants interact with several commonly used drugs, particularly barbiturates and anti-inflammatory analgesics.

c. Anticoagulants have not reduced the mortality from myocardial infarction to any great degree. This is not surprising now that it is appreciated that thrombosis of the coronary arteries is not the usual cause of myocardial infarction. Indeed, it appears that thrombus found in the coronary vessels in a patient who has had a myocardial infarct has usually formed after the incident and is not the precipitating cause.

Anticoagulants will not remove thrombi once they have formed, but fibrinolytic agents are effective (see p. 169). However, anticoagulants may prevent extension of a thrombus and thereby reduce the risk of release of emboli. It is probably by this latter effect that anticoagulants have a marginally beneficial effect on the mortality from myocardial infarction.

Mode of action

Anticoagulants fall into two main groups:

1. Direct acting. The main example is *heparin* which interferes with the enzymic reactions in the earlier stages of the clotting cascade.

2. Indirect acting. These, the *indanediones* and *coumarins*, prevent the formation of clotting factors in the liver, mainly those synthesised from vitamin K.

Heparin. This is given intravenously; its action is immediate but persists only for about 6 hours and so must be given repeatedly. When prolonged anticoagulation is wanted an oral anticoagulant (e.g. warfarin) is given at the same time and the heparin stopped when the oral anticoagulant takes effect about 24–36 hours later.

The short-lived action of heparin means that overdose rarely needs treatment, but heparin can be antagonised by protamine sulphate. Repeated small doses of heparin may be administered subcutaneously in order to prevent postoperative venous thrombosis.

The coumarins. These agents, of which the most widely used is probably *warfarin*, are given by mouth and have an effect after 12–16 hours (i.e. after the normally formed vitamin K-dependent clotting factors have been used up) and this persists for 2–5 days.

The indanediones, e.g. *phenindione*, have the same actions as the coumarins but are more prone to have allergic and other toxic effects and are less favoured as a consequence.

Control of oral anticoagulant treatment

Clotting function is maintained using the prothrombin time test and dosage should be adjusted to raise the prothrombin time to about twice that of the normal control. At such levels there is little risk either of spontaneous bleeding or of seriously prolonged bleeding after dental extractions.

Uses of anticoagulants

1. Myocardial infarction. The main group which seems to benefit are young patients, particularly men, after the first infarct. Treatment may be continued for a year or more. Older patients with arrhythmias and heart failure may be helped by the prevention of venous thrombosis and embolism.

2. Atrial fibrillation. Anticoagulants reduce the dangers of thrombus formation and release of emboli.

3. Deep vein thrombosis. This is a common complication affecting elderly patients who are in bed for long periods. Fragments of thrombus break off and may cause pulmonary embolism. Anticoagulants help prevent development of thrombosis in these circumstances.

4. Renal dialysis. Heparin is given to prevent thrombotic complications temporarily during the extracorporeal circulation of the patient's blood.

5. Pulmonary embolism. This is usually secondary to atrial fibrillation or deep vein thrombosis, is frequently recurrent and can be fatal. The mortality is significantly reduced by immediate anticoagulation.

6. During cardiac surgery.

7. To prevent thrombosis around prosthetic heart valves (together with an antiplatelet drug such as dipyridamole).

8. Multiple cerebral (little strokes).

Adverse effects of anticoagulants

The main complications are:

1. Bleeding as a result of (a) overdose, irregular tablet taking or inadequate laboratory control;

(b) existing haemorrhagic disease or from bleeding lesions such as piles, and (c) interaction with drugs which displace anticoagulants from plasma protein binding sites. These include chloral, trichloroethanol and sulphonamides. Other drugs such as aspirin potentiate the anticoagulant effect by affecting other aspects of the haemostatic mechanism such as inhibition of platelet aggregation. Severe bleeding can be controlled by giving vitamin K.

2. Diminished anticoagulant effect. Barbiturates in particular accelerate hepatic metabolism by enzyme induction. If such drugs are taken at irregular intervals anticoagulant action can fluctuate widely.

3. Allergic effects. Phenindione is the main culprit and warfarin or similar agents (coumarins) are preferable.

Antiplatelet drugs

These drugs, of which aspirin is the prototype, act mainly by interfering with platelet adhesion and aggregation and may therefore lessen the tendency to thrombosis in the arterial circulation, particularly on prosthetic heart valves.

Dipyridamole is used, together with anticoagulants, for this purpose.

The effectiveness of regular aspirin taking in the prevention of, or lowering the mortality from, myocardial infarction has been investigated. At the time of writing, analysis of the aggregate findings of six clinical trials suggests that reinfarction rates and mortality are significantly lowered. It seems probable that the optimal effect is obtained with a low daily dose (50–100 mg) of aspirin.

Surgical treatment of ischaemic heart disease

In angina resistant to drugs, and in many patients who have had myocardial infarcts, the blood supply to the heart can be improved by a coronary aortic bypass graft. Approximately 160 000 such operations were carried out in 1981 in the USA alone where these bypasses have become the most common major operation. It is, however, a remarkable comment on the evaluation of treatment methods that for several years after its introduction and after many hundreds of thousands of operations, there

was no evidence of increased life expectancy and little objective benefit of any sort. Even now, after 15 years of experience, the benefits of this operation remain controversial and an official enquiry has had to be made as to why so many men suffered the hazards and discomfort – not to mention the expense – of this operation with so little expectation of benefit.

Heart failure

Left ventricular failure

Left ventricular failure may be caused by hypertension, myocardial infarction or chronic valve disease (such as aortic stenosis or regurgitation). Acute left ventricular failure causes severe breathlessness due to interstitial and alveolar pulmonary oedema. The patient is, in effect, drowning in his oedema fluid.

1. To save life, oxygen must get into the alveolar capillaries. One hundred per cent oxygen is given by face mask. Oedema is removed as quickly as possible by using a powerful diuretic such as frusemide, ethacrynic acid or bumetamide.

2. If possible, the cause of the heart failure should be treated. If hypertension precipitated the heart failure, the blood pressure should be lowered with a fairly rapidly acting hypotensive drug such as diazoxide.

3. The patient is severely distressed and frightened. Morphine has for long been used to calm the patient and remove the compulsion to make excessive respiratory efforts. Diazepam is being increasingly used instead of morphine.

4. Slow intravenous injection of glyceryl trinitrate may be given to reduce oedema in resistant cases.

Right ventricular failure

This may be a secondary effect of left ventricular failure or may be a consequence of lung disease. Heart failure secondary to lung disease is known as *cor pulmonale* and is usually due to the common combination of longstanding chronic bronchitis and emphysema. An acute exacerbation of chronic bronchitis may precipitate respiratory failure, which in turn leads to right ventricular failure.

1. The patient is given oxygen (up to 30%) via a Venturi mask and is encouraged to cough forcibly.

2. Sputum is sent for bacteriological examination and in the interim a broad-spectrum antibacterial such as co-trimoxazole or amoxycillin is given but changed if necessary.

3. Sedatives, hypnotics or narcotic analgesics are absolutely contraindicated because of their depressant effect on respiration.

4. A bronchodilator such as salbutamol aerosol or injection of aminophylline is given.

5. Digoxin and a diuretic such as chlorothiazide may be given in the acute stage but there is usually no great urgency to start this aspect of treatment.

In the long term, heart failure is traditionally treated with a cardiac glycoside such as digoxin (p. 148) and a diuretic. In addition, however, vasodilators can substantially improve cardiac performance either by reducing peripheral resistance (hydralazine) or by causing dilatation of veins and reducing venous pressure (long-acting nitrates). Other drugs such as prazosin cause both arteriolar and venous dilatation and combinations of drugs can be tested until the optimal benefit is obtained. The ACE inhibitors are probably the most beneficial.

Cardiac glycosides have been shown to have less effect on cardiac performance in long-term use and digoxin can often be withdrawn once the acute phase of failure has been controlled.

Diuretics

Diuretics are drugs which increase the rate of urine production by the kidney to eliminate oedema. The clinically useful diuretics are so powerful that they can produce a negative extracellular fluid balance – in other words they can dehydrate the patient. The most powerful (frusemide and ethacrynic acid) can induce an output of over 10 litres of urine in a few hours. Most commonly, diuretics are given to eliminate oedema caused by heart failure but are often also effective in oedema due to kidney or liver failure. Another common use of diuretics is in the treatment of hypertension.

Diuretics are also useful to relieve localised oedema – such as in the lungs or brain.

The diuretics most often used are:

1. Thiazides (e.g. chlorothiazide, bendrofluazide).

2. Powerful short-acting ('loop') diuretics (e.g. frusemide, ethacrynic acid, bumetanide).

3. Aldosterone antagonists (spironolactone).

4. Potassium-retaining diuretics (e.g. triamterene, amiloride).

1. The thiazides are effective orally. They block sodium reabsorption in the distal renal tubule. Their action comes on after 1 hour and lasts about 6 hours. The thiazides aggravate diabetes and cause loss of potassium, but in general are free from other serious side-effects. Occasionally light-sensitivity dermatitis and gout may be precipitated.

2. Frusemide and ethacrynic acid can be given by mouth and injection. They act on the loop of Henle and distal tubule causing Na, Cl and K loss. Diuresis begins 2 minutes after intravenous administration of frusemide and is completed after 2 hours.

These drugs produce a massive loss of water, sodium and potassium from the body and can reduce the blood volume so severely as to precipitate hypovolaemic shock. More commonly potassium loss develops and may enhance the toxicity of the cardiac glycosides. Uric acid excretion is inhibited and this can cause an attack of gout. Frusemide can interfere with glucose tolerance and in large doses can cause deafness.

3. Spironolactone produces diuresis only in those patients who have oedema and sodium retention due to hyperaldosteronism. Excessive amounts of aldosterone are secreted by patients suffering from renal or hepatic failure.

4. Potassium-retaining diuretics. The thiazides, frusemide and ethacrynic acid can cause potassium deficiency. This may manifest itself as muscle weakness, atony of the gut, increased sensitivity of the heart to cardiac glycosides and cardiac arrest. This complication is countered by giving potassium salts or by using a potassium-retaining diuretic such as *amiloride* and *triamterene*.

Triamterene does not lead to hypokalaemic states and in fact potentiates reabsorbing mechanisms in the kidney tubules. In the treatment of oedema due to congestive heart failure triamterene may be given with a potassium-losing diuretic, and thereby both potentiate the diuretic effect and avoid potassium loss.

Abnormalities of cardiac rhythm

The normal cardiac impulse arises in the sinoatrial node. The nodal tissue consists of modified cardiac muscle, which repeatedly generates a wave of depolarisation which spreads in an orderly manner over the atria. The conducting tissue – the atrioventricular bundle (the bundle of His) – then carries the depolarisation wave into the ventricles.

Depolarisation in the atria and ventricles results from a transient change in ionic permeability of the muscle cell membrane. These ionic changes activate the contraction mechanism of the muscle by increasing the amount of free intracellular calcium necessary for this process.

Abnormalities of rhythm of the heartbeat may consist of:

1. Abnormal rate of discharge of the sinoatrial node.

2. Cardiac impulses arising elsewhere in the heart than the sinoatrial node.

3. Abnormal conduction of the cardiac impulse.

1. Since the normal cardiac impulse arises in the sinoatrial node, abnormalities of rhythm originating in this nodal tissue are spoken of as sinus or supraventricular tachycardia, (i.e. excessive rapidity) or sinus bradycardia, (i.e. excessive slowing) of the heart rate.

2. Extra beats may arise because of impulses arising sporadically from an abnormal focus in the atria or ventricles (atrial or ventricular extrasystoles). Such an abnormal focus may repeatedly discharge and produce episodes of increased heart rate (paroxysmal atrial or ventricular tachycardia).

If many variable abnormal foci discharge in the atria, atrial contraction will be uncoordinated and irregular. As a consequence, the ventricle will be stimulated irregularly and usually rapidly. This is known as atrial fibrillation and causes the pulse to be irregular in both rhythm and volume.

Similarly, multiple varying ectopic foci in the ventricle cause uncoordinated contraction of the ventricle. This is ventricular fibrillation in which the myocardium is doing no more than twitching

rapidly. When this happens, cardiac output immediately falls to zero and the patient becomes unconscious. Death follows within a few minutes.

3. Failure of the atrioventricular bundle to conduct the cardiac impulse from the atria to the ventricles is known as heart block. Conduction defects can also develop within the atria and impede the cardiac impulse from reaching the ventricles. In either event, extreme bradycardia may result; this causes a sudden lowering of cardiac output and attacks of unconsciousness.

Attacks of sinus tachycardia and atrial extrasystoles are not unusual in healthy persons. Atrial fibrillation can be the result of several diseases including rheumatic heart disease and thyrotoxicosis. Ventricular fibrillation may develop in the course of myocardial infarction or after cardiac surgery, or may be produced by drugs such as the cardiac glycosides, the halogenated hydrocarbon anaesthetics and adrenergic stimulants (such as isoprenaline or adrenaline).

Arrhythmias arising in the atria do not usually immediately threaten life. By contrast, ventricular extrasystoles and ventricular tachycardia are dangerous because they may lead to ventricular fibrillation.

Sinus bradycardia and heart block may follow myocardial infarction or may be the result of an excessive dose of a cardiac glycoside.

Anti-arrhythmic drugs

The following classification of anti-arrhythmic agents is suggested for the non-specialist:

1. Cardiac glycosides.
2. Quinidine-like drugs.
3. β blockers.
4. Drugs used for slow dysrhythmias; amiodarone and calcium blockers.

1. The cardiac glycosides, of which digoxin is the most commonly used, have two therapeutic uses – heart failure and rapid arrhythmias arising in the atria. Their main actions are (i) to increase the force of cardiac contraction, (ii) to slow the heart by stimulating the vagus, (iii) to slow conduction down the atrioventricular bundle, (iv) to prolong the effective refractory period of the heart.

The beneficial effect of a cardiac glycoside on heart failure is by stimulating the force of contraction of the myocardium. The antiarrhythmic action is due to the other properties, and the most important of these is slowing conduction down the atrioventricular bundle. The ventricles are thereby protected from excessively rapid stimulation coming from abnormal rhythms arising in the atria, such as atrial fibrillation.

The therapeutic dose of the cardiac glycosides is close to its toxic dose – and even when used at optimal levels may cause side-effects such as nausea and vomiting. With increasing dosage there is severe slowing of the heart due to vagal stimulation. Heart block is another dose-dependent undesirable effect. In large doses, on the other hand, the excitability of the myocardium is increased and this can produce dangerous ventricular arrhythmias.

Because of these different toxic effects, the cardiac glycosides are contraindicated in sinus bradycardia and heart block, and in ventricular arrhythmias.

In the presence of a low blood potassium or a high blood calcium the toxic action of the cardiac glycosides may follow even modest doses.

*2. Quinidine** is a drug which decreases the excitability of the myocardium, slows atrioventricular conduction and decreases the force of myocardial contraction. One practical disadvantage of quinidine is that it depresses the force of contraction of the heart, lowers the cardiac output and can precipitate heart failure. It is now little used.

There are several drugs which have qualitatively similar actions to quinidine, but they produce significant inhibition of myocardial excitability with relatively little depression in force of contraction. These include lignocaine, procainamide, mexiletine, flecainide, tocainide and disopyramide. They are used mainly in the treatment and prevention of ventricular arrhythmias (such as ventricular extrasystoles and tachycardia). These drugs may also be effective in rapid atrial arrhythmias but are contraindicated in heart block and in heart failure.

Lignocaine This is one of the safest and most useful agents for the control of fast arrhythmias in the early management of myocardial infarction. In order to get a quick but sustained effect, 50–100 mg of lignocaine is given intravenously. This can be followed if necessary by an infusion of 1.5–3 mg/min for up to 3 hours.

Side-effects are uncommon but most often affect the nervous system. There may be confusion or excitability going on to convulsions. These effects are dose related.

Flecainide and *tocainide* belong to the same general class of drugs as lignocaine.

3. Blockers of the β actions of the sympathetic transmitter and of sympathomimetic drugs include propranolol, oxprenolol and many others. As well as being used in the treatment of angina pectoris, hypertension and anxiety neurosis, these blocking agents are used to decrease the electrical excitability of the heart. The β blockers are used to treat ventricular arrhythmias but are also effective in controlling atrial arrhythmias.

Propranolol has β_2, (bronchial) as well as β_1, (cardiac) blocking properties and can therefore cause bronchospasm. Propranolol also has some quinidine-like properties and decreases the force of cardiac contraction. Metoprolol and atenolol have partial β_1, selectivity – but can still produce bronchospasm in many asthmatics.

4. Miscellaneous. Isoprenaline is a β agonist (i.e. stimulator) and therefore has all the actions on the heart of the catecholamines – including stimulation of rate of discharge of the sinoatrial pacemaker tissue and facilitating conduction in the bundle of His. Isoprenaline is used to treat excessive ventricular slowing due to failure of initiation or conduction of the cardiac impulse.

An excessively slow heart (sinus bradycardia) can be treated with *atropine*. This acts by blocking the parasympathetic nerve supply to the heart (the vagus) which, when unopposed, has a slowing action on the rate of nodal discharge.

Amiodarone is an anti-arrhythmic drug which

---

* Quinidine is one of the few drugs discovered (in effect) by a patient. At the turn of the century the famous cardiologist Wenckebach was visited by a patient who complained that none of his doctors knew how to treat the irregular beating of his heart. Nevertheless he himself had found that it was ameliorated by taking quinine (quinine in those days was often taken as a tonic, hence 'tonic water'). Wenckebach was shrewd enough to take the information seriously and confirmed this effect of quinine, but found that its isomer, quinidine, was more effective. It is a pity patients' ideas about how their complaints are best treated are rarely so useful. Alternatively it may be that patients should be listened to more carefully. Well, some of them!

may be effective for abnormalities of cardiac rhythm which are resistant to other agents. In particular, it will usually control paroxysmal atrial fibrillation which has not responded to digoxin. Amiodarone is often effective in ventricular tachyarrhythmias but is not indicated for heart block or bradycardia.

Verapamil is an agent which acts by impeding calcium flow across membranes. It is effective in angina as well as supraventricular tachycardia and is now the drug of choice for rapid rhythms arising in the atria, particularly paroxysmal atrial tachycardia.

Summary

The main points regarding arrhythmias and their control by drugs can be summarised as follows, although it must be appreciated that this is a considerable over-simplification of the clinical and therapeutic problems:

1. Some atrial arrhythmias such as extrasystoles and mild overactivity of the nodal tissue (sinus tachycardia) are harmless and happen in normal subjects.

2. Rapid atrial arrhythmias may result in a fall in cardiac output, because of a reduction in the time available for diastolic filling of the ventricles. It is often a feature of the failing heart, but is not an immediate threat to life. Atrial fibrillation and atrial flutter usually indicate underlying cardiac disease. The cardiac glycosides such as digoxin are particularly useful in rapid supraventricular tachycardias, because they protect the ventricle from excessive stimulation by slowing conduction down the atrioventricular bundle. β blockers are also used to treat atrial arrhythmias.

3. Extreme slowing of the heart (bradycardia) may be severe enough to cause loss of consciousness because of a fall in cardiac output. When this is due to a conduction defect (heart block), the situation may be improved by the use of isoprenaline or adrenaline.

Sinus bradycardia is treated with atropine, which blocks vagal activity. In heart block and sinus bradycardia the cardiac glycosides and β blockers are contraindicated.

4. Arrhythmias arising in the ventricle are always dangerous, as they can lead to ventricular fibrillation. Ventricular arrhythmias, which are a common consequence of, and one of the main causes of death after a myocardial infarct, may be treated with lignocaine followed by β blocking agents. The most reliable way of controlling ventricular arrhythmias due to ectopic foci is by giving a DC shock across the chest.

Cardiac pacemakers

In some disorders the sinus impulses reach the ventricle so slowly or irregularly that the patient can lose consciousness in the intervals between heartbeats (Stokes Adams attacks). Disorders such as this may be more satisfactorily treated by insertion of an electrical pacemaker than by drugs. Pacemakers act by delivering an electrical stimulus to the heart either at regular intervals or 'on demand' when the natural stimulus fails.

Treatment of ventricular fibrillation

This otherwise lethal condition is treated by electrical defibrillation. Electrodes and a conductive jelly are put over the sternum and near the apex of the heart, and a brief high voltage shock given. If a defibrillator is not available, an intravenous injection of lignocaine (1 mg/kg) may be tried.

If nothing better is available, one or two heavy blows on the sternum with the side of the fist has occasionally been successful.

SUGGESTED FURTHER READING

Anon 1987 Management of hyperlipidaemia. Drug and Therapeutics Bulletin 25: 89
Anon LA 1987 Beta-blockers and lipophilicity. Lancet i: 900
Anon 1987 Antibiotic treatment of infective endocarditis. Drug and Therapeutics Bulletin 25: 49
Anon 1988 Primary prevention of ischaemic heart disease with lipid-lowering drugs. Lancet i: 333
Anon 1988 Thrombolytic therapy for acute myocardial infarction – round 2. Lancet i: 565
Anon 1988 The treatment of mild hypertension. Drug and Therapeutics Bulletin 26: 5
Anon 1988 Fibrinolytic drugs in acute myocardial infarction. Drug and Therapeutics Bulletin 26: 45
Breckenridge A 1988 Angiotensin converting enzyme inhibitors. British Medical Journal 296: 618
The CONSENSUS Trial Study Group 1987. The effects of enalapril on severe congestive heart failure. New England Journal of Medicine 316: 1429
Desilivio A, Barlattani M P 1988 How best to use nitrates. British Medical Journal 295: 1163
Feely J, Pringle T, Maclean D 1988 Thrombolytic treatment

and new calcium antagonists. British Medical Journal 296: 705

Goldenberg I F 1987 New inotropic drugs for heart failure. Journal of the American Medical Association 258: 493

Ferlinz J 1986 Nifedipine in myocardial ischemia, systemic hypertension and other cardiovascular disorders. Annals of Internal Medicine 105: 714

Frohlich E D 1988 Beta-blockers and mental performance. Archives of Internal Medicine 148: 777

ISIS-1 Collaborative Group 1988 Mechanisms for the early mortality reduction produced by beta-blockades started early in acute myocardial infarction: ISIS-1. Lancet i: 291

Jones R M 1987 Calcium, its agonists and antagonists, past, present and future. Journal of the Royal Society of Medicine 80: 136

Mason J W 1987 Amiodarone. New England Journal of Medicine 316: 455

Moser M 1986 Treating hypertension. A review of clinical trials. American Journal of Medicine 81 (suppl 6C): 25

Oates J A, Wood A J J (1987) Mexiletine. New England Journal of Medicine 316: 29

Orme M 1988 Aspirin all round? British Medical Journal 296: 307

Peters R W 1987 Beta-blockers and mortality after myocardial infarction. Archives of Internal Medicine 147: 33

Peto R, Gray R, Collins R et al 1988 Randomised trial of prophylactic daily aspirin in British male doctors. British Medical Journal 296: 313

Relman A S 1988 Aspirin for the primary prevention of myocardial infarction. New England Journal of Medicine 318: 245

Robertson J I S 1987 The large studies in hypertension: what have they shown? British Journal of Clinical Pharmacology 24: 3S

Smith T W 1988 Digitalis. Mechanisms of action and clinical use. New England Journal of Medicine 318: 358

Somberg J C, Tepper D 1986 Flecainide: a new antiarrhythmic agent. American Heart Journal 112: 808

Woosley R L 1988 Indications for antiarrhythmic therapy: a wealth of controversy, a dearth of data. Annals of Internal Medicine 108: 450

UK-TIA Study Group 1988 United Kingdom transient ischaemic attack (UK-TIA) aspirin trial: interim results. British Medical Journal 296: 316

11. The respiratory system

Breathing is an apparently simple process by which oxygen is taken in and carbon dioxide eliminated by the lungs, but its control is complex. Drugs may affect the central nervous control of respiration or they may act on the lung itself.

Drugs which depress respiration

The narcotic analgesics (opioids)

Central depression of respiration is caused by the narcotic (opioid) analgesics to a varying degree. Thus, morphine, heroin and pethidine produce a considerable reduction in the rate and depth of respiration and inhibition of the cough reflex. Codeine is a weaker analgesic and cough suppressant but is nevertheless useful in clinical practice. Methadone, pentazocine and phenazocine when first used were thought to cause less respiratory depression, but using doses equi-analgesic to the older drugs have been found to produce a similar degree of respiratory inhibition.

The respiratory effects of these drugs appear to be due to their action in diminishing the sensitivity of the respiratory centre to carbon dioxide. Normally, carbon dioxide is a very potent physiological stimulus to breathing and the opioid drugs reduce its effectiveness at this site in the brain.

Depression of respiration caused by the narcotics is an undesirable side-effect when these drugs are being used as analgesics. This side-effect can be used to advantage, however, when the narcotic analgesics are used to diminish respiratory effort in acute pulmonary oedema due to left ventricular failure or during assisted respiration with mechanical ventilators. Severe respiratory depression due to morphine and pethidine and also that due to pentazocine and phenazocine is reversed by naloxone.

Hypnotics

Respiratory depression is also caused by many of the hypnotic drugs – particularly barbiturates. Any central nervous depressant, including intravenous diazepam, may lead to a dangerous degree of hypoxia in patients suffering from respiratory insufficiency due to chronic lung disease such as asthma or chronic bronchitis and emphysema.

Respiratory stimulants

Carbon dioxide is the most important respiratory stimulant but occasionally drugs are used to stimulate breathing. If respiratory depression is due to opiate overdose, nalorphine or naloxone is normally effective. Respiratory depression due to overdose of hypnotic drugs or serious lung disease does not respond to or is made worse by the narcotic antagonists (such as nalorphine or naloxone), but nikethamide or doxapram may stimulate respiration to some degree. Nevertheless, the proper treatment of respiratory depression due to hypnotics, anaesthetics and tranquillisers, is positive pressure artificial respiration.

BRONCHIAL ASTHMA

Asthma is a disease characterised by attacks of reversible airway obstruction. Spasm of the bronchiolar smooth muscle contributes to the obstruction but there is also a considerable degree of

153

mucosal oedema and swelling together with plugging of bronchi by mucus.

Several factors may precipitate attacks of asthma in susceptible individuals. These include allergy, infection and psychological influences. The relative importance of each of these varies in different patients, but treatment may include the elimination of allergens, antibiotic therapy and palliation of psychological stresses. In addition, most asthmatic patients are treated with drugs which directly relieve the bronchial obstruction.

An important mechanism by which these factors produce airway obstruction is by the release of mediators from sensitised mast cells in the lungs. When these cells are exposed to specific antigens or other harmful stimuli, they release histamine, SRS-A (slow reacting substance anaphylaxis type – a mixture of leucotrienes, particularly LTC_4 and LTD_4), 5HT (serotonin) and some prostaglandins. Such chemicals produce bronchospasm, mucosal oedema and increased mucus secretion, all of which contribute to obstruction of the airways.

The drugs currently used for asthma include:

1. Sympathomimetic agents.
2. Anticholinergic agents.
3. Theophylline.
4. Sodium cromoglycate (Intal).
5. Corticosteroids.

Sympathomimetic agents

Sympathomimetic drugs of the β stimulator type – such as adrenaline and isoprenaline – are effective in relaxing bronchial smooth muscle, reducing submucosal oedema and reducing the liberation of mediators from mast cells.

Adrenaline is obsolete in asthma therapy because it has to be injected (subcutaneously) and also causes severe cardiac effects.

Isoprenaline can be absorbed from a sublingual tablet, but is more usually inhaled as an aerosol. By this route, even small doses are effective, little is absorbed into the circulation and the effect comes on quickly. However, isoprenaline stimulates not only β receptors in the bronchi (β_2 and thus relieves asthma) but also stimulates β receptors in the heart (β_1 and may thus cause tachycardia and increased myocardial excitability). A considerable overdose of

isoprenaline follows repeated use of an aerosol inhaler over a short space of time. Large amounts of isoprenaline thus absorbed into the circulation can precipitate dangerous cardiac arrhythmias and death has resulted from ventricular fibrillation.

Isoprenaline is rarely used now as a major drug in asthma and has been replaced by drugs which have a selective β_2 stimulant (bronchodilator) action and little effect on the heart. Such drugs are safer than isoprenaline in the treatment of asthma and include salbutamol (Ventolin) and terbutaline (Bricanyl).

Salbutamol is usually given as an aerosol in the control of chronic asthma. It can also be given intravenously for severe attacks when its relatively slight β_1 effects on the heart are an advantage.

Anticholinergic agents

Atropine-like drugs have long been used for the management of asthma until superseded by newer agents such as salbutamol which is both effective and lacks the unpleasant side-effects of anticholinergic drugs. *Ipratropium* (isopropyl atropine, Atrovent), however, is approximately as effective a bronchodilator as salbutamol and, unlike other anticholinergic drugs, does not appear to have a drying effect on the bronchial mucosa.

Ipratropium is useful, particularly in those patients who do not respond to sympathomimetic drugs such as salbutamol, in asthma associated with chronic bronchitis (p. 154).

Ipratropium is taken from an inhaler but its onset of action is delayed for 30–60 minutes. The duration of action is 3–4 hours and a dry mouth can be a troublesome side-effect.

Theophylline

Theophylline is a xanthine, similar to caffeine. It is a mild diuretic, a central stimulant and a cardiac stimulant; it also relaxes smooth muscle. Theophylline is very effective in terminating an attack of asthma when given by slow intravenous injection. Like the sympathomimetic drugs, theophylline relaxes smooth muscle and decreases mediator release from mast cells by raising their intracellular concentration of cyclic 3′, 5′-adenosine monophosphate (cAMP). The effects of theophylline on the heart are similar to those of adrenaline and when given rapidly can precipitate ventricular fibrillation which can be quickly fatal.

Theophylline is absorbed by mouth, but it is a gastric irritant and causes vomiting. When the substance is combined with another molecule – such as choline (as in choline theophyllinate, Choledyl) much more theophylline can be given by mouth without causing nausea.

Theophylline itself is poorly soluble in water and is combined with ethylene diamine in the preparation used for intravenous administration (aminophylline).

Theophylline has no theoretical advantages over more selective agents such as salbutamol and may be more dangerous. It has, however, withstood the test of time and many regard it apart from steroids as still the most effective drug for severe asthma. Experience has however confirmed that theophylline is less useful than newer drugs.

Sustained release preparations of aminophylline or theophylline are popular for the control of less severe but chronic asthma. The tablets are taken every 12 hours and are often effective for controlling nocturnal asthma when sodium cromoglycate fails.

The dose must be limited to the minimum needed to get the desired effect as these preparations can cause gastric irritation or mild central stimulation. There is an additive effect as well when selective β_2 adrenoreceptor stimulators such as salbutamol are also taken and there then may be a risk of producing severe cardiac arrhythmias.

Sodium cromoglycate (Intal)

This substance is not used to terminate an attack of asthma, but is taken prophylactically several times a day and is effective in reducing the frequency and severity of attacks. It acts by preventing release of chemical mediators of asthma and preventing other bronchoconstrictor mechanisms by stabilising mast cell vesicles and by blocking irritant-receptors in the respiratory mucosa. Thus, even when the patient is exposed to a specific allergen or to a chemical or physical irritant, histamine and leukotrienes (SRS-A) are not released and parasympathetic outflow is not increased. The drug is inhaled as a powder or solution. Side-effects seem to be negligible.

Ketotifen (Zaditen) is an antihistamine which has some sodium cromoglycate-like activity. It is taken orally and produces a dry mouth and sedation, and may have to be taken for 4 weeks or more before it produces its full prophylactic affect.

Corticosteroids

When asthma is so severe that no other agent gives relief, steroids such as hydrocortisone or prednisolone are used. These may be given in large doses for a short period to terminate a severe, prolonged and refractory attack or in small doses for a long period to reduce the frequency and severity of attacks. Hydrocortisone is administered intravenously in an emergency, while for acute or chronic therapy prednisolone is given in tablet form orally.

Prolonged use of steroids produces side-effects including oedema, hypertension, peptic ulceration, a moon-shaped face and aggravation of diabetes. In children, growth may be arrested. Treatment longer than 3 or 4 weeks may produce long-lasting adrenal suppression with consequent inability to withstand physical stress for up to 2 years after treatment is stopped. ACTH does not appear to arrest growth and does not cause adrenal suppression, but has to be injected and may produce sensitisation.

Local administration of corticosteroids to the lungs by inhalation of an aerosol reduces the severity of chronic asthma and greatly decreases systemic absorption of these drugs. Beclomethasone dipropionate, budesonide and betamethasone valerate are given in this way from pressurised, metered aerosol sprays and have helped in the management of severe chronic asthma. Proliferation of fungi, particularly candida (thrush), in the oropharynx and upper airway may complicate this type of treatment but this does not often seem to cause trouble.

It should be noted that there are about 2000 deaths a year from asthma in Britain, mainly as a result of undertreatment or of failing to recognise and deal with worsening of the disease. A few of these deaths may be accounted for by cardiac complications resulting from combined treatment with theophylline and β agonists.

Chronic bronchitis and emphysema

These two very common lung diseases frequently co-exist. They are the most common cause of chronic obstructive pulmonary disease (COPD), a term which well describes their main effects. In effect, the patient suffers from chronic inflammatory disease of the bronchi, varying degrees of airways obstruction due to progressive fibrosis and loss of effective alveolar diffusing surface. Bronchospasm is typically associated. This chronically progressive picture is punctuated by acute exacerbations of lung infection.

Chronic bronchitis is not curable, but the progress of the disease can be slowed by stopping smoking, avoiding cold and damp environments and treating the infection and bronchospasm.

Acute infections of the lungs superimposed on chronic disease can precipitate right-sided heart failure (cor pulmonale) and respiratory failure.

Respiratory failure develops when lung function is so severely disturbed that the blood oxygen content falls, the carbon dioxide content rises and the blood pH falls. The patient is in danger of dying from lack of oxygen and yet, paradoxically, giving 100% oxygen may dangerously depress respiration. This is because anoxia is the only remaining stimulus these patients have to breathe. Chronic intoxication with carbon dioxide, however, reduces the effectiveness of anoxia as a respiratory stimulant. In practice, the patient is encouraged to breathe deeply and cough forcibly – using stimulants such as nikethamide when necessary. Sedatives, hypnotics and opiates are absolutely contraindicated. Oxygen is given either intermittently or at a controlled concentration of 24–30% by using a Venturi mask.

The precipitating cause of this crisis is usually an infection. Sputum should be taken for culture and in the interim a broad-spectrum antibacterial such as co-trimoxazole, ampicillin, amoxycillin or tetracycline is given.

If there is bronchospasm, salbutamol or prednisolone is given. The presence of heart failure is an indication for giving a diuretic (such as chlorothiazide).

It is important to encourage the patient to cough up sputum, and physiotherapy can greatly assist this process. There is no clear evidence that expectorant drugs or mucolytics such as carbocisteine (carboxymethylcysteine) are of benefit.

Chronic obstructive pulmonary disease with its associated hypoxia is one of the few contraindications to the use of intravenous diazepam because it is a mild respiratory depressant.

Cardiac asthma

This is mentioned only to differentiate it from bronchial asthma. Cardiac asthma is an acute medical emergency since there is usually terrifying difficulty in breathing caused by waterlogging of the lungs (acute pulmonary oedema) which is the result of acute left ventricular failure. This in turn is often caused by a myocardial infarct, hypertension or valvular disease of the heart (see Ch. 10). The patient can (as with bronchial asthma) often only manage to breathe when sitting upright and an attempt to make a patient with cardiac asthma lie down is likely to be disastrous.

Cough suppressants

Suppression of coughing in patients with incipient respiratory failure or with excessive amounts of secretion in the lungs is harmful. Antitussive drugs may be indicated when the cough is painful or unproductive. The most commonly used drugs for this purpose are codeine and *pholcodine*; codeine linctus is very widely used to control an irritating cough remaining after a respiratory infection has subsided. Morphine, diamorphine, methadone and pethidine are very powerful cough suppressants but are not usually used for this purpose because of their high risk of dependence. Many sedatives, such as promethazine, are cough suppressants.

Expectorants are drugs which facilitate the production and expectoration of sputum. Although ammonium salts, potassium iodide, ipecacuanha and squill increase bronchial secretion when given in near emetic doses, they probably play no useful role in lung disease apart from a placebo effect.

Mixtures of sedatives and expectorants are widely used in the treatment of cough. A popular mixture is Benylin Expectorant, which contains the sedative antihistamine *diphenhydramine*, with ammonium chloride, sodium citrate and menthol in syrup and chloroform water.

SUGGESTED FURTHER READING

Anon 1988 Asthma in the preschool child. Drug and
  Therapeutics Bulletin 26: 21
Anon 1987 Antibiotics for exacerbations of chronic bronchitis?
  Lancet ii: 23
Drugs and Therapeutics Bulletin 1988 Chemotherapy of
  pulmonary tuberculosis in Britain. 26: 1
Flenley D C 1987 Should bronchodilators be combined in
  chronic bronchitis and emphysema? British Medical Journal
  295: 1160
Nelson H S 1986 Adrenergic therapy of bronchial asthma.
  Journal of Allergy and Clinical Immunology 77: 771
Newhouse M T, Dolovich M B 1986 Control of asthma by
  aerosols. New England Journal of Medicine 315: 870

Petty T L 1986 Rational respiratory therapy. New England
  Journal of Medicine 315: 317
Reed C E 1986 Aerosols in chronic airways obstruction. New
  England Journal of Medicine 315: 888
Reed C E 1986 New therapeutic approaches in asthma.
  Journal of Allergy and Clinical Immunology 77: 537
Scadding J G 1987 Asthma and bronchial reactivity. British
  Medical Journal 294: 1115
Sharp J T 1986 Theophylline in chronic obstructive
  pulmonary disease. Journal of Allergy and Clinical
  Immunology 78: 800
Sheller J R 1987 Review: asthma: emerging concepts and
  potential therapies. American Journal of the Medical Sciences
  293: 298

12. The blood

ANAEMIA

Anaemia is a group of disorders of which the essential feature is deficiency of haemoglobin. It is a common and important cause of oral symptoms, particularly sore tongue, angular stomatitis and occasionally recurrent aphthae. Oral symptoms may give the first hint of the presence of a deficiency state, but the mechanism of oral changes is unknown.

Iron

Iron deficiency is the most common cause of anaemia in the Western world.

Absorption and metabolism

The chief source of iron is meat and offal. It is mostly as ferric iron but ferrous iron is better absorbed. A reducing agent such as ascorbic acid helps to convert dietary iron into the ferrous form but must be given in large amounts to be useful.

Absorption of iron is chiefly from the upper small intestine where it is favoured by a relatively low pH.

Iron is actively transported through the intestinal mucosal cells to reach the plasma where it becomes bound to a globulin (transferrin) and carried to the bone marrow.

When the body iron levels are adequate, further absorption is inhibited. Iron absorption is also impaired by lack of gastric acid, by defects of intestinal absorption (malabsorption syndrome and coeliac disease) and by drugs which have a chelating action, particularly tetracycline.

Causes of iron deficiency

1. Chronic blood loss is the most common cause.
2. Defective absorption (as described above).
3. Pregnancy.
4. Dietary deficiency may contribute to these conditions, but is rarely the sole cause of hypochromic anaemia.

Effects of iron deficiency

Most obvious are a low haemoglobin (less than 12 g/100 ml) together with overt signs and symptoms common to all types of anaemia. The anaemia is characteristically hypochromic and microcytic and is preceded and accompanied by depletion of storage iron in the marrow, a low serum iron (sideropenia) and a raised total iron binding capacity (TIBC) in the serum.

Surprisingly perhaps, symptoms – particularly soreness of the tongue – can be caused by sideropenia before the haemoglobin level falls below the lower limit of normal. In more severe cases there may be atrophy of the epithelium of the dorsum of the tongue which becomes smooth and red. This form of glossitis is characteristic of severe anaemia and, although it may be associated with angular stomatitis, the rest of the oral mucosa usually appears normal. This change is a striking illustration of the way iron deficiency (and sometimes other types of anaemia) has an atrophic effect on the oral epithelium and that this effect is remarkably selective.

Iron deficiency also increases susceptibility to infection and should always be looked for in patients with persistent *Candida albicans* infection of the mouth or elsewhere.

Iron therapy

Iron should be given only when there is a demonstrable deficiency. It is not otherwise a tonic, as was at one time thought.

Oral iron preparations. Ferrous salts are used. They may cause gastrointestinal discomfort or constipation and should be taken after a meal. Ferrous sulphate is the traditional preparation, but other salts such as the gluconate and fumarate are used in the hope of reducing gastrointestinal irritation.

The response to oral iron is slow, as only a relatively small proportion is absorbed; treatment should always be continued for several months.

It should go without saying that in addition to giving iron, the cause of the deficiency – particularly any source of bleeding – must be sought.

Injectable iron preparations. These are used when oral administration fails. The response is rapid and the depleted iron stores are replenished.

Intramuscular iron (iron dextran) sometimes causes reactions such as nausea, dizziness and headaches. There is also suspicion that it may be carcinogenic and (rarely) sarcomas have been reported several years after its administration.

Intravenous iron preparations do not have this danger but, unless given in a slow infusion, can cause severe and occasionally fatal reactions resembling anaphylaxis.

Toxic effects. Heavy doses of iron can cause severe gut irritation. Absorption of larger amounts can cause cardiovascular collapse and damage to brain and liver. This may happen to a child who takes a handful of brightly coloured iron tablets. The results can be fatal.

Vitamin B_{12}; cyanocobalamin

Vitamin B_{12} is essential for normal blood formation and deficiency causes pernicious anaemia ('pernicious', because, in the past it was fatal). In addition to anaemia, this disease is characterised by atrophic changes in the gastric mucosa and, if untreated, degenerative changes in the spinal cord and peripheral nerves (subacute combined degeneration).

As in the case of iron deficiency, early deficiency of B_{12} can occasionally cause soreness of the tongue before the haemoglobin falls. The reason for this curiously selective effect is not known.

The main source of B_{12} is meat and particularly liver if not too well cooked. Dietary deficiency can develop, but surprisingly rarely, in total and uncompromising vegetarians (vegans) who eat no animal products of any sort.

Apart from this last case and some other rare exceptions, vitamin B_{12} deficiency anaemia is not a dietary deficiency but a defect of absorption. As a result of atrophic changes in the stomach in pernicious anaemia, Intrinsic Factor is not secreted. Extrinsic Factor (vitamin B_{12}) is not therefore absorbed. Since this is the basis of the disease, B_{12} is not effective orally and has to be given by intramuscular injection. Gastric mucosal atrophy also causes absolute failure of acid secretion and this is one of the diagnostic criteria of the disease.

Deficiency of vitamin B_{12} affects all blood cells and, although the effect on the red cells is the most prominent and important, the formation of white cells and platelets is also depressed.

Vitamin B_{12} therapy

Hydroxycobalamin should be given only when the diagnosis of pernicious anaemia has been confirmed, by marrow biopsy, by detecting low serum vitamin B_{12} levels, by testing gastric function and by testing the absorption of a minute dose of B_{12}. This is necessary as B_{12} will produce some response in folic acid deficiency and once given interferes with diagnosis for some time.

Hydroxycobalamin is given intramuscularly since it is excreted less quickly and is preferable as it reduces the frequency of administration. Injections are given twice weekly at first, then when the body stores have been made up, maintenance doses are given at intervals of 2–4 weeks for the rest of the patient's life.

Folic acid

Folic acid deficiency is, in Britain, the next most common cause of macrocytic anaemia to B_{12} deficiency.

Folic acid is present in plant leaves (*folium* = a

leaf) but has to be converted into a biologically active product after absorption. It is an essential requirement for production of DNA by man, animals and microorganisms. Some of the latter, however, synthesise folic acid from simpler compounds and it is by interference with this process that sulphonamides and trimethoprim have their antibacterial effect.

Causes of folic acid deficiency

1. **Pregnancy.**
2. **Malabsorption syndromes.**
3. **Drug-induced.** The main example is prolonged use of phenytoin, but only a small minority of patients so treated seem to be susceptible. Cotrimoxazole can in theory, and on rare occasions does, cause folic acid deficiency.

Some folic acid antagonists (e.g. methotrexate) are cytotoxic drugs given to suppress white cell production in the treatment of acute leukaemia.

4. **Alcohol.** An important cause of folate deficiency is alcoholism, which should be suspected in any adult where no other cause can be found. Liver function tests should also be carried out, as disordered function as a result of cirrhosis may be associated and, if so, alcohol is almost certain to be the cause.

Conversely, if a patient is suspected of being an alcoholic, macrocytosis should be looked for as it is a very early sign.

Folic acid therapy

Folic acid should be given (a) when there is evidence of folic acid deficiency and (b) when pernicious anaemia has been excluded. Both pernicious anaemia and folic acid deficiency produce a macrocytic anaemia with similar changes in the peripheral blood and marrow. One means of distinguishing them is to assay the plasma B_{12} and folic acid levels. This is important because, if folic acid is mistakenly given to a patient with pernicious anaemia there is at first partial improvement in the blood picture, but degenerative changes in the nervous system due to B_{12} deficiency are accelerated. Folic acid should not therefore be given to a patient with pernicious anaemia. On the other hand, when there is severe malabsorption due to

gastrointestinal disease both B_{12} and folic acid deficiency may develop. In this case both drugs have to be given.

As with iron and B_{12}, latent folic acid deficiency can cause oral symptoms, particularly sore tongue and sometimes angular stomatitis or recurrent aphthae.

Drug-induced anaemia

Anaemia alone is a rare, direct toxic effect of drugs but is common as a secondary consequence of drugs such as aspirin, which frequently cause chronic blood loss with prolonged use.

Drug-induced anaemia is more commonly only a component of pancytopenia (aplastic anaemia) caused by a variety of marrow poisons as discussed later.

Methyldopa can however cause haemolytic anaemia and the antiviral drug zidovudine can cause megaloblastic anaemia. Nitrous oxide also interferes with vitamin B_{12} metabolism but even with very prolonged usage nervous system damage rather than anaemia is the chief effect (see Ch. 8).

As mentioned earlier, phenytoin and (largely theoretically) co-trimoxazole can interfere with folic acid metabolism and also cause megaloblastic anaemia.

DISORDERS OF WHITE CELLS

Leukaemia

Leukaemia is a malignant tumour of immature leucocytes.

The overproduction of immature and defective leucocytes overwhelms the normal functions of the marrow and production of other blood cells is depressed. The main effects differ in degree according to the type of leukaemia and stage of the disease, but are as follows:

1. **Anaemia.** This is invariable and is a common cause of death.
2. **Infection.** This is the consequence of defective function of the immature or primitive granulocytes. The effects are sometimes seen strikingly in the mouth because the leukaemic patient may be unable to resist the low-grade infection at the

gingival margins and this can cause severe necrotising ulceration. As described below, the risk of infection is often made worse by the effects of treatment.

3. Bleeding. This is the result of platelet deficiency, causing purpura, and in some cases haemorrhage is severe.

Drugs used in the treatment of leukaemia

Antitumour agents are cytotoxic and are described in more detail in Chapter 14. It must also be emphasised here, however, that these drugs are not specific in their actions and are toxic to all dividing cells in varying degree. These drugs are therefore an important cause of leucopenia. Since many are also immunosuppressive in their cytotoxic action on lymphocytes, they can severely depress cell mediated immunity. As a consequence infection (particularly fungal infection) is now one of the main causes of death.

Cytotoxic chemotherapy, usually with a combination of agents, nevertheless often induces at least a remission of symptoms and in the case of acute lymphocytic leukaemia in childhood has apparently achieved cures.

Patients with acute leukaemia, particularly monocytic leukaemia, are prone to severe oral infections. These may be the first sign of the disease, but the problem is also made worse in many cases by treatment with antitumour drugs.

The main principles of treatment of leukaemia in general are therefore:

1. Antitumour agents. These are selected according to the cell type involved (see Ch. 14).

2. Antibiotics and antifungal agents.

3. Blood transfusions to combat anaemia and haemorrhage.

Leucopenia and agranulocytosis

Leucopenia is an abnormally low white cell count, usually of polymorphonuclear leucocytes (neutrophils).

Agranulocytosis is a clinical term used to describe a condition characterised by severe necrotising infections typically of the mouth and throat second-ary to a severe deficiency of neutrophil leucocytes.

The most common cause of neutropenia is severe infection but the main causes can be summarised as follows:

1. Certain infections (typhoid, viral, rickettsial or overwhelming bacterial infections).

2. Acute leukaemia. Neutrophil production may be overwhelmed by invasion of the marrow by leukaemic cells. In myelogenous leukaemia neutrophils are overproduced but there are few mature functional granulocytes, the vast bulk of the cells being primitive and defective. In any type of leukaemia there may also be a phase of arrest of release of white cells from the marrow into the blood (aleukaemic leukaemia).

3. Irradiation. Lymphocytes are the most sensitive cells. Heavier dosage can cause neutropenia or total arrest of marrow activity.

4. Drugs. These are usually the same as those which may cause aplastic anaemia.

5. There is increasing evidence that aplastic anaemia can be autoimmune in nature.

The Acquired Immune Deficiency Syndrome (AIDS)

AIDS is an increasingly common cause of leukopenia, immunodeficiency and lethal opportunistic infections. Increasing numbers of antiviral and other drugs are used for its treatment. As yet only zidovudine (see Ch. 3) has been convincingly shown to be of benefit, but it too can cause bone marrow depression and anaemia.

Drug-induced leucopenia and aplastic anaemia

The main groups of drugs which depress marrow function include the following:

1. Antitumour (cytotoxic) and immunosuppressive agents. These, in large doses or in susceptible patients, can cause widespread marrow damage. In higher dosage many of these drugs are used as immunosuppressive agents by depressing antibody synthesis or by a lymphocytotoxic action (see Ch. 14).

Corticosteroids cause lymphocytopenia (and hence are used in the treatment of acute lymphocyte leukaemia) and by contrast a neutrophil leuco-cytosis.

2. **Antibacterial agents.**
   Chloramphenicol.*
   Sulphonamides (rarely).
   Co-trimoxazole.
   Arsenicals.
3. **Analgesics.**
   Amidopyrine.*
   Phenylbutazone* and its analogues (amido-pyrine derivatives).
4. **Antidiabetic and antithyroid agents** (often sulphonamide derivatives).
   Tolbutamide (rarely).
   Thiouracil and its analogues.
5. **Metals.**
   Gold salts (used in the treatment of rheumatoid arthritis).

Those drugs marked* are particularly dangerous. Amidopyrine is now no longer used in Britain while chloramphenicol is (or should be) used only where there is no safer substitute.

Until recently therefore, the most common cause of agranulocytosis, in Britain, was the anti-inflammatory analgesic phenylbutazone and its analogues. As a consequence they are no longer generally prescribable.

Co-trimoxazole is reported to be the most common cause of agranulocytosis (neutropenia) in Britain. This however may be to some extent a reflection of its scale of use, as (paradoxically) it is also widely regarded as the prophylactic antimicrobial of choice in deeply immunosuppressed bone marrow transplant patients.

The line of white cells which respond earliest to these toxic effects is unpredictable. When neutropenia is the first sign, it may be reversible by stopping the drug.

If the white cell count starts to fall it may be possible to arrest the process by immediate withdrawal of the drug. In other cases, particularly with chloramphenicol, purpura due to platelet deficiency is often the first sign of pancytopenia (aplastic anaemia) which follows rapidly and is often irreversible.

The mechanism of production of aplastic anaemia, whether due to chloramphenicol or of unknown cause, remains obscure but appears to be immunologically mediated in some cases.

Management of drug-induced leucopenia or aplastic anaemia

The main principles are:

1. To stop all drugs being taken or at least to stop that which is most likely to be the cause.
2. To give non-toxic antibiotics as necessary to deal with any infections.
3. To give blood transfusions, to combat anaemia or haemorrhagic tendencies.
4. Possibly to give androgenic steroids. Their usefulness is not certain.
5. Possibly to give a marrow transplant.

HAEMORRHAGIC DISEASE

Normal haemostasis

The blood has self-protective properties which prevent or help to prevent excessive loss after injuries.

Haemostasis is a complex process but has two chief components:

1. **Formation of a platelet plug.** This takes place very rapidly. The adherence of the platelets to the damaged endothelium at the edges of the wound and to one another to form thrombus, together with contraction and retraction of the vessel, stop bleeding from a puncture wound within a few minutes.

It is this mechanism which enables the haematologist to take blood from a haemophiliac without starting intractable haemorrhage. Defects in the mechanism are caused by deficiency or defective function of platelets. Defects of the vessels themselves are a rare cause of purpura.

2. **Clotting.** Final arrest of bleeding depends on the conversion of circulating fibrinogen to solid fibrin. This is a relatively slow process, but effectively seals relatively large wounds and provides the scaffolding in which granulation tissue forms.

The clotting process depends on a cascade of interactions, a slightly simplified view of which is shown in Figure 12.1.

Systemic causes of haemorrhagic tendencies can be summarised as follows:

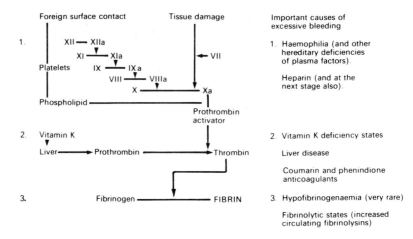

The diagram indicates the complexity of the sequence of events leading up to clotting to show
in particular the main areas where deficiencies or drugs may interfere with the process.
(The precise sequence of interaction of the individual plasma factors is of little importance
in the present context.)

Fig. 12.1   The clotting mechanism and areas of action of some hereditary and acquired haemorrhagic diseases

1. **Purpura.**
   a. Idiopathic thrombocytopenic purpura (some-times an effect of AIDS).
   b. Leukaemia.
   c. Drug-induced purpura.
   d. Vascular defects: (i) hereditary; (ii) toxic (drugs, infections, immune mechanisms).
2. **Clotting defects.**
   a. Hereditary deficiency of plasma clotting factors.
   b. Prothrombin deficiency: (i) vitamin K deficiency; (ii) liver disease; (iii) anticoagulants
   c. Fibrinogen deficiency.
3. **Fibrinolytic syndromes.**

In addition to those listed, there are other conditions which (like hypofibrinogenaemia) are very rare and will not be considered further.

The fibrinolytic system

In addition to the haemostatic mechanisms, there is another system having the reverse effect. This is the activation of plasminogen to plasmin which serves primarily to lyse small clots within the vessels to maintain their patency. Occasionally activation of the fibrinolytic system may cause or contribute to excessive bleeding as discussed in more detail later.

Dental haemorrhage

By far the most common cause of prolonged bleeding after dental extractions is excessive tissue damage, which is local in origin. Although local causes account for most cases of dental haemorrhage, systemic causes are more important, in that bleeding may be intractable and endanger life (as in haemophilia) or may be due to a disease such as leukaemia which is itself lethal.

DRUGS WHICH AFFECT HAEMOSTASIS

Dental procedures frequently result in the shedding of blood and in the case of extractions, control of bleeding can be difficult. Knowledge of the effects of drugs on haemostasis are therefore particularly important in dentistry.

Since haemostasis is an essential mechanism to protect against excessive blood loss, it would seem to be highly desirable that it should work with maximal efficiency. However, there are occasions when clotting or the build-up of platelet thrombi needs to be limited to prevent (for example) blockage of the coronary arteries or to prevent pulmonary embolism. Otherwise, depressed haemostasis is an unwanted and sometimes dangerous toxic effect of a variety of drugs.

Drugs can therefore depress haemostasis or, in other cases, improve it.

Drugs can be used either:

1. To improve haemostasis when there is a haemorrhagic tendency as in haemophilia or purpura.

2. To interfere with haemostasis, particularly to combat thrombotic disorders (see also Ch. 10). Such drugs (as discussed later) comprise three main groups, namely:
   a. Anticoagulants.
   b. Antiplatelet drugs.
   c. Fibrinolytic agents.

Yet other drugs can interfere with haemostasis as an undesired side-effect.

PURPURA

Although there is a considerable degree of interaction between platelets and clotting factors, purpura and the coagulation defects typically form distinct entities which have to be managed in different ways.

Purpura is characterised by subcutaneous bleeding which forms minute petechiae or gross ecchymoses. These tend to form where there is pressure – often very slight – on the skin. Alternatively, there may be complaint of spontaneous bruising. In the mouth ecchymoses may form under a denture, especially under the post-dam line, or there may be gross gingival bleeding either spontaneous or following toothbrushing.

1. Idiopathic thrombocytopenic purpura (ITP)

This disease is characterised by increased destruction of platelets and is autoimmune in nature. The platelets are probably sensitised by circulating platelet-specific IgG, making them susceptible to destruction and removal by splenic macrophages. The most satisfactory method of treatment is splenectomy and this is curative in 70–80% of cases.

Corticosteroids are also effective, but are used for ITP only if splenectomy is ineffective or contraindicated, and for preoperative assessment.

If both splenectomy and corticosteroids fail, then immunosuppressive agents can be used. However, in a minority of patients (10–20%) the disease is unresponsive to any of these forms of treatment.

It is important not to give aspirin (because of its ability to inhibit platelet aggregation) to patients with ITP.

ITP can also be a manifestation of AIDS in which autoimmune complications can be a feature.

2. Acute leukaemia

Suppression of all other marrow cells by the proliferating stem cell can lead to gross platelet deficiency. Purpura may be an early sign of acute leukaemia and the combination of purpura with anaemia in a young person is a clinical picture which should cause serious concern. When purpura is a major feature the bleeding tendency may respond to cytotoxic therapy (see Ch. 14) but transfusion is likely to be necessary if bleeding becomes severe.

3. Drug-induced purpura

There are two main ways by which purpura can be caused by drug treatment.

There may be:

a. Thrombocytopenia (alone). This is probably immunologically mediated.

b. Aplastic anaemia in which there is total depression of the bone marrow but where the deficiency of platelets may often be the cause of early signs or be so severe that bleeding dominates the clinical picture.

a. Drug-dependent thrombocytopenia. Examples of drugs capable of causing purpura as a toxic effect include
   Apronal (Sedormid – an obsolete hypnotic)
   Sulphonamides
   Some beta-lactam antibiotics
   Quinine and quinidine
   Sulphonamides
   Thiazide diuretics

The probable mechanism in most cases is that a drug–antibody complex binds to the platelet surface and leads to immunologically mediated platelet destruction.

Antibiotics which can interfere with platelet

aggregation are the antipseudomonal penicillins, carbenicillin and ticarcillan, and the cephalosporin, latamoxef.

Corticosteroids can often lessen the severity of the purpura by interfering with the effects of the antigen–antibody reaction, but it is necessary also to stop giving the drug.

b. Purpura in drug-induced aplastic anaemia. Marrow aplasia is a dangerous complication which in some cases proves to be irreversible. The important causes of drug-induced aplastic anaemia and leucopenia have been described earlier. Haemorrhage due to platelet deficiency is sometimes an early sign of marrow damage due to chloramphenicol for example and is often an indication of rapidly progressive aplasia with the probability of a fatal termination. The management is also as described earlier, namely to stop the causative drug immediately and to give whole blood or platelet concentrates if bleeding is severe.

4. Vascular defects

True vascular defects are a very rare cause of significant purpura. Vascular purpura is probably most common in patients, particularly the elderly, on prolonged corticosteroid therapy. Depression of protein production by the steroid causes weakening of the vessel walls.

Purpura is one of the main features of scurvy – an exceedingly rare disease – but vitamin C deficiency affects platelet function to at least as great a degree. Purpura can also be an allergic reaction to drugs.

DISORDERS OF CLOTTING

1. Hereditary defects

These for all practical purposes affect only the plasma factors which interact to activate prothrombin, i.e. the earlier stages of the cascade. Haemophilia A (factor VIII deficiency) and B (factor IX deficiency – Christmas disease) are by far the most common and most important of this group of diseases. In haemophilia the specific plasma factor is formed but is defective in structure and unable to function normally.

Haemophilia

Both haemophilia A and B are inherited as sex-linked recessive traits and are clinically identical. The gene is transmitted on the X chromosome but only males show the disease. Haemophilia A ('classical' haemophilia) is more common and more difficult to manage.

Management of haemophilia. Extractions are a major hazard in haemophilia and an essential aspect of the management of haemophilia is regular, meticulous dental care to reduce the need for extractions. However, local anaesthetic injections, especially inferior dental blocks, can also be a hazard, particularly for severe haemophiliacs. The needle can tear the wall of a small vessel and cause a deep, spreading haematoma which can threaten the airway. Although submucous infiltrations are frequently given without complications, the risk is still there and it may be safer as a general policy, to use nitrous oxide analgesia and avoid the use of local anaesthetics.

Management of extractions. Surgery must be carefully planned to avoid complications and preoperative radiographs must be taken to show any unsuspected disease which may add to the problems.

The severity of the disease must also be assessed by laboratory tests of haemostatic function and factor VIII assay. Haemoglobin estimation, blood grouping and cross-matching should also be carried out.

For the operation the patient should be admitted to hospital and reconstituted freeze-dried or synthetic factor VIII concentrate given intravenously 1 hour before the operation. Enough factor VIII should be given for dental extractions to raise the level to 50–75% of normal. In addition, the antifibrinolytic drug tranexamic acid (see below) is given intravenously or by mouth 24 hours preoperatively. More factor VIII may need to be given if there is an unusual degree of trauma and administration of factor VIII also needs to be continued postoperatively for more major surgery.

Usually the patient should be kept in hospital for a week after extractions and given oral tranexamic acid four times a day. To avoid the risk of infection and breakdown of the clot, oral penicillin should also be given. If bleeding starts again, more factor VIII has to be given.

Factor VIII concentrate is, incidentally, heat-treated to prevent the transmission of hepatitis and HIV. However, as a result of previous administration of blood or untreated factor, many haemophiliacs have impaired liver function or are carriers of hepatitis B. The more unfortunate ones have acquired or died from AIDS or are carriers of this virus.

Management of haemophilia B (Christmas disease). Clinically, Christmas disease does not differ from haemophilia A and the management is along the same principles. Replacement is by factor IX concentrate given intravenously.

Von Willebrand's disease

Von Willebrand's disease which is heritable as an autosomal dominant trait is less common than haemophilia. It is a complex disorder in which there is a deficiency of factor VIII as well as a platelet defect. Usually, however, the main clinical manifestation is purpura and the clotting defect is insignificant. In those cases where the factor VIII deficiency is severe, replacement with factor VIII concentrate is necessary, as in haemophilia, but less frequent infusions are required. In many cases, desmopressin alone may be adequate.

Fibrinolysis and antifibrinolytic drugs

The clotting process is an essential mechanism to prevent excessive loss of blood. At sites of intravascular endothelial damage however, minute thrombi form but are normally prevented from propagating and occluding vessels, by the fibrinolytic system. Fibrinolysis is brought about by the proteolytic enzyme, plasmin, produced by activation of circulating plasminogen. In normal haemostasis therefore, there is balance between the haemostatic and fibrinolytic processes.

Excessive fibrinolytic activity can occasionally cause severe haemorrhage. It is most often a complication of some major surgical or obstetric procedures, some chronic illnesses, snake bite or, rarely, drugs. Fibrinolysis alone, however, is rarely a cause of excessive bleeding but a case has been reported of gingival bleeding as the first sign of fibrinolytic disease, due (in that case) to alcoholism. Treatment with an antifibrinolytic agent was successful.

In haemophilia however, even normal fibrinolytic activity may be undesirable as there is a tendency for lysis of such little clot as forms. Antifibrinolytic agents which act by inhibiting the activation of plasmin, are therefore useful supplements to and lessen the requirements for factor replacement, as mentioned earlier.

Tranexamic acid is a synthetic antifibrinolytic agent. It is more potent and has fewer side-effects than its earlier but now obsolete analogue, aminocaproic acid. Tranexamic acid alone may be adequate for simple extractions in haemophilia or von Willebrand's disease but is more widely used to supplement replacement of the missing factor.

Antifibrinolytic agents have also been used with varying success for a variety of other haemorrhagic disorders, such as menorrhagia, cerebral haemorrhage and severe epistaxis as well as in fibrinolytic states.

Desmopressin

Desmopressin (DDAVP), an analogue of posterior pituitary vasopressin, corrects the haemostatic defect in mild haemophilia by inducing the release of endogenous factor VIII C (procoagulant factor VIII) and von Willebrand factor. Desmopressin is being increasingly used, therefore, in some centres for the management of mild haemophiliacs and patients with von Willebrand's disease for such operations as dental extractions.

Desmopressin is given by slow intravenous injection, but since it also liberates plasminogen activator from endothelial cells it should be followed immediately by tranexamic acid to inhibit the enhanced fibrinolytic activity.

Desmopressin is also useful for patients who have developed antibodies against factor VIII and has the very important advantage that it can often replace blood products which can transmit hepatitis or AIDS.

The other use of desmopressin is for the treatment of diabetes insipidus.

2. Prothrombin deficiency

Vitamin K (phytomenadione) is a fat-soluble vitamin synthesised naturally by the bacteria of the gut. It is necessary for the formation of prothrombin and other clotting factors by the liver. Acetomenaphthone is a synthetic water-soluble analogue which can be given by mouth.

Deficiency of vitamin K or defective prothrombin synthesis can develop in or as a consequence of:

a. The newborn where the normal gut microflora has not yet established itself (haemorrhagic disease of the newborn).

b. Suppression of gut flora by prolonged broad spectrum antibiotic treatment.

c. Certain malabsorption syndromes.

d. Obstructive jaundice. Absence of bile from the intestine prevents vitamin K absorption.

e. Chronic liver disease where synthesis of clotting factors is impaired (described below).

f. Treatment with anticoagulants.

Vitamin K deficiency

True deficiency (as opposed to failure of absorption) of vitamin K is for all practical purposes a problem affecting only the newborn. It is hardly ever the result of destruction of the gut flora by broad spectrum antibiotics. Hypoprothrombinaemia in the newborn is treated by giving vitamin K (phytomenadione) by injection.

For deficiency due to malabsorption, vitamin K is given orally in the form of *menadiol*, daily.

Liver disease

The liver is the site of production of prothrombin and other clotting factors but not antihaemophilic factor. Hepatic disorders affecting clotting function fall into two main groups; (i) vitamin K-dependent functions, and (ii) hepatocellular disease which affects all synthetic activities.

Vitamin K-dependent functions. Obstructive jaundice with lack of bile salts prevents absorption of fat-soluble vitamin K. This causes reduced synthesis of prothrombin and some other clotting factors (VII, IX and X). When vitamin K cannot, for such a reason as this, be absorbed from the gut a water-soluble analogue, acetomenaphthone, can be given by mouth and is effective.

Liver disease. When liver function is severely impaired by hepatocellular disease such as advanced cirrhosis, synthesis of many clotting factors, including that of prothrombin from vitamin K, is depressed. The administration of vitamin K is ineffective when the liver is no longer capable of prothrombin synthesis. Bleeding tendencies can be counteracted only by giving whole blood which contains the missing factors.

Anticoagulants

As discussed earlier (p. 144), anticoagulants are used to prevent thrombotic complications in a variety of circumstances but particularly deep vein thrombosis and for cardiovascular surgery. The coumarin derivatives (especially warfarin) are the main drugs used for long-term anticoagulation and act by antagonising the effects of vitamin K. The formation of prothrombin (and some other clotting factors) in the liver is thus depressed. When excessive doses are given the patient may have spontaneous bleeding. In addition, several drugs potentiate the action of anticoagulants in a variety of ways. Chloral and sulphonamides are examples of drugs which increase the level of active anticoagulant by displacing it from plasma protein binding sites.

Dental management of patients on anticoagulants. Dosage of anticoagulants seems usually to be kept to relatively modest levels (about $2 \times$ the control prothrombin time or, more strictly, the International Normalised Ratio or INR). Dental bleeding from this cause is rarely a problem unless the patient takes the tablets irregularly and has a widely fluctuating response. When clotting is delayed by the action of anticoagulants, but dental surgery has to be carried out, the dose should be reduced by the physician only if the prothrombin time is excessively prolonged. The patient should not be told to stop treatment entirely. This carries with it at least a theoretical risk of 'rebound' thrombosis. For the same reasons vitamin K, which antagonises the anticoagulants, should not be given. The only indication for its use in patients on anticoagulants is for otherwise uncontrollable, life-threatening bleeding after surgery.

Tranexamic acid may be adequate to control minor external bleeding and allows anticoagulant treatment to be continued.

Anticoagulant therapy is a contraindication to the prescribing of aspirin. It may also be (with other haemorrhagic defects) one of the few indications for giving antibiotics for minor acute dental infections such as a periapical abscess to allow extractions to be postponed until the haemorrhagic tendency can be controlled.

By contrast other drugs, particularly carbamazepine, lead to increased metabolism and diminished activity of anticoagulants such as warfarin. This is because such drugs stimulate metabolising enzymes in the liver. Hence the dose of warfarin may have to be increased to achieve the same effect. Alternatively, if the administration of the interacting drug is stopped the anticoagulant action will be suddenly enhanced.

Heparin is a complex mucopolysaccharide which, when injected, has an immediate anticoagulant effect by inhibiting the activation of factor X and formation of thrombin. It is not antagonised by vitamin K or its analogues.

Heparin acts for only about 6 hours. Dental surgery can therefore be carried out on a renal dialysis patient on the day after heparin was given and dialysis performed The benefits from the dialysis are then almost maximal and the effects of the heparin will have completely worn off.

Antibiotic-associated hypoprothrombinaemia

Antibiotics such as tetracycline and metronidazole can destroy the gut bacteria responsible for synthesizing vitamin K if dosage is heavy and prolonged. Hypoprothrombinaemia from this cause is rare.

Hypoprothrombinaemia and bleeding can also result from interference with vitamin K metabolism by some of the newer cephalosporins such as cephamandole and latamoxef. Those mainly at risk are the elderly and those with impaired renal function, malnutrition or who have had recent intestinal surgery. If these antibiotics have to be used in such patients vitamin K supplementation may be necessary.

Anticoagulants and antiplatelet drugs

The uses of drugs, such as heparin, the coumarins, aspirin and dipyridamole in thrombotic disease have been discussed in Chapter 10 in relation to thrombotic disorders.

Fibrinolytic agents

Fibrinolytic agents are used for life-threatening thrombotic events or emboli but to be effective must be given immediately after the diagnosis has been made.

Enzymes such as streptokinase and urokinase act by activating circulating plasminogen to form plasmin which is fibrinolytic. Allergic reactions are a hazard and the drug has an anticoagulant effect as a result of neutralisation of circulating plasmin and some clotting factors.

A recent advance is the introduction of *tissue plasminogen activator* which acts locally at the site of thrombus formation since it has a low affinity for circulating plasminogen but a high affinity in the presence of fibrin. More effective still is *acylated plasminogen streptokinase activated complex (AP-SAC)*, which if given intravenously within 6 hours of a heart attack may reduce the mortality by nearly 50%.

SUMMARY: EFFECTS OF DRUGS ON HAEMOSTASIS

As mentioned earlier drugs can interfere with haemostasis, often as an undesirable toxic effect, and precipitate or worsen bleeding. Specific defects of haemostasis, notably haemophilia, can be controlled by replacement of missing haemostatic factors, and other types of haemorrhagic disease such as idiopathic thrombocytopenic purpura may also be controllable with appropriate drugs.

The main examples of drugs affecting haemostasis can be summarised as follows:

I. Drugs interfering with haemostasis
   1. Interference with prothrombin production (anticoagulants and some antibiotics).
   2. Interference with platelet function (aspirin and related drugs, and some antibiotics).
   3. Depression of platelet production (drugs which depress the bone marrow).
   4. Damage to vessel walls (corticosteroids).
   5. Fibrinolytic agents.
II. Drugs enhancing haemostasis
   1. Antihaemophilic and other clotting factors.

2. Vitamin K.
3. Antifibrinolytic agents.
4. Desmopressin.
5. Corticosteroids (for autoimmune thrombocytopenia).

Most of the agents which enhance haemostasis are specific in their action and only counter the corresponding defects.

Agents used locally to assist haemostasis

Mechanical aids. Cellulose, alginate, gelatine and fibrin foams are absorbable foams which provide a meshwork and an increased surface and help activate the clotting mechanism. They are not a substitute for suturing a persistently bleeding socket but a piece of one of these foams, cut to size, can be tucked gently into the socket before suturing.

Oxidised regenerated cellulose (Surgicel) is regarded as being the most generally useful of these products. It is easily handled and seems to have minimal toxicity or irritant properties. An important application is the arrest of primary haemorrhage from vessels in the socket wall. A piece of Surgicel is cut to size and layered against the bleeding area. Bleeding usually soon stops and there should be no need to suture the socket margin. In extreme cases it may be necessary to fill the socket lightly with Surgicel and suture the socket margins to prevent it from being extruded.

When bleeding is mainly from torn tissues at the socket margins, as is commonly the case, trimming the damaged bone edges and suturing the gum margins is the most effective management. Under such circumstances a layer of absorbable foam beneath the sutures probably contributes little.

Vasoconstrictors, adrenaline and noradrenaline

Submucous injection of vasoconstrictors will reduce bleeding from small vessels and may control superficial soft tissue haemorrhage. They are also used to obtain a 'bloodless field' for oral surgery. This may cause complications when halothane is used as the anaesthetic because this increases the sensitivity of the heart to catecholamines. Never-

theless the dangers are not quite so severe as they might seem, and if arrhythmias prove troublesome they can usually be controlled by giving a β blocker.

Vasoconstrictors will not control bleeding from the depths of an extraction socket and it is far quicker and more effective, as described earlier, to give a local anaesthetic and suture the socket. Superficial application of adrenaline on gauze to the wound is ineffective as the adrenaline is simply washed away and has no deep effect on the vessels. Adrenaline on silk floss is sometimes used to control gingival haemorrhage by tying the floss silk round the neck of the tooth and pushing it as deeply as possible under the gingival margin.

Astringents

Astringents, particularly tannic acid, are (or were) described as haemostatics since they precipitate protein from blood to form a semisolid mass. In an attempt to control dental bleeding of local origin tannic acid powder can be put on a pad of gauze under pressure. The usual result is that a sticky mass forms in and around the socket and is then pulled off with the pad. Rather than messing about in this way, the socket should be sutured under local anaesthesia.

SUGGESTED FURTHER READING

Anon 1988 Management of venous thromboembolism. Lancet i: 275
Anon 1986 Analgesics, agranulocytosis and aplastic anaemia: a major case-control study. Lancet ii: 899
Chapman P J, Macleod A W G 1987 The effects of diflunisal on bleeding time and platelet aggregation in a multidose study. International Journal of Oral and Maxillofacial Surgery 16: 448
Choay J, Petitou M 1986 The chemistry of heparin: a way to understand its mode of action. Medical Journal of Australia 144: HS7
Fitzgerald G A 1987 Dipyridamole. New England Journal of Medicine 316: 1247
Gralnick H R, Maisonneuve P, Sultan Y, Rick M 1985 Benefits of danazol treatment in patients with hemophilia A (classic hemophilia). Journal of the American Medical Association 253: 1151
Mohr D N, Ryu J H, Litin S C, Rosenow E C. Recent advances in the management of venous thromboembolism. Mayo clinic Proceedings 63: 281
Roeser H P 1987 Drug-bone marrow interactions. Medical Journal of Australia 146: 145

13. Drugs affecting allergic reactions and the immune response

Inflammation is the vascular and exudative response of the tissues to injury. This injury is often, of course, infective or physical but it may also be due to a clearly recognisable allergic reaction (e.g. contact dermatitis) or to less well-defined immunological mechanisms as in rheumatoid arthritis and other collagen diseases.

Nevertheless, whatever the stimulus, the repertoire of inflammatory changes in tissue is limited. These characteristically include vasodilatation and increased capillary permeability, oedema, and polymorph and macrophage infiltration of tissues. Some of the clinical consequences of these include pain, swelling, redness and impaired function of the inflamed region.

Inflammation due to allergy differs in its overt manifestations from allergy due to infection only because of the degree with which one or other components of the reaction predominates and as a result of direct tissue damage by the microbes themselves.

Inflammation in response to a bacterial infection is mediated by similar factors to those which mediate allergic responses. A 'simple' infection such as a boil, goes on to localised tissue destruction and suppuration. The early vascular and exudative changes are not, however, essentially different from those in allergic bronchial asthma where vasodilatation, increased capillary permeability and localised oedema contribute considerably to the airways obstruction. In many infections it is far from clear how great a part the infection plays and how much of the reaction is allergic. In other infections, particularly some due to viruses, it is believed that much of the trouble may be caused less by the microorganism than by a combination of antigen (virus) and antibody.

Figure 13.1 illustrates some of the mechanisms involved.

A stimulus sufficient to injure cells provokes the release of chemical mediators into the extracellular space. These substances include histamine, kinins, 5-hydroxytryptamine, prostaglandins and leukotrienes (SRS-A, Slow Reacting Substance Anaphylaxis type). Such chemicals produce the observable changes of inflammation. An injection of histamine, for instance, is painful and there is localised oedema and redness due to increased capillary permeability and arteriolar dilatation.

Histamine and leukotrienes (SRS-A) are important mediators of inflammation due to allergic reactions, whilst a wider range of mediators is involved in inflammation caused by infections and physical agents. Antihistamines, however, do not always have a useful effect on inflammation of allergic origin.

The treatment of inflammation due to infection is ideally by removal of the initial cause, i.e. the destruction of the invading organisms. Similarly, some immune reactions can be avoided by preventing antigen–antibody interactions by the use of immunosuppressive agents.

Allergy and autoimmune disease

Allergy is a term used loosely to describe a wide variety of conditions where the immune response becomes harmful to the patient. Allergy has been succinctly described as 'immunity gone wrong'.

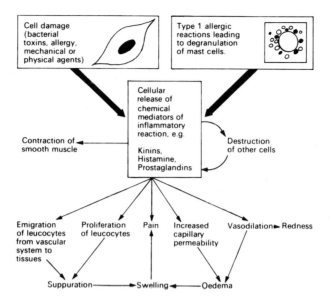

Fig. 13.1 Diagrammatic representation of the mechanisms and interactions involved in allergic and other inflammatory reactions

These reactions may be acute or chronic and have been classified into four main types.

Type I response (anaphylactic)

Examples are (i) acute anaphylaxis; (ii) hay fever, urticaria and asthma (atopic allergy).

Here the specific antibody (IgE) is cell bound, particularly to mast cells. Contact with the antigen triggers the release of substances causing vasodilatation and increased capillary permeability or constriction of bronchial muscle, or all together.

Type II response (cytotoxic or cytolytic)

In this type of reaction the antibody (usually IgG or IgM) reacts with antigen bound to the cell surface. Complement often takes part and the cells are damaged or lysed. Examples are (i) autoimmune haemolytic anaemia; (ii) blood transfusion reactions.

Type III response (immune complex disease)

Here the antigen and antibody are free, but under certain conditions react in the circulation or tissue spaces and fix complement. Precipitation of this complex causes damage to small blood vessels.

Examples of Type III reactions are serum sickness and the renal lesions of infective endocarditis.

Type IV response (cell-mediated immunity, delayed hypersensitivity)

Sensitised lymphocytes react with antigen at some local site and cytotoxic substances are liberated.

Examples are (i) the Mantoux (tuberculin) and similar skin reactions; (ii) contact dermatitis; (iii) homograft rejection.

Immunologically mediated diseases however fall into two main groups, namely:

1. Reactions to exogenous allergens. These give rise to the common allergies such asthma, urticaria and hay fever (collectively known as atopic disease) as well as acute anaphylaxis. They are Type I reactions mediated by IgE and release of mediators from mast cells.

2. Autoimmune diseases. Many of these diseases are uncommon. They are characterised by formation of autoantibodies to host cell components. Rheumatoid arthritis is the most common example; others are lupus erythematosus, thyroiditis, Addison's disease and pemphigus vulgaris.

Generally speaking, there are considerable

differences between the managements of these two groups of diseases and the drugs used in their treatment can also act at a variety of sites.

Histamine and allergy

It has been recognised for many years that histamine produces some of the features of an acute inflammatory response – particularly that due to an allergic reaction. The reason for this became apparent when the mechanism of allergy began to be investigated. In a reaction of the immediate type, the components may be represented diagrammatically as shown in Figure 13.2.

Repeated injection of a foreign protein (antigen) into an animal stimulates the production of protein antibodies which combine with the foreign compound in a highly specific manner. The foreign protein is initially ingested by macrophages which send out information to lymphocytes. These store the information until a subsequent exposure to the same antigen, when the B-type lymphocytes transform into plasma cells. These then secrete specific antibody capable of combining with the antigen.

The antibodies involved in the immediate type of allergic response are immunoglobulins of the IgE type – reaginic antibodies. Reaginic antibodies produce the asthmatic response, urticaria, hay fever and anaphylaxis. The IgE molecules stick to the surface of mast cells. This produces no clinical disturbance until the appropriate antigen comes into contact with these sensitised mast cells. The storage granules in their cytoplasm then discharge their contents. Amongst these are histamine (in the skin and nasal mucosa) and leukotrienes (in the lungs).

Although histamine is found in high concentrations in mast cells, it is also found in other cells.

Injection of histamine into the skin produces the triple response. This consists of a central pale area of swelling due to localised oedema. Surrounding the pale area is a well-defined zone of dusky erythema due to dilatation of venules, arterioles and capillaries. Around this is a diffuse bright flare due to reflex arteriolar dilatation. Local application of histamine into the skin or subcutaneous tissues is painful and irritating.

Certain basic drugs such as morphine, pethidine and tubocurarine liberate free histamine from cells

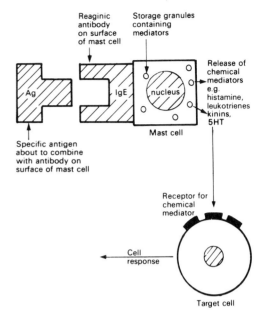

Fig. 13.2 Diagrammatic representation of the specific way in which antigen binds to antibody, triggering the release of chemical mediators which act in turn on the target cell

and can produce histamine reactions such as skin flushing or bronchospasm in asthmatic individuals.

Histamine and the antihistamines

Histamine is an important chemical mediator of many allergic reactions. It is present in an inactive, bound form in cells, but becomes active and is released in response to antigen–antibody reactions and to a variety of insults. These include physical injury, drugs (e.g. morphine) and irritant chemicals.

The main actions of histamine include the following:

1. Smooth muscle. Histamine causes most types of smooth muscle to contract. For example, bronchospasm is one of the characteristic (and disabling) features of allergic asthma. The smooth muscle of the arterioles behaves differently however.

2. Arterioles and capillaries. Histamine causes these vessels to dilate; this leads to a fall in blood pressure which in anaphylactic reactions can be rapid and severe. Capillary permeability also increases allowing fluid to escape from the circulation, intensifying the fall in blood pressure.

3. The skin. Histamine causes itching which is characteristic of most allergic skin reactions such as urticaria (nettle rash; hives).

4. Gastric secretion. Histamine stimulates gastric acid and pepsin secretion but the histamine receptors involved are different from those which are stimulated in the reactions listed above.

Histamine receptors

These are of two types:

H₁ receptors. These are involved in the reactions listed above, but not gastric secretion.

H₂ receptors. These are mainly related to gastric and other secretions. Their existence has been confirmed by the development of agents which specifically block these sites and inhibit gastric acid secretion. These are discussed further in Chapter 17.

Antihistamines

The effects of histamine can be countered in various ways, but the term 'antihistamines' (when unqualified) refers to a large group of drugs which block H₁ histamine receptors. These drugs share a wide variety of other properties – notably sedation and atropine-like effects – which are irrelevant to their antihistamine action. Examples are *chlorpheniramine, diphenhydramine, mepyramine and promethazine.*

There are no significant differences between these antihistamines apart from their duration of actions. However, a newer group of H₁ antihistamines, *astemizole, oxatomide* and *terfenadine,* usually cause significantly less sedation as a result of their poor penetration of the blood–brain barrier.

The H₁ receptor blockers, however, control only a few allergic diseases, partly because histamine is not always the sole cause and other active substances are released. They are most effective in urticaria, angio-oedema (angioneurotic oedema) and hay fever (seasonal allergic vasomotor rhinitis).

Actions of antihistamines

The antihistamines are taken by mouth, are quickly absorbed and act in about half an hour. Their effects last several hours but some, such as promethazine, may be effective for a day or more.

Since the antihistamines are receptor blockers and compete with histamine for the receptor sites, they are most effective as preventive agents. They are therefore useful for continued control of seasonal hay fever, urticaria and angio-oedema in patients subject to frequently recurring attacks.

Antihistamines are of no value in asthma where leukotrienes (not histamine) are the important mediators of the reaction.

Antihistamines are available as creams for local application for relief of itching and for insect or plant stings. They are of little value (at least one manufacturer takes the precaution of adding a local anaesthetic to the preparation) but are effective sensitisers. Their use should be discouraged. Parenteral injection of antihistamines is often suggested for the control of severe hypersensitivity reactions such as anaphylactic shock but adrenaline and hydrocortisone are the first line of treatment.

Other actions of antihistamines

These drugs vary in the relative intensity of their many possible effects:

1. Sedation. With few exceptions the antihistamines depress the CNS and the degree of sedation is roughly related to the potency of antihistamine effect. Some, such as promethazine (Phenergan) and trimeprazine (Vallergan) are also used as sedatives, particularly as premedication for children. Promethazine used as a hypnotic has prolonged after-effects – particularly persistent drowsiness the following day.

As mentioned earlier, some newer antihistamines such as astemizole and terfenadine penetrate the blood–brain barrier to a lesser degree and cause less CNS depression and drowsiness.

2. Antiemetic and antitussive actions. These are also a consequence of CNS depression. The antiemetic action is effective for the control of motion sickness for which antihistamines are widely taken. It is one of their most useful applications.

Adverse effects

These are common.

1. Sedation is an almost invariable accompaniment of effective doses. As with other CNS depressants the effect is potentiated by alcohol. This however applies less to the newer antihistamines such as terfenadine.

2. Sensitisation is liable to follow topical application and dermatitis can be troublesome. Overdosage is dangerous and leads to coma or occasionally convulsions. Rarely, use of some of the antihistamines has been followed by agranulocytosis.

3. Atropine-like effects. Antihistamines cause dry mouth and reduce lacrimal and nasal secretions.

Sodium cromoglycate (Intal)

Sodium cromoglycate is widely used to decrease the frequency of attacks of asthma or hay fever. It is inhaled as a powder and is effective as a preventive agent when taken in a continuous course but has no useful effect in the treatment of an acute attack.

It is generally more effective in children than adults but may control exercise-induced as well as allergic asthma in some patients.

Sodium cromoglycate acts by inhibiting the release of histamine and synthesis of leukotrienes from sensitised mast cells, apparently by stabilising mast cell vesicles.

Sodium cromoglycate is obtainable as insufflation capsules (Rynacrom) for hay fever and has the advantages of being more effective than and lacking the sedating effect of antihistamines.

Sodium cromoglycate is remarkably non-toxic but may cause irritation and coughing on inhalation.

Nedocromil has similar actions to cromoglycate but, after inhalation, is absorbed into the circulation and has, as a consequence, a more widespread action on mast cells. It also appears to be more effective than cromoglycate for adults but, as a result of its absorption, may cause transient headache or nausea.

Ketotifen has actions like those of sodium cromoglycate as well as those of an antihistamine. Its main advantage is that it is taken orally but its antihistaminic action causes drowsiness.

Adrenaline and related agents

Many of the commonly used drugs in allergic reactions act at mediator level. Thus the β agonists such as adrenaline and isoprenaline act as physiological antagonists of the mediator activity on smooth muscle. An example of this is the use of these drugs in asthma. Here the mediators are leukotrienes (SRS-A) and histamine. The sympathomimetic agents appear to act on specific receptors and relax bronchial smooth muscle by a completely different mechanism from that of the mediators, namely by increasing the intracellular concentration of cyclic adenosine monophosphate (cAMP). This is known as physiological antagonism.

Adrenaline is valuable in some acute allergic emergencies particularly if life-threatening, and is the first line of treatment for acute, allergic angiooedema and anaphylaxis.

Adrenaline combats the effects of allergic reactions mainly because of its ability to cause:

1. Bronchial relaxation (β_2 effect).
2. Vasoconstriction particularly in the mucosa, skin and viscera (α effect) and decreased capillary permeability.
3. Reduction in mucosal oedema – partly by diminishing mediator release.

The advantage of adrenaline in these situations is that it acts within a few minutes. However, its effects are short-lived and it may have to be given again after 30–60 minutes.

It is given subcutaneously or, in anaphylactoid reactions where the circulation is failing, by intramuscular injection.

The main danger of adrenaline is that if the injection is made accidentally into a vessel, or if too much is absorbed from an intramuscular injection, it can cause dangerous cardiac arrhythmias. These can terminate in ventricular fibrillation.

The direct (β) effects of adrenaline on the heart, i.e. increased rate and force of contraction (β_1) are helpful if the patient is acutely hypotensive, but since the extensive vasculature of the muscles is relaxed (β_2 effect) the peripheral resistance falls slightly and the overall effect on the blood pressure may be small. The systolic pressure is slightly raised but the diastolic pressure tends to fall.

The effects of adrenaline in acute anaphylaxis are probably not entirely due to these β adrenergic effects on heart and circulation, since it also has direct anti-allergic actions. Adrenaline will suppress the histamine-induced triple response and histamine release from the lungs of sensitised animals. It appears that these actions are mediated by the formation of cyclic AMP from ATP, and adrenaline and other β adrenergic agents suppress mediator release from IgE-sensitised human mast cells.

In the case of asthma, longer-acting agents which have a more selective effect in relieving bronchospasm, such as salbutamol, are now available and can be taken orally, by inhalation or intravenously.

Adrenaline is useful for acute angio-oedema (particularly when it involves the larynx with the risk of asphyxia) by causing vasoconstriction and reduced capillary permeability. In addition, corticosteroids should be given intravenously. Adrenaline and related drugs are also discussed in Chapter 5.

Aminophylline, which produces a sympathomimetic effect by a different mechanism from that of adrenaline, is also useful for the control of asthma. Some regard it as still the most effective agent for control of an acute severe attack.

Anticholinergic drugs

Ipratropium (isopropyl atropine) is in many cases as potent a bronchodilator as salbutamol. Ipratropium is therefore particularly useful for maintenance therapy when bronchitis and asthma are associated with heart disease since it has no sympathomimetic actions. The anticholinergic actions of ipratropium, however, cause a dry mouth and may cause urinary retention in elderly men with enlarged prostates.

IMMUNOSUPPRESSIVE DRUGS

Immunosuppressive treatment has its main applications in the treatment of severe autoimmune diseases and for organ transplantation. The most widely used immunosuppressive and anti-inflammatory drugs are the corticosteroids. The latter are also used for asthma unresponsive to other drugs.

Immunosuppressive drugs, particularly the cytotoxic agents, have serious side-effects, notably, susceptibility to infection as a result of suppression of normal immune responses. Infections are the

most common cause of death resulting from the use of these drugs.

Drugs which have major immunosuppressive effects fall into two main groups namely:

1. Non-cytotoxic agents:
   Corticosteroids and cyclosporin.
2. Cytotoxic agents:
   Azathioprine, methotrexate and others.

An arbitrary and misleading distinction is often made between corticosteroids and immunosuppressive agents (cytotoxic drugs). Both are immunosuppressive and increase susceptibility to infection. However, corticosteroids differ from the cytotoxic agents in their wide range of other (hormonal) actions (see Ch. 15) unrelated to their immunosuppressive effects. Cytotoxic drugs, by contrast, can induce severe bone marrow depression and their use may be followed by tumour formation (see Ch. 14).

Corticosteroids

The adrenocorticosteroids have their widest application in the management of acute and chronic conditions which have an allergic basis. Although the many actions of corticosteroids are considered in more detail in Chapter 15, their mode of action in allergic conditions is due to inhibition of interleukin secretion. Corticosteroids do not appear to inhibit antigen–antibody interaction and it is probable that another action is by protecting the target cells from the effects of the mediators released as a result of such reactions. The integrity of cell membranes is stabilised and capillary permeability is decreased. Leakage of fluid from the circulation is diminished in shock-like states and oedema is reduced in areas of inflammation.

Corticosteroids are often of great benefit in conditions such as acute anaphylactic shock or severe bronchial asthma as described earlier (see Ch. 11) as well as in certain inflammatory conditions as described later.

Corticosteroids are also effective in Type II reactions where there are circulating antibodies as in autoimmune haemolytic anaemia, blood transfusion reactions and thrombocytopenic purpura.

The management of acute anaphylactic reactions is discussed in Chapter 19.

Immunosuppressive and anti-inflammatory actions of corticosteroids

Several mechanisms are involved; all may result from intracellular receptor binding leading to the synthesis or activation of *lipocortin* but include the following:

1. Lipocortin inhibits phospholipase A2 and the release of arachidonic acid from phospholipids. The result is that the synthesis of leukotrienes, prostaglandins, thromboxane and prostacyclin is blocked.
2. Production of interleukin 2 is depressed. This in turn, leads to reduced T lymphocyte proliferation.
3. Lymphokine release is lessened.
4. The response to lymphokines is diminished.

The immunosuppressive actions of corticosteroids are therefore complex and are by no means fully understood, but the overall effect is to depress cell-mediated responses predominantly. Antibody production and antigen–antibody interactions do not appear to be inhibited. However, corticosteroids are often effective in Type II reactions such as idiopathic thrombocytopenic purpura associated with anti-platelet antibodies, probably by protecting the target cells.

In the case of asthma or anaphylaxis, it is probable that the benefits of corticosteroids are mainly (a) to lessen the output of mediators and (b) to protect target cells from such mediators. The integrity of cell membranes is stabilised and capillary permeability is reduced. Oedema is thus reduced in the inflamed areas (the bronchi in asthma) and in anaphylactic reactions, leakage of fluid from the circulation is diminished.

As a result of depression of cell-mediated immunity, however, viral and fungal infections are common complications of longer-term use and are a major hazard for organ transplant patients. Fungal infection (oropharyngeal thrush), for example, is a common consequence even of local deposition of potent corticosteroids from inhalers for asthma.

Cyclosporin

Cyclosporin (Sandimmun) is a fungal product which has weak antibiotic actions but was found to be an effective immunosuppressive drug.

The mode of action of cyclosporin appears to be quite different from other immunosuppressant drugs in that it selectively inhibits the early stages of T lymphocyte activation, by interfering with the synthesis of the soluble transmitter substance interleukin 2 (IL2) which mediates lymphocyte interaction.

Since cyclosporin is not toxic to the bone marrow and therefore causes less severe side-effects than cytotoxic drugs, it has been valuable in organ transplantation where it has been mainly used.

The chief adverse effect of cyclosporin is that it is nephrotoxic and dosage has to be regulated accordingly.

Another side-effect of cyclosporin is to induce gingival hyperplasia similar to that caused by phenytoin (p. 212).

Immunosuppressive cytotoxic agents

One approach to the problem of undesired immune responses in the treatment of graft rejection or severe autoimmune disease is the use of cytotoxic drugs such as azathioprine or methotrexate. One action of these drugs is to prevent nucleic acid synthesis and thus block protein production and cell division. The result is that antibodies (which are proteins) are not manufactured. The proteins (lymphokines), which are otherwise produced by sensitised lymphocytes and which damage cells, are also not synthesised.

This form of treatment of immune reactions is not without risk as the agents used are toxic and are also used as cytotoxic drugs, as described in the next chapter.

These immunosuppressive drugs have proved valuable in the treatment of severe Type IV (cell-mediated) reactions and have made transplant surgery possible by depressing the graft rejection reaction and are often used with large doses of corticosteroids. Other diseases treated in this way include the more severe collagen diseases such as disseminated lupus erythematosus, and there is some evidence that survival is increased by such treatment.

Drugs which have major immunosuppressive effects can therefore be divided into two main groups as follows:

1. Non-cytotoxic agents:
   Corticosteroids and cyclosporin (p. 177).
2. Cytotoxic agents.

These are discussed more fully in the next chapter.

Non-steroidal anti-inflammatory agents (NSAIAs)

There are many drugs which are not corticosteroids but have an anti-inflammatory action. Examples are aspirin, indomethacin and ibuprofen. These agents act by inhibiting synthesis of the mediators of the inflammatory response, mainly prostaglandin E_2 (PGE_2). Anti-inflammatory agents are useful for painful conditions secondary to inflammation. They are widely used for arthritis. Like the steroids, the anti-inflammatory activity of these analgesics is associated with a tendency to cause gastric haemorrhage from acute mucosal erosions. This results from lowering the local concentration of prostaglandin E_2 (PGE_2) which normally maintains submucosal vasodilatation and nourishes the mucosa.

SUGGESTED FURTHER READING

Brandon M L 1985 Newer non-sedating antihistamines will they replace older ones. Drugs 30: 377
Calne R Y, White D J G 1982 The use of cyclosporin A in clinical organ grafting. Annals of Surgery 196: 330
Cameron S (1982) Immunosuppression after transplantation. Hospital Update 8: 835
Council on Scientific Affairs 1987 Introduction to the management of immunosuppression. Journal of the American Medical Association 257: 1781

Cupps T R, Fauci A S 1982 Corticosteroid-mediated immunoregulation in man. Immunological Reviews. 65: 133
Currie G 1982 Modes of action of immunosuppressive agents. Hospital Update 8(1): 1101
European Multicentre Trial Group 1983 Cyclosporin in cadaveric renal transplantation. Lancet ii: 986.
Fritz K A, Weston W L 1983 Topical glucocorticosteroids. Annals of Allergy 50: 68
Hodges J R 1984 The hypothalamo-pituitary-adrenocortical system. British Journal of Anaesthesia 56: 701
Kolata G 1983 Cyclosporin obviates rejection problems with organ transplants and may also be used to treat autoimmune diseases and parasitic infections. Science 221: 40.
Lewis L D, Cochrane G M 1986 Systemic steroids in chronic severe asthma. British Medical Journal 292: 292
Meuleman J, Katz P 1985 The immunologic effects, kinetics and use of glucocorticoids. Medical Clinics of North America 69: 805
Miller J A, Levene G M 1982 Steroids in dermatology. British Journal of Hospital Medicine 28: 331
Patterson R 1988 Diagnosis and treatment of drug allergy. Journal of Allergy and Clinical Immunology 81: 380
Pauwels R 1986 Mode of action of corticosteroids in asthma and rhinitis. Clinical Allergy 16: 281
Pitt P I, Sultan A H et al 1987 Association between azathioprine therapy and lymphoma in rheumatoid disease. Journal of the Royal Society of Medicine 80: 428
Salaman J R 1983 Steroids and modern immunosuppression British Medical Journal 286: 1373
Savin J A 1985 Some guidelines to the use of topical corticosteroids. British Medical Journal 290: 1607
Schleimer R P 1985 The mechanisms of anti-inflammatory steroid (sic) action in allergic diseases. Annual Review of Pharmacology and Toxicology 25: 381
Slapak M 1987 Triple and quadruple immunosuppressive therapy in organ transplantation. Lancet ii: 958
Slocumb C H, Polley H F 1980 Adrenocortical steroids – then and now. Mayo Clinic Proceedings 55: 774
Spector R G 1981 Pharmacological properties of the glucocorticoids. International Dental Journal 31: 152
Spiro H M 1983 Is the steroid ulcer a myth? New England Journal of Medicine 309: 45
Thomson A W, Webster L M 1988 The influence of cyclosporin A on cell-mediated immunity. Clinical and Experimental Immunology 71: 369
White D J G 1982 Cyclosporin A. Clinical pharmacology and therapeutic potential. Drugs 24: 322
Whitehouse J M A 1983 Cytotoxic drugs for non-neoplastic disease. British Medical Journal 287: 79

14. Antitumour drugs and cytotoxic chemotherapy

Cytotoxic chemotherapy is the use of drugs to destroy tumour cells. Antibacterial chemotherapy has been very successful in the treatment of many types of infections. In this case, the invading bacterial cell is physically and chemically different from animal (host) cells and antibacterial chemotherapeutic agents specifically attack features peculiar to the invading organisms. The great difficulty in producing antitumour chemotherapeutic drugs is that tumours arise from tissues of the body and usually remain similar to their cells of origin. Antitumour agents do not possess a high degree of specificity, and concentrations sufficient to destroy all the tumour cells would generally also produce unacceptably severe toxic effects.

One of the most important differences between tumour cells and normal cells is that in tumours there is excessive and uncontrolled cell division and the effectiveness of many antitumour drugs depends on their antimitotic action. Unfortunately, some tissues in the body too are constantly in a state of repeated cell division and are particularly vulnerable to damage by cytotoxic drugs. Thus antimitotic drug action on the marrow can cause anaemia, leucopenia (including agranulocytosis) and thrombocytopenia. Actions on the gonads may cause sterility and effects on the intestine may cause haemorrhage and diarrhoea. Inhibition of hair follicle cell proliferation can lead to baldness.

Antitumour drugs are usually used to act systemically and their main applications are against leukaemia and the malignant lymphomas, including Hodgkin's disease and myeloma. In the great majority of cases no more than temporary remissions in the disease are attained but in some types of acute leukaemia in children and in Hodgkin's disease cytotoxic treatment has greatly improved the prognosis.

Cytotoxic agents can also be given by regional perfusion to achieve a high local dosage to the tumour. This method has been used for advanced cancers of the mouth, for instance, but it is a treatment of last resort and has had little success.

The main groups of antitumour drugs (of which there are now very many) are:

1. Alkylating agents.
2. Antimetabolites.
3. Miscellaneous (including antitumour antibiotics).
4. Hormones.

Alkylating agents

These bind firmly to both strands of DNA in the cell nucleus and prevent their separation. Separation of the strands of nuclear DNA is a necessary preparatory step to cell division and without it cell division cannot take place.

Examples of alkylating agents are *cyclophosphamide*, *chlorambucil* and *melphalan*. They include the chemical group of nitrogen mustards which in turn were derived from war gases. Cyclophosphamide is mainly used in the treatment of lymphomas, myelomas and some carcinomas. Chlorambucil is active by mouth and is used to treat lymphomas, chronic lymphatic leukaemia and Hodgkin's disease. Melphalan is used in the treatment of myelomatosis and seminoma.

All the alkylating agents suppress cell division in the marrow and in this way cause leucopenia (particularly granulocytopenia), anaemia and thrombocytopenia.

The alkylating agents are also immunosuppressive due to their inhibition of cell division in lymphoid tissue and their destructive action on circulating lymphocytes.

Antimetabolites

Antimetabolites block metabolic steps in the synthesis of purines and pyrimidines from folic acid. Antimetabolites are structurally similar to a natural component in the synthetic pathway and the drug combines with the enzyme responsible for synthesizing the natural substance. The important action of all the antimetabolites used in tumour therapy is that they block the synthesis of nucleic acids. The result is that nuclei cannot divide, cytoplasm cannot grow and cell division is prevented.

An important anti-folate antimetabolite is *methotrexate*. This is used in the treatment of Hodgkin's disease and acute leukaemia. The anti-purine substance *mercaptopurine* is also used to treat acute leukaemia.

Miscellaneous antitumour drugs and X-rays

Actinomycin blocks the synthesis of messenger RNA and thus prevents protein synthesis and cell growth. Actinomycin is an antibiotic but is too toxic (for the reason given) for antibacterial use. *Vinblastine* and *vincristine* (from *Vinca rosea*, the periwinkle) arrest cell division at the metaphase stage by preventing movement of the chromosomes on the mitotic spindle.

X-rays and other forms of radiation used in the treatment of tumours have a complex action on dividing cells. Amongst the observable effects are chromosomal breakages and abnormalities in cell division.

X-rays are used in the treatment of some skin tumours, Hodgkin's disease and lymphomas. They are used to treat a wide variety of carcinomas and have almost entirely displaced surgery in certain sites such as the mouth.

Interferons

The potential use of interferons for the control of tumour growth has been discussed earlier (see Ch. 3).

Hormones

Oestrogens. A variety of hormones affects the growth of individual tumours. Oestrogens such as stilboestrol may delay the extension of carcinoma of the prostate.

Before the menopause, oestrogens may accelerate the growth of breast carcinoma – but after the menopause the same hormones sometimes slow down proliferation of this tumour.

Corticosteroids. Very high doses of glucocorticoids – such as hydrocortisone or prednisolone – affect immune responses in various ways and potentiate the action of other immunosuppressive drugs. These hormones are used with success in producing a remission in acute lymphatic leukaemia and in Hodgkin's disease.

Hormone antagonists

Hormone antagonists may be effective for the management of hormone-dependent tumours.

Tamoxifen blocks oestrogen receptors in target organs and currently is the drug of choice for breast cancer with metastases in postmenopausal women, but is being increasingly used as the first line of treatment for breast cancer in younger women.

Combination cytotoxic chemotherapy

Because of their serious toxic effects, antitumour drugs should only be used for malignant diseases where there is a reasonable chance of a response. These drugs have little selectivity of action and are often used in combinations of up to four at a time as such combinations have been found empirically to be most effective for particular tumours. A typical example is the use of mustine, Oncovin (vincristine), prednisolone and procarbazine (MOPP) for the treatment of Hodgkin's disease and which has been found to be highly effective.

Although assumptions are frequently made that 'cancer can be cured' by methods such as these, it has to be accepted that significant successes in this field are limited. However, cure is possible in many cases of Hodgkin's disease and childhood lymphocytic leukaemia. Other antitumour treatments are not curative but may prolong life for variable periods or provide valuable palliation of symptoms.

Complications of antineoplastic chemotherapy

The main problems are the result of the non-specific cytotoxic action of these drugs upon the marrow and of their immunosuppressant action. These effects tend to act together to make the patient highly vulnerable to infection even by organisms which are not otherwise pathogenic

The main adverse effects from cytotoxic drugs include the following;

1. Gastrointestinal tract. Anorexia, distressingly severe nausea, vomiting or diarrhoea are common. The cells lining the gastrointestinal tract are vulnerable since they are constantly replaced and hence are rapidly dividing.

2. The bone marrow. Anaemia, leucopenia or agranulocytosis are common and the last contributes to an increased susceptibility to infection.

3. Immunosuppression. The corticosteroids and azathioprine are frequently used in combination and together suppress lymphocyte production, are lymphocytotoxic and depress lymphocyte function in other ways. Cell-mediated immunity is greatly impaired or abolished. Viral and fungal infections are a common consequence and infection is the chief cause of death during cytotoxic or immunosuppressive treatment.

The susceptibility to infective complications is compounded in patients with leukaemia or lymphomas – diseases where cytotoxic agents are usually used. In this situation both the disease itself and also cytotoxic agents impair resistance to infection. The mouth is often the first or main site where these infections develop. The oral bacteria of the gingival margins, for instance, can become pathogenic to these patients causing oral ulceration or septicaemias.

4. Teratogenic effects. Cytotoxic agents are among the few drugs in clinical use that have been shown to be capable of damaging the developing fetus.

5. The development of new tumours after cytotoxic chemotherapy is well recognised and is discussed below.

6. Sterility.

7. Hair loss. The rapidly dividing cells of hair follicles are vulnerable to cytotoxic drugs such as cyclophosphamide. Complete baldness can result and is distressing, particularly for women. However the hair eventually grows again.

Oral complications of cytotoxic treatment

1. Ulceration. Methotrexate and other antibiotics in particular cause oral ulceration, and other types of cytotoxic drugs also have this effect to varying degree. Oral ulceration may be the first sign of toxicity and may be so severe as to make it necessary to stop chemotherapy.

2. Infections. Cytotoxic drugs promote oral infections particularly by *Candida albicans* and also by unusual organisms such as staphylococci and Gram-negative bacilli.

3. Bleeding. Drug-induced thrombocytopenia can cause excessive gingival bleeding or other signs such as mucosal purpura.

4. Neoplasms, particularly lymphomas, associated with the use of cytotoxic agents for immunosuppression may develop in the mouth.

Oral infections can be controlled with varying degrees of success by keeping the mouth very clean – including removal of bacterial plaque – and by frequent irrigations of the mouth with an antibiotic antifungal preparation such as tetracycline with amphotericin (Mysteclin syrup). Such blunderbuss treatment is justified in this case as the infections are mixed in character and antibiotics alone tend to promote fungal infection if it is not already present. If an identifiable pathogen can be isolated, specific antibacterial or antifungal treatment should, of course, be given.

The use of cytotoxic drugs as immunosuppressive agents

The immune response, whether humoral (antibody) or cell mediated, depends on division and differentiation of lymphoid cells, and protein synthesis. The anticancer drugs which act by interfering with cell division, growth and protein synthesis have immunosuppressive actions. In fact, illogical though it may be, these same drugs are called 'immunosuppressives' when they are used for such purposes as the prevention of rejection of a graft or transplant, and 'cytotoxic' when they are used in cancer chemotherapy.

In the prevention of graft rejection, adrenal cortical steroids – particularly semi-synthetic analogues such as prednisolone – are used in large doses.

Drugs also used to suppress or prevent rejection reactions include:

1. Alkylating agents: e.g. cyclophosphamide and chlorambucil.

2. Antimetabolites: (i) antipurines e.g. mercaptopurine, azathioprine and thioguanine (ii) antifolates e.g. methotrexate. A common combination is prednisolone and azathioprine.

The other uses of these drugs as immunosuppressive agents include some types of nephritis, otherwise uncontrollable rheumatoid arthritis, asthma, systemic lupus erythematosus and Wegener's granulomatosis. Pemphigus vulgaris which may start as a vesiculating stomatitis is one of the few diseases where immunosuppressive treatment has been clearly shown to be life-saving. These drugs are dangerous, and the enormous doses required for immunosuppression mean that toxic effects always appear.

The advantages of cyclosporin over cytotoxic drugs for immunosuppression have been discussed earlier. It is somewhat less potent in its immunosuppressant effects and is usually supplemented with other agents. However, it is now increasingly used.

Cancer as a complication of cytotoxic chemotherapy

There is an increased incidence of cancers, particularly lymphomas and leukaemias, as a complication of cytotoxic chemotherapy. At one time this was believed to result from cytotoxic drugs impairing the (so-called) immune surveillance function of the immune system. The latter was thought to have a protective function by recognising and destroying malignant cells as they appear. However if this were the case, then an increased incidence of the common types of cancer (such as the lung, breast and gastrointestinal tract) rather than the relatively uncommon lymphoreticular tumours, should be expected. Moreover, several immunosuppressive drugs are mutagenic and, under experimental conditions, some of them have been shown to be carcinogenic.

It may be noted incidentally that irradiation, a well-established form of cancer treatment, is also potentially carcinogenic and second neoplasms can follow such treatment. Cancer of various types has been a long-term effect on the immediate survivors of the atom bombs dropped on Japan at the end of the Second World War.

SUGGESTED FURTHER READING

Anon 1987 Adjuvant tamoxifen in early breast cancer. Lancet ii: 191

Anon 1987 Short-term intensive therapy for childhood non-Hodgkin lymphoma. Lancet ii: 1410

Anon 1988 Treatment of childhood acute lymphoblastic leukaemia. Lancet i: 683

Foon K A 1986 Interferon of lymphoproliferative disorders. Seminars in Haematology 23 (suppl 1): 10

Kearsley 1986 Cytotoxic chemotherapy for common adult malignancies: 'the emperor's new clothes' revisited? British Medical Journal 293: 871

Macleod R I, Welbury R R, Soames J V 1987 Effects of cytotoxic chemotherapy on dental development. Journal of the Royal Society of Medicine 80: 207

Mauer A M 1986 New directions in the treatment of acute lymphoblastic leukaemia in children. New England Journal of Medicine 315: 316

Mead G M, Whitehouse J M A 1986 Modern management of non-Hodgkin's lymphoma. British Medical Journal 293: 577

Porzosolt F, Digel W, Jacobsen H et al 1988 Different antitumor mechanisms of interferon-alpha in the treatment of hairy cell leukaemia and renal cell cancer. Cancer 61: 288

Walsh T D, West T S 1988 Controlling symptoms in advanced cancer. British Medical Journal 296: 477

15. Hormones and the skeleton

Hormones are used in a wide variety of ways in clinical practice. Only a few examples are dealt with in this chapter where stress is laid on some of the more commonly used agents

SEX HORMONES

In both sexes the adrenal cortex produces oestrogens, progestogens and androgens. The testes are the main site of androgen production, while the ovaries produce oestrogens and progestogens.

Androgens, such as testosterone propionate, methyltestosterone and testosterone are used in the treatment of hypogonadism in the male. Androgens are also used as anabolic agents in wasting diseases and in chronic renal failure.

Oestrogenic substances used in therapeutics include stilboestrol, ethinyl oestradiol and mestranol. Some of the progestogens in use are given to prevent osteoporosishave been used to suppress lactation. Oestrogen-progestogen mixtures are effective in a wide range of gynaecological disorders – particularly of the menstrual cycle.

Destruction of the pituitary leads to gonadal hypofunction because of failure of production of luteinising hormone and follicle stimulating hormone. This may be treated with gonadal steroid replacement or by administration of gonadotrophins – such as human menopausal gonadotrophin, which has both luteinising and follicle stimulating properties.

Partial destruction of the pituitary may be followed by excessive production of prolactin. This results in galactorrhoea, amenorrhoea, impotence and infertility. One form of treatment is with the ergot alkaloid, bromocriptine, which inhibits the release of prolactin and is the drug of choice to stop normal lactation.

Important uses of sex hormones are as follows:

1. Replacement treatment of gonadal failure.
2. Menstrual disorders.
3. Oral contraception.
4. Treatment of hormone-dependent cancers (see Ch. 14).

ORAL CONTRACEPTIVES

The most effective oral contraceptive is an oestrogen-progestogen combination. It acts mainly by inhibiting ovulation due to a suppression of pituitary gonadotrophin release. Additional mechanisms which contribute to their high contraceptive effectiveness are by increasing the viscosity of the cervical mucus, and by depressing tubular motility and endometrial development.

The patient takes the combined pill for 20 or 21 days, leaves a 7-day gap and then starts to take the pill again for a further 20 or 21 days. During the 7-day gap there is usually uterine haemorrhage.

Adverse effects

Serious side-effects are rare with steroidal contraceptive agents, but minor toxic effects are common. These include nausea, breast discomfort, headache or migraine, aggravation of diabetes, ankle swelling, weight gain, bleeding in mid-cycle and failure to bleed during the 7-day gap. The progestogen appears to be mainly responsible for changes such as lethargy and depression. The oestrogen component is related to the complication of venous and arterial thrombo-embolism. A large scale survey carried out over several years has shown that the risk of cerebrovascular disease and deep vein thrombosis is five to six times higher than in non-users. In one extensive survey women who used oral contraceptives experienced an excess of hospital referrals for cerebrovascular disease, cervical erosions, skin disorders, self-poisoning, migraine, venous thrombosis and embolism (especially in those with blood group A), hay fever, gallbladder disease, amenorrhoea and sterility. They showed fewer than expected hospital referrals for cancer, benign lesions of the breast, menstrual disorders other than amenorrhea, duodenal ulcer and retention cysts of the ovary.

There is also an increased risk of mortality from cardiovascular disease due to myocardial infarction about three to five times greater than in non-users. The risk increases with age, pre-existing hypertension and cigarette smoking. The use of oral contraceptives after the age of 35 may therefore be inadvisable. The risk of cancer from oral contraceptives is discussed later. After stopping this form of contraceptive, fertility may be subnormal for several cycles but in most individuals fertility is not affected.

The benefits of oral contraceptive treatment have to be balanced against the risks, and it is generally agreed that their level is acceptable, bearing in mind that the hazards of pregnancy and labour may be higher.

Some women may, however, continue to take these agents for 20 or more years and the effects of such long-term treatment are uncertain.

Dental aspects of oral contraceptive use

Mild deterioration of gingivitis with increased gingival oedema and, possibly also, of periodontitis may result from the use of oral contraceptives. The increased risks associated with hypertension and ischaemic heart disease, particularly in older women who are smokers and use oral contraceptives, also need to be considered if general anaesthesia is to be given.

The broad spectrum antibiotics, such as amoxycillin, slightly diminish the action of oral contraceptives but this effect is not likely to be significant clinically.

Note: Those with a passion for accuracy may have noticed that *the* pill is not *a* pill. Pills consist of the agent made up in a pasty mixture that sets hard: they are now obsolete because of the variability of dissolution and absorption. The pill is, in fact a tablet, i.e. highly compressed powder.

Associations between oral contraceptives and cancer

A study which showed an association between long-term use of oral contraceptive preparations with a high progestogenic activity and an increased incidence of breast cancer has not been confirmed in more recent surveys.

Another extensive study has shown an increased risk of cervical carcinoma among users of contraceptive drugs compared with those who used intra-uterine contraceptive devices.

Prolonged use of the pill is associated with an increased risk of endometrial cancer.

Neither of these studies establishes a cause and effect relationship between use of the pill and cancer. Nevertheless, it has been suggested that oral contraceptive agents with low oestrogen and low progestogenic content should be chosen for long-term use.

THE THYROID HORMONES

The thyroid gland secretes thyroxin (T4) and tri-iodothyronine (T3). These hormones stimulate the metabolism of tissues and increase their rate of utilisation of glucose and oxygen. The metabolic rate is partly dependent on the thyroid hormones and in hypothyroidism (myxoedema) the basal metabolic rate (BMR) is abnormally low, whilst in hyperthyroidism (thyrotoxicosis) the BMR is high.

Hypothyroidism

The thyroid hormones are needed during development for growth of the skeleton and for normal brain maturation. Congenital absence or hypofunction of the thyroid, due for instance to iodine deficiency, leads to dwarfing, mental deficiency and other consequences due to the low BMR. This clinical entity is known as cretinism.

In the adult or child hypothyroidism is treated by oral administration of T4. In the adult the smallest dose of thyroxin which will raise the metabolic rate to normal is used. Cretinism is treated by giving the largest tolerable dose of thyroxin as soon as the condition is recognised to prevent mental deficiency and dwarfing.

Patients suffering from severe myxoedema may have such a low metabolic rate that they become comatose. T4 takes about 48 hours before it starts to raise the metabolic rate and therefore may not be suitable for such an emergency. Under these circumstances T3 is often used. Not only is it about five times more active than T4 but it raises the metabolic rate within 6 hours.

Hyperthyroidism

In addition to the raised metabolic rate the increased secretion of T3 and T4 enhances responsiveness of the tissues to sympathetic activity. Therefore, severely thyrotoxic patients often have cardiac arrhythmias and may be more sensitive to adrenaline. There is, however, no *clinical* evidence to support the belief that the use of adrenaline in dental local anaesthetics is contraindicated in patients with hyperthyroidism. A β blocker such as propranolol is often effective in treating fast arrhythmias in hyperthyroidism.

The treatment of thyrotoxicosis may be by operation (partial thyroidectomy) or by destruction of some of the thyroid cells by radioactive iodine (^{131}I). Alternatively, drugs may be used. Two drugs used in this way are *carbimazole* and *propylthiouracil*. Both of these drugs block the synthesis of T3 and T4 in the thyroid by preventing the incorporation of iodine into their organic precursors. Side-effects of these drugs include rashes (common) and agranulocytosis (rare).

Calcitonin

Calcitonin (thyrocalcitonin) is a third hormone secreted by the thyroid gland. It is not secreted by the follicular cells but by the C cells in the parafollicular regions. This hormone is also secreted by the thymus and parathyroids. Calcitonin does not affect the metabolic rate, but is concerned with calcium homeostasis. It lowers plasma levels of calcium and phosphate and enhances renal excretion of phosphate. The main action of calcitonin is to inhibit the removal of calcium from bone, i.e. it opposes the action of parathyroid hormone which increases reabsorption of calcium from bone and raises plasma calcium. The interaction of these hormones and other factors affecting calcium metabolism is discussed later.

However, the physiological function of calcitonin is not understood. Neither removal of the thyroid nor overproduction of calcitonin by a tumour (medullary carcinoma of the thyroid) appears to have any significant effect on bone metabolism.

At present the main clinical indication for calcitonin has been Paget's disease of bone, but it may also be useful in the management of hypercalcaemia particularly when secondary to malignant disease.

DIABETES AND ANTIDIABETIC AGENTS

Insulin is the antidiabetic peptide secreted by the β cells of the islets of Langerhans of the pancreas. If insufficient insulin is produced by the pancreas, diabetes mellitus develops. In this condition glucose cannot be fully used by cells so that there is excessive breakdown of glycogen and fats within cells. Fats are not completely oxidised but are broken down to acetoacetate, acetone and β-hydroxybutyrate (the so-called acetone or ketone bodies). When these substances enter the circulation they are excreted on the breath and in the urine, and ketosis is said to be present.

In diabetes the blood glucose is raised. Large amounts of glucose therefore enter the renal tubules by way of the glomerular filtrate and cause an osmotic diuresis. Polyuria leads to dehydration and thirst.

The diabetic patient is excessively susceptible to infection – particularly by staphylococci or *Candida albicans*. Serious degenerative arterial disease frequently leads to retinopathy, occlusive coronary artery disease and peripheral occlusion of limb vessels. Acute episodes of ketosis, acidosis and loss of consciousness (diabetic coma) may punctuate the course of this chronic illness.

There are two major types of diabetes, namely insulin-dependent diabetes mellitus (IDDM), which is typically of early onset, and non-insulin dependent diabetes mellitus (NIDDM), which is typically late in onset. Juvenile-onset diabetes starts in adolescence or early adult life and is characterised by weight loss, ketosis and inability of the pancreas to produce insulin. In the second type (maturity-onset diabetes) the patient is usually obese and has raised levels of circulating insulin. However, lack of exercise, obesity and age produce insulin resistance in the tissues, thus leading to a relative lack of insulin.

Young, thin diabetics with ketosis usually need insulin to correct their metabolic abnormalities. Obese, maturity-onset diabetes may be corrected by dietary measures and weight loss only, but many elderly diabetics require in addition to diet, oral hypoglycaemic agents such as sulphonylureas or biguanides. Any diabetic who develops ketosis, acidosis or hyperglycaemic coma needs insulin.

Insulin

Insulin is a peptide which is traditionally crystallised out from acid extracts of beef or pig pancreas but human insulin is now also synthesised using recombinant DNA technology. It is not effective orally because it is destroyed by proteolytic digestive enzymes; it is given by injection – usually subcutaneously. In diabetic coma, insulin may be injected intramuscularly or intravenously.

When a rapid action is needed, especially for treatment of diabetic coma, soluble insulin is used. For a more prolonged effect, protamine zinc insulin slowly releases insulin from the protein–insulin complex. Insulin zinc suspension is in the form of crystals, the size of which determines the duration of effect.

A diabetic often needs a combination of insulins in an attempt to keep the blood sugar at a steady level in the face of varying demands.

The action of insulin in a diabetic is to lower the blood sugar by enhancing uptake and utilisation of glucose by cells and thereby abolish glycosuria and polyuria. There is also decreased breakdown of fat to form ketone bodies – thus leading to cessation of ketosis and correction of acidosis. Protein and fat anabolism increase relative to catabolism.

Monocomponent and human insulins. Allergy to insulin can develop against such substances as insulin precursors remaining in the solution or to insulin from a particular animal – usually bovine insulin. These reactions can often be prevented by the use of newer, highly purified insulins obtained from a single species of animal and monocomponent insulins from which allergenic substances such as pro-insulin have been removed.

Insulin indistinguishable from human insulin but produced from bacteria by recombinant DNA technology ('genetic engineering') is available.

Toxic effects of insulin

Hypoglycaemia. If too much insulin is given either by accidental overdose or relative to a reduced dietary carbohydrate intake, hypoglycaemia may result. Mild hypoglycaemia causes excessive hunger. More severe hypoglycaemia may produce signs similar to fainting or drunkenness. The patient may become confused, ataxic, argumentative and eventually develops convulsions and coma.

If recognised in its early stages, hypoglycaemia can be reversed by giving sugar by mouth. Once consciousness is lost glucose must be given intravenously and is usually quickly effective. Hypoglycaemia which does not respond adequately to glucose alone may be reversed temporarily with injections of glucagon. This is another peptide hormone secreted by the islets of Langerhans of the pancreas. It is produced by the α cells and has a hyperglycaemic action by accelerating hepatic breakdown of glycogen.

Hypoglycaemia may develop in a dental patient who is prevented by treatment from eating at the proper time, while the diabetic who needs a general anaesthetic has to have carefully arranged dosage of insulin and glucose to tide him over the period of starvation and unconsciousness and to prevent either hypoglycaemia or ketosis. Prolonged hypoglycaemia can lead to death or permanent brain damage.

Allergy. Allergic reactions to insulin consist of localised itching and swelling at the site of injection, or generalised urticaria. In general, pig insulin is less allergenic than beef insulin. A common expression of immune reactions to insulin is insulin resistance. Allergy to monocomponent or even to human insulin can occasionally develop. Nevertheless, newly diagnosed diabetics are usually given human insulin.

Localised fat atrophy. This is another reaction at the site of repeated subcutaneous injections and appears as localised depression of the skin.

Oral hypoglycaemic agents

These agents are principally used for maturity-onset, non-ketotic diabetes which cannot be adequately controlled by diet alone. There are two main groups of orally active hypoglycaemic drugs: (a) the *sulphonylureas* and (b) the *biguanides*.

a. *Sulphonylureas* act by increasing the release of insulin from the pancreas. Thus they are only effective in the presence of functioning islet tissue. Two commonly used members of this group are *tolbutamide* (Rastinon) and *chlorpropamide* (Diabinese). Tolbutamide is rapidly destroyed in the liver and has to be taken two or three times a day. Its action is greatly enhanced and prolonged in the presence of severe liver disease. Chlorpropamide is not metabolised, but is excreted unchanged via the kidney. It can be effective for over 24 hours when given only once daily. Its action is potentiated in patients with renal failure. *Glibenclamide* has an action intermediate in duration between tolbutamide and chlorpropamide, but like the latter can be taken once daily. Glibenclamide or tolbutamide are preferable for use by the elderly in whom chlorpropamide can cause prolonged hypoglycaemia. These drugs can produce hypoglycaemia – but this is usually easily managed by giving glucose or sugar by mouth. Another disadvantage of the sulphonylureas is that they tend to increase appetite. This may be troublesome, in that it may add to the patients' difficulties in keeping to their carbohydrate and calorie restricted diets.

b. *Biguanides* such as metformin (Glucophage) have similar uses to the sulphonylureas but they have the advantage for obese diabetics that they tend to diminish appetite. Biguanides appear to act at tissue level and enhance the action of circulating insulin. Like the sulphonylureas they do not have a hypoglycaemic action in the total absence of functioning islet cells.

The most serious side-effect particularly of phenformin is lactic acidosis. This presents as malaise, impairment of consciousness and acidosis. The mortality is over 50% and there is no effective treatment. This very dangerous complication is uncommon, but is usually seen in patients taking phenformin who are elderly or have renal or cardiac failure.

The biguanides and sulphonylureas have a synergistic action and the two types of drug may be given together. Both phenformin and metformin are rapidly absorbed from the gut and rapidly excreted unchanged by the kidneys. They are given twice or three times daily.

In adult-onset diabetes, the overall mortality rate in patients treated with tolbutamide and phenformin was in one trial slightly higher than in patients treated with diet alone, or diet plus insulin. Other trials have failed to confirm these findings.

ADRENAL CORTICAL HORMONES: CORTICOSTEROIDS

The adrenal cortex secretes cortisol (hydrocortisone), aldosterone and some of the sex hormones. Cortisol is a *glucocorticoid*, and raises the blood glucose by accelerating the breakdown of tissue glycogen.

The glucocorticoids have powerful anti-inflammatory actions. It is because of this that drugs such as hydrocortisone and prednisolone can be life-saving in severe refractory asthma and anaphylaxis. The mechanism of this effect is via a mediator substance, lipocortin. The steroid enters many types of cell, binds to cytoplasmic receptors and then the combination enters the nucleus which is stimulated to produce the specific mRNA for lipocortin synthesis. The lipocortin mediates several actions, which include:

1. Inhibition of phospholipase and thus reducing the synthesis of prostaglandins and leucotrienes. The prostaglandins cause the pain, oedema and vasodilatation of acute inflammation and the leucotrienes mediate cellular infiltration, mucosal secretion and bronchoconstriction in more prolonged inflammation.

2. Inhibition of the production of interleukin 2. This is a substance secreted by lymphocytes which stimulates the proliferation of T-lymphocytes. Because steroids block proliferation of T-cells in this way, cell-mediated immunity is reduced.

3. Inhibition of the release of and the response to lymphokines. The lymphokines are proteins released from killer lymphocytes in severe inflammation (such as rejection of a foreign tissue graft or necrosis in a granuloma) which destroys tissue cells.

Aldosterone is a *mineralocorticoid* and controls sodium and water excretion.

If cortisone is administered it is inactive until it is converted in the liver to cortisol.

Clinical applications of glucocorticoids

There are two main applications for glucocorticoids, namely, (1) as replacement of the steroid in patients with adrenal insufficiency (due to adrenal or pituitary disease) and (2) the more common use is in the suppression of inflammatory and immunologically mediated diseases such as rheumatoid arthritis, eczema and asthma.

Corticosteroids enter the general circulation when given orally or by injection. Alternatively, the drug may be applied locally to skin or mucous membranes. This gives a high concentration at the site of inflammation with relatively little systemic absorption.

Cortisol has mineralocorticoid activity as well as glucocorticoid and anti-inflammatory effects. Mineralocorticoids promote retention of sodium and water, and loss of potassium by the kidney. These actions help to restore blood pressure, and fluid and electrolyte balance in cases of adrenal insufficiency but play no part in anti-inflammatory effects.

Corticosteroids are used in physiological amounts in replacement therapy and successfully reverse the tendency to hypoglycaemia, dehydration and hypotension due to adrenal insufficiency in such conditions as Addison's disease.

Table 15.1 Equivalent anti-inflammatory doses of glucocorticoids

Bethamethasone	3 mg
Cortisone acetate	100 mg
Dexamethasone	3 mg
Hydrocortisone	80 mg
Methylprednisolone	16 mg
Prednisolone	20 mg
Triamcinolone	16 mg

When anti-inflammatory activity is required, it is necessary to use a steroid with predominantly glucocorticoid (anti-inflammatory) actions and thus avoid oedema and hypertension. Such steroids include *prednisolone, triamcinolone, betamethasone* and *dexamethasone*. Prednisone is inactive until it is converted in the body to prednisolone. The latter is used instead of prednisone.

The relative potencies of the different corticosteroids are shown in Table 15.1.

Adverse effects

When used as an anti-inflammatory agent, very large doses are used and this causes a variety of toxic effects. These include:

1. Feedback inhibition of the pituitary-adrenal system.
2. Glucocorticoid actions.
3. Mineralocorticoid actions.

1. Pituitary-adrenal inhibition. Prolonged steroid therapy in childhood can arrest growth, presumably because of inhibition of pituitary growth hormone release, but other actions probably contribute.

Another important consequence of prolonged steroid treatment is adrenal cortical suppression. During corticosteroid treatment and for up to 2 years after cessation of steroid administration, the adrenal cortex cannot produce its normal outpouring of cortisone in response to stress. Under these circumstances, if the patient for instance breaks a leg, develops a severe infection, undergoes an operation under general anaesthesia or goes into status asthmaticus, acute adrenal insufficiency with severe hypotension may develop. This can be prevented by giving large doses of steroids.

2. Glucocorticoid actions. The toxic effects of cortisone due to its glucocorticoid (and anti-inflammatory) actions include aggravation of pre-existing diabetes, development of diabetes in a pre-diabetic individual, peptic ulceration and gastric haemorrhage, loss of bone density and loss of collagen in the skin. Resistance to infections is reduced and bacterial, fungal and viral infections may be acquired.

3. Mineralocorticoid actions. Sodium and water retention lead to oedema and hypertension. Potassium loss causes muscular weakness.

Treatment of adrenal insufficiency

Both the glucocorticoid and mineralocorticoid properties of the steroids are needed. The glucocorticoid action is provided by hydrocortisone. In addition to combat hyponatraemia, dehydration and hypotension, a pure mineralocorticoid steroid is also given. Aldosterone is the natural mineralocorticoid secreted by the adrenal cortex, but this is not readily available. A synthetic steroid – fludrocortisone – has very powerful mineralocorticoid activity with negligible glucocorticoid and anti-inflammatory effects and is an effective substitute.

In the body cortisone is converted to hydrocortisone (cortisol). When a very rapid action is needed – as in hypotensive and Addisonian shock, anaphylactic shock or status asthmaticus – hydrocortisone in large doses is injected intravenously. Cortisone may be given for chronic conditions, usually orally or intramuscularly. However, hydrocortisone is also preferred in chronic illness because of individual variation in the ability of the liver to activate cortisone to cortisol.

Actions of adrenal corticosteroids: summary

The actions of corticosteroids have been considered from the viewpoint of their pharmacological actions. Their clinical usefulness and also their adverse effects can, however, be summarised as follows:

1. Carbohydrate metabolism (glucocorticoid effects)

Gluconeogenesis increases and the peripheral utilisation of glucose may be depressed. The blood sugar is thereby raised and diabetes may be precipitated or exacerbated.

2. Protein metabolism

Anabolism (conversion of amino acids to proteins) is depressed but catabolism is not. There is therefore muscle wasting, loss of bone matrix (causing osteoporosis) and increased capillary fragility, causing purpura. Healing and fibrosis are also inhibited.

3. Inflammation and allergy

The inflammatory response is suppressed. This can be useful, but may be dangerous since infection may progress unchecked.

Anaphylaxis and other consequences of allergic reactions are suppressed, but the antigen–antibody reaction itself is apparently unaffected. Antibody production is depressed only when large doses of steroids are given.

High concentrations of adrenal cortical steroids depress cell-mediated immunity. These immunosuppressive actions account for the main usage of corticosteroids clinically (See Ch. 13).

4. Mineral metabolism

Sodium retention by the renal tubule is promoted, leading to water retention. The increased plasma volume may in turn lead to oedema and raised blood pressure.

5. Fat deposition

Fat is deposited in particular sites, notably face, shoulders and abdomen. The face becomes 'moon shaped' and this is one of the characteristic signs of prolonged corticosteroid therapy.

6. Mood changes

A feeling of well-being is not uncommon, but may go on to euphoria or, rarely, psychotic states.

7. Anti-vitamin D action

Absorption of calcium from the gut is impaired and hypercalcaemia in diseases such as sarcoidosis (but not hyperparathyroidism) is reversed.

8. Adrenocortical suppression

Prolonged administration of corticosteroids depresses cortical function by a feedback mechanism. After a time the cortex becomes unable to respond to stressful conditions by production of cortisol and dangerous hypotensive collapse can result.

Growth in children may be arrested. The overall mechanism is unknown, but the epiphyses fuse prematurely. Pituitary growth hormone release may be inhibited. Depression of protein formation and calcium absorption are presumably also contributory.

In addition to the moon face appearance (which often passes for healthy plumpness), the complexion is often of very good colour. This, with the subjective feelings of well-being, often effectively masks serious disease with a spurious and dangerously misleading appearance of good health. It is important to bear this in mind when assessing a patient for surgery and general anaesthesia.

Uses of corticosteroids in oral disease

Topical application

Corticosteroids are used for non-infective, inflammatory conditions, such as recurrent aphthae and lichen planus, where there is no identifiable cause that can be removed.

The actions of corticosteroids under these circumstances are not clear, but they are probably mainly anti-inflammatory.

The preparations available are Corlan pellets (hydrocortisone hemisuccinate 2.5 mg) and triamcinolone paste (Adcortyl in Orabase).

Recurrent aphthae

Since there is no reason to suppose that corticosteroids hasten the healing of ulcers, they are probably most effective during the initial inflammatory changes. It is not easy even for the patient to know when these are starting and the only practical way of dealing with the problem is to take the pellets whether or not ulcers seem to be present. For this purpose Corlan pellets are used and allowed to dissolve as slowly as possible in the mouth. Two or three a day are taken. Such a course of treatment is only justified for patients who have very frequent ulceration (a week or so between the healing of one crop and the outbreak of another). There is no evidence that this level of dosage (i.e. up to 7.5 mg of hydrocortisone a day) has any

harmful effect such as adrenal suppression. In any case, since the disease is subject to natural remissions and the effectiveness of treatment difficult to assess, this course of treatment should be continued for no more than 2 months, then stopped for a month to reassess the position. If results seem to have been satisfactory, another course of treatment can be given.

Triamcinolone paste (Adcortyl in Orabase) is triamcinolone acetonide (0.1%) in a vehicle consisting of gelatin, pectin and methyl cellulose. This takes up water and forms a gel which adheres firmly to the oral mucosa. This forms a protective covering and keeps the corticosteroid in contact with the lesion.

The chief problem is the great difficulty patients inevitably have in applying a pin-head amount of the paste in precisely the right place within their own mouth and then getting the paste to gel. If it fails to imbibe enough water, the paste simply wipes off. If this preparation is to have any value at all, the patient has to be shown exactly how to apply it but, because of the inherent difficulties, may still fail to get any benefit. These difficulties restrict the usefulness of triamcinolone paste to cases where the lesions are accessible, i.e. near the front of the mouth, and are relatively infrequent.

The usefulness of corticosteroids for aphthous stomatitis is limited. Only a minority of patients respond well; stronger corticosteroids or systemic administration achieve no better results.

Lichen planus

Corlan pellets and triamcinolone paste can also be used for atrophic or erosive lesions of lichen planus, but with limited effect. The more powerful anti-inflammatory corticosteroids are more useful, but preparations for topical oral use are not generally available. Severe and otherwise intractable cases of oral lichen planus respond to systemic corticosteroids. Triamcinolone paste is sometimes helpful in the management of gingival lichen planus (so-called desquamative gingivitis).

Bullous stomatitis

Mucous membrane pemphigoid can often be treated with topical corticosteroids while the lesions remain localised to the mouth. The most suitable preparations are the more potent corticosteroids such as beclomethasone dipropionate or betamethasone valerate, but the only available preparations of these that can be conveniently used in the mouth are the sprays used for the treatment of asthma. Such sprays deliver a metered dose of 100 μg per puff but this can be repeated several times until there is an adequate amount of the corticosteroid deposited on the lesion. If, however, ocular bullae develop then systemic corticosteroids become necessary.

Pemphigus vulgaris is an autoimmune disease where the epithelial cells lose their normal adherence to one another causing oral ulceration and disintegration of the skin surface with fatal effects if untreated. Antibodies both localised to the region of the intercellular attachments and systemically in the circulation can be demonstrated and the disease responds well to immunosuppressive treatment but very large doses (100 mg of prednisolone a day) of corticosteroids are needed to control the disease. To lessen the dose azathioprine is given in addition, but even so, a typical regimen would be prednisolone 40–60 mg/day plus azathioprine 100–150 mg/day. After prolonged treatment of this sort patients have a sustained remission.

Management of dental patients on systemic corticosteroids

When patients have been on long-term corticosteroid therapy (and possibly for up to 2 years after its withdrawal) adrenocortical function is depressed. A stressful situation such as an injury or operation under general anaesthesia can then precipitate acute hypotension and circulatory failure. This may be fatal. Protection must therefore be provided by giving adequate amounts of hydrocortisone as it is less difficult to prevent than to treat a crisis of this sort.

Short-term use of corticosteroids in this way has no significant ill-effects and it is safer to err on the side of giving too much rather than too little for this dangerous condition.

If such a patient needs dental surgery under general anaesthesia or even multiple extractions under local anaesthesia at least 100 mg of hydrocortisone should be given beforehand. Hydrocortisone

succinate can be given intravenously at the start of the operation or at induction. This immediately raises the blood level of cortisol and is usually adequate if the operation is not too long. If signs of a falling blood pressure appear the injection should be repeated as often as necessary.

When hypotensive collapse develops in an inadequately prepared or unprepared patient 100–500 mg of hydrocortisone succinate should be given intravenously immediately and the patient admitted to hospital. Even with continued administration of hydrocortisone and intravenous fluid infusion, it may take 24 hours for the blood pressure to recover fully, but occasionally the condition proves irreversible and fatal.

Routine conservative dentistry under local anaesthesia probably requires no special precautions. But if there is any sign of incipient collapse intravenous hydrocortisone should be given without hesitation.

Steroid antagonists

A few drugs block steroid synthesis. The main example is *metapyrone*, which controls the symptoms of and is used for the preoperative management of Cushing's disease. *Aminoglutethimide* inhibits steroid production in the adrenals and also blocks conversion of androgens to oestrogens in the tissues. It is used as a hormone antagonist in the treatment of breast cancer.

PARATHYROID HORMONE AND CALCITONIN

The control of body calcium

Calcium plays several essential roles in the body. These include formation and maintenance of the skeleton, the control of secretory processes and the functioning of excitable tissues such as nerve and muscle. Calcium in trace quantities is also essential for blood clotting and various other enzymic reactions. The amounts needed for these latter processes are, however, so small that they are not affected by the blood calcium level. If the blood calcium level fell sufficiently low, death due to cardiac arrhythmia would come long before clotting or other enzymic processes were impaired.

The concentration of calcium in the plasma and other body fluids is dependent on:

1. The amount of calcium absorbed from the intestine.

2. The amount of calcium excreted in the urine.

3. The equilibrium between mobilisation from, and deposition of calcium into bone.

The skeleton forms the main bulk of calcium salts in the body and acts as the reservoir of calcium.

Several factors influence these basic processes. These include vitamin D, parathyroid hormone and calcitonin (see Fig. 15.1).

Vitamin D

Vitamin D exists in several forms. The natural fat-soluble vitamin is cholecalciferol (vitamin D_3). Calciferol (vitamin D_2) is a semisynthetic product which is used therapeutically. When ultraviolet light acts on the skin it converts an inactive precursor, 7-dehydrocholesterol, into vitamin D_3.

Vitamin D_3 is absorbed from the gut. Cholecalciferol is then converted by the liver and kidney into a metabolite which acts on intestinal absorption of calcium, renal handling of calcium and phosphate, calcification of skeletal tissue and contractility of voluntary muscle. Thus, the active vitamin en-hances calcium absorption from dietary sources by potentiating intestinal transport of the ion. Calcium and phosphate enter the kidney in the glomerular filtrate. Vitamin D increases reabsorption of renal tubular calcium into the circulation and decreases the reabsorption of phosphate. If there is a relative or absolute lack of vitamin D there is failure of the organic matrix of replacement bone to calcify and this results in a bone disease known as osteomalacia, in which there is skeletal weakness.

Vitamin D deficiency in children causes rickets. The mechanism of the disease process is similar but, in developing bones, rickets causes disorganisation of the zone of provisional calcification of the epiphyseal cartilage and the epiphyseal plates become thickened, wide and uneven.

Malabsorption syndromes are also potential causes of vitamin D deficiency while chronic renal disease (either hereditary or inflammatory) can also cause excessive bone mineral loss. The latter condition is known as renal rickets and is relatively resistant to vitamin D.

Vitamin D deficiency also causes muscular weakness.

An important consequence of vitamin D

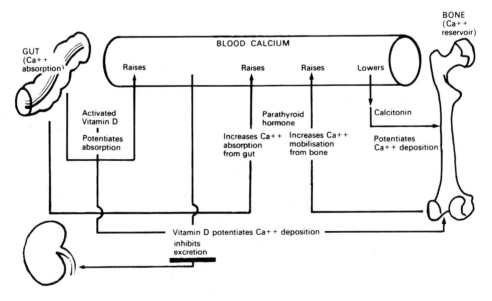

Fig. 15.1 Diagram indicating the way in which calcium balance is maintained by the interaction of three main agents (vitamin D, parathyroid hormone and calcitonin) on calcium absorption and deposition or resorption from bone

deficiency is hypocalcaemia which may be severe enough to result in tetany or convulsions.

Parathormone

The parathyroid gland secretes the peptide hormone, parathormone (PTH). This hormone is released when the blood calcium falls, while a raised blood calcium inhibits release of PTH.

PTH acts on bone, intestine and excretory mechanisms. PTH mobilises calcium from bone and thus raises plasma calcium at the expense of bone calcium. This is the most important action of the hormone. Excessive activity of the parathyroid glands due to hyperplasia or a PTH-producing tumour causes excessive bone resorption, enhances osteoclastic activity and disappearance of bone matrix. Advanced disease is characterised by osteitis fibrosa cystica but this is now rare.

Osteitis fibrosa cystica consists of areas of bone destruction which resemble cysts in radiographs. These are not cysts but solid aggregations of soft tissue consisting mainly of osteoclasts.

PTH potentiates the action of vitamin D in mediating the absorption of calcium by the intestine. PTH decreases excretion of calcium into the urine, faeces, sweat and milk.

Hypofunction of the parathyroid is characterised by a lowering of blood calcium, which may lead to tetany.

Calcitonin

This hormone is produced by the thyroid gland. It has actions which are, in general, opposite to those of PTH and injection of calcitonin produces an immediate fall in blood calcium. It acts principally by increasing uptake of calcium by bones.

Clinical applications of calcitonin. Salmon and human calcitonin have been used. At present the usual preparations for treatment are porcine and synthetic salmon calcitonin. As might be expected, the preparations of animal origin can provoke antibody production which interferes with treatment.

The main uses of calcitonin so far are in the treatment of hypercalcaemia and Paget's disease.

Hypercalcaemia. The causes include immobilisation, vitamin D intoxication, sarcoidosis, multiple myeloma, malignancy of bone and hyperparathyroidism. Calcitonin acts rapidly and can reverse severe hypercalcaemia which might otherwise be fatal due to renal failure or cardiac arrhythmias.

Paget's disease

In the early stages especially, osteoclastic activity predominates and may cause hypercalcaemia and severe bone pain. These can both be corrected by giving calcitonin but there is usually antibody production after a time. Salmon calcitonin is less strongly antigenic than porcine but antibody production is a limiting factor in the prolonged treatment necessary for Paget's disease.

Disodium etidronate. Etidronate is adsorbed onto hydroxyapatite crystals and slows both their rate of growth and resorption. This reduces the rate of bone turnover characteristic of Paget's disease and etidronate is probably the treatment of choice since it can be given in repeated courses without diminished activity.

Summary

Some of the factors controlling blood calcium can be summarised as follows:

1. Dietary intake of vitamin D and calcium.

2. Parathormone secretion promotes removal of calcium from the bones and raises the blood calcium level. PTH also potentiates the action of vitamin D by increasing absorption and decreasing renal excretion of calcium.

3. Calcitonin opposes the action of parathormone and lowers the blood calcium mainly by increasing deposition of calcium in the bones.

4. Absorption of calcium may also be depressed in intestinal diseases characterised by malabsorption, i.e. steatorrhoea.

5. Excretion of calcium is enhanced in some chronic renal diseases.

6. Increased demands for calcium are made during pregnancy and lactation and may be excessive if intake is poor.

7. Ionisable calcium is depressed when there is alkalosis. This in turn may be due to overbreathing (losing CO_2) or vomiting (losing gastric acid) and can lead to tetany.

SUGGESTED FURTHER READING

Anon 1987 LHRH analogues for contraception. Lancet i: 1179
Anon 1987 Problems when withdrawing corticosteroids. Drug and Therapetics Bulletin 25: 73
Ferner R E, Neil H A W 1988 Sulphonylureas and hypoglycaemia. British Medical Journal 296: 949
Hughes I A 1987 Steroids and growth. British Medical Journal 295: 684
Kubba A A, Guillebaud J P 1986 Clinical algorithms. Contraception. British Medical Journal 293: 1491
Nattrass M 1986 Treatment of type II diabetes. British Medical Journal 292: 1033
Nordstrom R E A, Nordstrom R M 1987 The effect of corticosteroids on postoperative edema. Plastic and Reconstructive Surgery 80: 85

16. Nutrition: vitamins

Vitamins catalyse metabolic processes and are essential for normal health. Vitamins (apart from vitamin K which is synthesised in the gut) are supplied by the diet and vitamin supplementation (despite widespread beliefs to the contrary) is rarely needed.

Vitamin deficiencies result from:

1. Malnutrition.
2. Abnormal diets.
3. Disorders of absorption.

Vitamin deficiencies produce well-defined diseases but it is very rare for deficiency of a single vitamin to develop. Vitamin deficiencies are usually multiple and associated with malnutrition. As a consequence vitamin deficiencies are only seen in Britain or the rest of the Western world in special groups of people. These include food faddists, vegans (those who eat a pure vegetable diet with no meat or dairy products of any sort) and chronic alcoholics. In the past scurvy developed among the crews of sailing ships who, on journeys lasting many months, were completely deprived of fruit or green vegetables. Some vitamin deficiencies are due to failure of absorption rather than dietary deficiencies. The main examples are vitamin B_{12} deficiency causing pernicious anaemia and vitamin K deficiency causing hypoprothrombinaemia. These examples are discussed in Chapter 12 since their effect is on the functions of the blood.

Vitamin deficiencies have in the past been of considerable interest in dentistry because lack of vitamin C and members of the B group in particular can cause gingivitis or stomatitis. As a consequence it has been suggested that subclinical deficiencies of these agents can contribute to oral disease. There is in fact no evidence to support this view.

There is no purpose in arbitrarily giving or taking vitamins if the diet is adequate and in the absence of disease affecting absorption. Vitamins are not tonics and any effect they may have in healthy persons is purely subjective.

The taking of large quantities of multivitamin preparations is however sedulously promoted by the 'health food' industry with greater benefits to it than to the consumer.

The vitamins comprise two groups:

1. Fat-soluble vitamins A, D, E and K.
2. Water-soluble vitamin B group and C.

Fat-soluble vitamins (A, D, E and K)

Vitamin A

Vitamin A (retinol) is present in fish, milk, egg yolk and liver. It is also present in carrots and green vegetables as a precursor or provitamin. Vitamin A is essential for the formation of retinal pigment (visual purple) and deficiency of vitamin A leads to impaired vision in poor light (night-blindness).

Vitamin A also affects the behaviour of epithelium; deficiency causes glandular epithelium to undergo squamous metaplasia while squamous epithelium tends to become hyperkeratinised. It was thought, therefore, that vitamin A deficiency played a part in the development of chronic hyperkeratotic lesions of the mouth (so-called leukoplakia) but although this idea is still under consideration there is at the moment no proof that this is the case.

Overdose of vitamin A can have serious toxic effects including desquamation of the skin and hepatotoxicity.

There is some evidence that vitamin A may

possibly have a protective action against tumour formation.

Analogues of vitamin A (retinoids) are of considerable interest in dermatology and one of them (etretinate; Tigason) is available for the treatment of severe congenital disorders of keratinisation and of intractable psoriasis. Adverse effects are frequent however, and most patients develop dryness and cracking of the lips and many develop a dry mouth or nose. Etretinate is also teratogenic. Isotretinoin (Roaccutane) is another retinoid used in dermatology for the treatment of severe acne. As well as being teratogenic, this substance can cause hyperostosis, corneal opacities and premature fusion of the epiphyses.

Vitamin A is believed by some to be involved in some way with oncogenesis. In one retrospective study a group of men with cancers of the head and neck region appeared to have had less than average vitamin A intake. Vitamin A derivatives have also been used as adjuncts to other drugs in the treatment of various types of tumours and some benefits have been claimed. The role of vitamin deficiency in oncogenesis and of vitamin A analogues in cancer treatment is currently being investigated.

Vitamin D

The main source of vitamin D is in fish liver oils but small amounts are also present in eggs and butter. In strong sunlight vitamin D can be synthesised in the skin. In Britain margarine is fortified with vitamins A and D. The requirements are, however, small except during periods of bone growth and pregnancy.

Deficiency of vitamin D in the growing child causes rickets. This at one time was said to have disappeared from Britain but cases are still seen, especially among immigrants and particularly in Scotland and the North of England where lack of sunlight, a high carbohydrate diet and possibly also the use of wholemeal flour, containing factors which impair the absorption of calcium, appear to be contributory.

Another factor that is likely to contribute to rickets among those who use wholemeal flour is that the latter is the only form of flour to which calcium (as a result of the 'health food' lobby) is not added, as a legal requirement. Is rickets then one of the benefits of a wholesome, additive-free diet?

There is no basis for the idea that dental caries is due to poor calcification of the teeth resulting from vitamin D deficiency, and in fact countries where malnutrition is rife show a lower incidence of dental caries than in the West where the diet is often excessive particularly in respect of sugar. The giving of vitamin D and calcium for the prevention or reduction of dental caries is therefore valueless. In addition, there are dangers associated with increasing children's intake of vitamin D since they are likely to be having foods such as milk and cereals fortified with this vitamin. Some children are sensitive to the action of this potent drug and hypervitaminosis D causes hypercalcaemia and renal calcinosis.

The role of vitamin D in calcium homeostasis has been discussed in more detail in Chapter 15.

Vitamin K

Vitamin K is present in green leaves and fruit and is also synthesised by the microorganisms in the gut which probably provide the main source. Deficiency does not come from dietary causes but from malabsorption due to such diseases as obstructive jaundice.

Vitamin K, as discussed in Chapter 12, is a precursor of prothrombin, an essential clotting factor. Virtually the only condition in which true vitamin K deficiency is seen is in the newborn who are neither taking green vegetables nor have a fully developed gut flora which synthesises vitamin K. Hypothrombinaemia caused by deficiency of vitamin K is treated by giving acetomenaphthone by injection. This, however, is ineffective where there is severe liver disease since prothrombin cannot then be synthesised. Vitamin K is of no value whatsoever as a non-specific haemostatic agent when there is no deficiency.

Vitamin E

Vitamin E, an antioxidant, has for long been thought to be of no medical importance. However, in the USA in particular, vitamin E has been consumed on a considerable scale because of the pathetic and misplaced belief that, since it is necessary for normal reproductive activity of rats, it increases sexual vigour in humans. The effect of vitamin E in humans is quite different from this, but it has been difficult to establish whether vitamin E deficiency can genuinely affect humans, largely because of the very long time it takes to deplete the normal body stores.

However, vitamin E deficiency can result from syndromes where fat absorption is defective such as abetalipoproteinaemia and can lead to degenerative neurological disorders and retinal lesions in children. High doses of vitamin E can considerably improve neurological function in these conditions, especially if treatment is started early, but benefit even in affected adults has also been reported.

This rare neurological disorder is the only known effect of vitamin E deficiency in humans.

Water-soluble vitamins (B and C groups)

B group vitamins

Vitamin B₁ (thiamin, aneurin). The main source is in the husks of grain and in peas, beans and eggs. Deficiency of thiamin causes the disease known as beri-beri which is virtually only seen in the Far East, but a similar deficiency state may develop in chronic alcoholics. It is characterised by polyneuritis, cardiac failure and mental disorder.

Vitamin B₂ (riboflavin) is widely distributed in yeast products, meat, offal, milk and green vegetables. Riboflavin deficiency causes cracking of the lips (cheilitis), stomatitis, a sore tongue with a pebbly surface and dermatitis. As a consequence vitamin B (usually as a mixture of several B vitamins) is often given for stomatitis, cheilitis or a sore tongue but is almost never effective since the causes are elsewhere.

Vitamin B₆ (pyridoxine) is also widely distributed and the sources are similar to those of riboflavin. Pyridoxine acts as a coenzyme in many metabolic processes but it is not certain whether pyridoxine deficiency is a definable disease in man and no clinical syndrome has so far been ascribed to it apart from the peripheral neuropathy due to isoniazid treatment.

Nicotinamide. The main sources of nicotin-amide are again meat, offal and whole grains. Severe deficiency of nicotinamide produces pellagra (literally 'rough skin') with the classical features of glossitis, dermatitis, diarrhoea and dementia. Pellagra is usually a multiple deficiency state associated with malnutrition and rarely if ever a pure nicotinamide deficiency.

Ascorbic acid (vitamin C)

The main sources are fresh green vegetables and fresh fruit. The vitamin is easily oxidised and destroyed by cooking. If the sources of vitamin C are cut off, deficiency takes several months to develop. Scurvy is exceedingly rare in Britain and practically the only people who get it are the isolated elderly living on a restricted diet (e.g. tea and buns).

Vitamin C is concerned with collagen formation and deficiency also affects platelet function. Vitamin C deficiency (scurvy) is characterised by a rash, purpura and mental changes. Purpura may be severe and is a contributory factor in the production of the spongy, swollen and bleeding gums which are a sign only of advanced disease. Vitamin C has no beneficial effect on the treatment of the common forms of gingivitis.

Lest it be thought that scurvy is of historical interest only, a 24-year-old engineer was reported in 1983 to have the disease in classical form including swollen, bleeding gums. He had lived largely on peanut butter sandwiches, recalled having eaten an apple 4 years previously but could not recall *ever* having eaten an orange.

It has been suggested that massive doses of ascorbic acid prevent or are helpful in the treatment of the common cold. This is, however, unproven and the effect, if any, is marginal. Moreover, cessation of megadose intake of ascorbic acid can lead to rebound deficiency and scurvy. In one bizarre case, death followed the intravenous injection of no less than 80 g of ascorbic acid. This really does seem to be carrying prevention too far.

SUGGESTED FURTHER READING

Aggett P J 1979 Trace elements in medicine. Hospital Update 5: 981

Bieri J G, Corash L, Hubbard V S 1983 Medical uses of vitamin E. New England Journal of Medicine 308: 1063

Bollag W 1983 Vitamin A and retinoids. Lancet i: 860

Dworken H J 1983 Vitamin E reconsidered Annals of Internal Medicine 98: 253

Eastwood M A , Passmore R 1983 Dietary fibre. Lancet ii: 202

Goldfarb M T 1987 Retinoids in dermatology. Mayo Clinic Proceedings 62: 1161

Heath D A 1987 Treating Paget's disease. British Medical Journal 294: 1048

Herbert V 1980 The Vitamin craze. Archives of Internal Medicine 140: 173

Morley J E, Levine A S 1983 The central control of appetite Lancet ii: 398

Muller D P R, Lloyd J K, Wolff O H 1983 Vitamin E and neurological function. Lancet, i: 225

Orfanos C E, Ehlert R, Gollnick H 1986 The retinoids. Drugs 34: 459

Paterson C R, Feely J 1983 Vitamin D metabolites and analogues, diphosphonates, danazol, and bromocriptine. British Medical Journal 286: 1625

Peck G L 1980 Retinoids in dermatology. Archives of Dermatology 116: 283–284

Riggs L B, Kumar R 1981 Vitamin D in the therapy of disorders of calcium and phosphorus metabolism. Mayo Clinic proceedings 56: 327

Roberts H J 1981 Perspective on vitamin E as therapy. Journal of the American Medical Association 246: 129

Rudman D, Williams P J 1983 Megadose vitamins. New England Journal of Medicine 309: 488

Shah J P, Strong E W, DeCosse J J, Itri L, Sellers P 1983 Effect of retinoids on oral leukoplakia. American Journal of Surgery 146: 466

Yob E H, Pochi P E 1987 Side effects and long-term toxicity of synthetic retinoids. Archives of Dermatology 123: 1375a.

17. The alimentary system

Indigestion (dyspepsia)

Indigestion is not a disease but a variety of symptoms, often without organic cause. Typical symptoms of indigestion are a feeling of distension (flatulence), abdominal discomfort or pain, acid reflux (heartburn), intolerance of some foods and nausea. The same symptoms can however result from peptic ulcer, cancer of the stomach and many other gastrointestinal diseases and these must be excluded before dyspepsia is treated as such. Features strongly suggestive of functional dyspepsia is that the patient often has anxiety traits and, despite persistence of symptoms for long periods, the patient remains well and does not lose weight.

The treatment of functional indigestion is important because: (1) it is one of the most common complaints in medicine, (2) the cost of treatment runs into many millions of pounds annually and (3) patients need to be reassured of the absence of serious organic disease.

Management of dyspepsia. Organic disease must first be excluded by appropriate investigation. Non-drug treatment includes reassurance, stopping smoking and reducing alcohol intake, and exclusion of provocative foods such as fried foods. The main drugs effective for dyspepsia are antacids (the standard over-the-counter preparations, which are consumed on a vast scale) and H_2 receptor antagonists (see below).

Antacids. The most satisfactory formulation of antacids for indigestion or peptic ulcer pain is the combination of aluminium glycinate or hydroxide and magnesium trisilicate or hydroxide. These are effective buffers but do not cause alkalosis, and are long acting. In addition, the mildly constipating effect of aluminium compounds is counteracted by the mildly purgative action of the magnesium hydroxide. Liquid mixtures are more effective than tablets – the latter are simply more convenient to carry around.

Hiatus hernia and gastro-oesophageal reflux are a displacement of the oesophagogastric junction and part of the stomach into the thorax. Because the pinching action of the diaphragm has been lost, gastric contents repeatedly reflux into the oesophagus. This process causes heartburn and other symptoms. There seems, however, to be little relation between the physical changes and the symptoms, many of which are probably functional.

Frequent and regular administration of antacids suppresses symptoms by reducing the irritant action of gastric acid on the oesophageal mucosa. Local anaesthetics with antacids are sometimes used to diminish oesophageal pain.

An alternative approach is to increase the viscosity and solidity of the gastric contents in order to reduce reflux. Alginic acid is used in this way.

Metoclopramide has many actions on alimentary function and amongst these it increases the tone of the oesophagogastric sphincter and increases the magnitude of peristaltic waves down the oesophagus. Further benefit in hiatus hernia is provided by the action of the drug in increasing the rate of gastric emptying through the pylorus. Metoclopramide is often also used as an antiemetic.

Cimetidine and *ranitidine* (p. 201) are also effective in relieving the symptoms of gastro-oesophageal reflux.

Achalasia is a disorder of oesophageal motility due to deficiency in the autonomic nerve supply and causes difficulty in swallowing. Amyl nitrite helps the condition by relaxing the oesophago-gastric sphincter. Parasympathomimetic drugs such as methacholine also help.

Antiemetic drugs

Several drugs antagonise the vomiting response. These may act on the vomiting centre in the brain or on nervous connections with it. Alternatively drugs may have a direct action on the alimentary tract.

1. Hyoscine and most of the antihistamines (such as *cyclizine* and *diphenhydramine*) have a central antiemetic action and are useful in the prevention of motion sickness and vomiting associated with vertigo.

2. Chlorpromazine and *trifluoperazine* are major tranquilliser drugs which are also powerfully antiemetic. They are not effective against travel sickness, but are active against vomiting due to toxic and metabolic causes.

3. Metoclopramide has both peripheral and central antiemetic actions. It is not effective against travel sickness, but prevents vomiting due to a wide range of toxic and metabolic causes. Metoclopramide increases oesophageal and gastric motility. It also increases peristalsis in the small intestine. Like the phenothiazine drugs, metoclopramide has a central inhibitory action on the chemoreceptor trigger zone in the brain. This normally has a stimulatory effect on the vomiting centre when activated.

As discussed earlier, this action of metoclopramide on the chemoreceptor trigger zone of the vomiting centre is because it is a dopamine receptor blocker. It can thus cause involuntary muscular activity and, in particular, trismus.

Domperidone (Motilium) has a similar action to metoclopropamide but little of the drug penetrates the brain and thus it does not cause the involuntary movement and muscular spasm which result from metoclopropamide administration. However, domperidone also has a powerful inhibitory effect on the chemoreceptor trigger zone.

4. Cannabinoids (such as nabilone) are powerful antiemetics and may be helpful in treating nausea following irradiation or cytotoxic drug treatment.

5. Steroids (such as prednisolone) may act as antiemetics in terminal illness.

Vomiting or retching during dental procedures (such as impression taking) are mainly caused by anxiety and can often be prevented by giving diazepam.

Gastric secretion and peptic ulceration

Acid and pepsin are secreted by the gastric mucosal cells. The parasympathetic nerve to the stomach is the vagus. When this is activated gastric secretion is increased. When food enters the stomach, gastrin is secreted and further stimulates acid production

Substances released by the small intestine – cholecystokinin-pancreozymin and secretin – diminish gastric acid production. It is thought that gastrin acts by releasing histamine from the stomach wall, which in turn stimulates acid secretion.

Peptic ulceration is a localised area of inflammation and loss of epithelium in the alimentary tract. A peptic ulcer will only form at a site where acid and pepsin come in contact with the mucosa. The commonest sites involved are the lower end of the oesophagus, stomach and duodenum. The condition may present as pain or as a complication of the ulcer such as perforation or haemorrhage.

The following are some of the medical approaches to the treatment of peptic ulceration:

1. Bed rest not only diminishes peptic ulcer symptoms, but increases the rate of healing. It is not known why this is so effective, but it has been suggested that complete rest decreases autonomic nervous stimulation of secretion.

2. Stopping smoking is also a surprisingly effective means of accelerating ulcer healing.

3. H_2 receptor blocking drugs. Histamine has several actions. These can be divided into two groups: H_1 effects, which include vasodilatation, increased capillary permeability and bronchoconstriction; H_2 effects are stimulation of acid and pepsin secretion by the stomach, contraction of the uterus and stimulation of the heart. H_2 blocking drugs therefore inhibit acid and pepsin secretion by the stomach. In practice, such drugs are proving to be very effective in accelerating the healing of peptic ulcers. *Cimetidine* (Tagamet) and *ranitidine* (Zantac) are the H_2 blockers in current use.

Cimetidine rarely causes significant side-effects but there may occasionally be confusion or dizziness in the elderly and drugs such as oral anticoagulants, phenytoin and benzodiazepines may be potentiated by inhibition of their metabolism in the liver. Mild gynaecomastia and nephritis have also been reported. Ranitidine appears to be remarkably free from side-effects.

H_2 blocking agents produce gastric hypochlorhydria which may allow bacterial colonisation of the stomach and excessive production of nitrosamines. These substances are potentially carcinogenic but although gastric cancer has not been shown to be a clinical complication of H_2 blocker use, they should not be given for indefinite periods. Courses of 1–2 months are preferable. Needless to say, it should also be established that a gastric ulcer is not malignant before starting treatment with these drugs.

Cimetidine and ranitidine are particularly effective in accelerating the healing of duodenal ulcers (although a minority of these fail to respond) and are also valuable for reducing acid secretion in such conditions as severe reflux oesophagitis with ulceration or bleeding from erosive gastritis. Although these drugs are frequently highly effective in promoting the healing of peptic ulceration, the relapse rate after cessation of treatment is high.

4. Pirenzepine (Gastrozepin) is also a selective inhibitor of gastric acid secretion but does not act via H_2 receptors. It appears to inhibit the nervous stimulation of gastric secretion and to accelerate the healing of peptic ulcers. The mode of action of pirenzepine is a selective blockade of gastric muscarinic acetylcholine receptors (M_1).

5. Sucralfate is a salt of sucrose sulphate. This binds to the ulcer crater and exerts a local antacid action. It is as effective as H_2 blockers in promoting the healing of peptic ulcers.

6. Antacids such as sodium bicarbonate and aluminium hydroxide reduce gastric acidity and thus diminish the activity of gastric pepsin. Although antacid therapy may relieve the pain of peptic ulceration, it does not accelerate healing unless large doses are given frequently for a long period. Tripotassium dicitratobismuthate (De-Nol)

has also been shown to accelerate healing of peptic ulcers. Whether this is due to antacid effects or other properties of bismuth salts is not known.

In general, antacids are not toxic, but excessive administration can lead to side-effects. Large doses of sodium bicarbonate produce alkalosis, whilst calcium carbonate in excess can induce hypercalcaemia. Magnesium and aluminium compounds are therefore preferred.

Small frequent meals have antacid properties, due to the repeated exposure of the gastric contents to the amphoteric groups in dietary protein.

7. Anticholinergic drugs block the parasympathetic nerves to the stomach which mediate secretion. These drugs also diminish motor activity in the alimentary tract and are often called 'antispasmodics'. It is possible that smooth muscle spasm contributes to ulcer pain which these drugs could antagonise.

Drugs in this group used for the symptomatic relief of peptic ulcer include propantheline and dicyclomine. They may produce some symptomatic relief, but do not accelerate healing.

8. Carbenoxolone sodium is a derivative of one of the components of liquorice root. It effectively accelerates the healing of gastric ulcers. The drug is anti-inflammatory and also appears to protect the gastric mucosa from the effects of acid and pepsin attack. Water retention, hypertension, cardiac failure and pulmonary oedema can complicate treatment with this drug.

9. Metoclopramide reduces peptic ulcer symptoms, but does not affect healing.

10. Prostaglandins may accelerate the healing of peptic ulcers. This is because they decrease acid secretion and increase mucosal resistance. NSAIAs aggravate peptic ulceration because they inhibit prostaglandin synthesis. Examples of prostaglandin analogues under trial are misoprostol and enprostil.

Drugs used to control diarrhoea

Mild infections should not be treated with antibiotics, but symptomatic relief of non-infective diarrhoea may be given by drugs which decrease intestinal motility, or which reduce the fluid content of the stools.

1. Drugs which reduce peristalsis include atropine, diphenoxylate (in Lomotil) and mebeverine. Morphine and codeine reduce propulsive gut activity by producing a static spasm of the smooth muscle of the intestinal wall.

2. Increased viscosity of the gut contents may be achieved by agar, kaolin, methyl cellulose or bran.

3. Diarrhoea caused by the more virulent strains of shigella or enterotoxin-producing strains of *E. coli* should be treated by giving co-trimoxazole or trimethoprim, but the most important aspect of the treatment of severe infective diarrhoea is replacement of the electrolyte and fluid loss, if necessary by intravenous infusion.

Other treatments for specific illnesses include steroids and sulphasalazine for ulcerative colitis and Crohn's disease.

Infections of the gastrointestinal tract

Infective diarrhoea

Infective diarrhoea is a common hazard particularly affecting tourists in hot countries (travellers' diarrhoea, turista). It is caused by a variety of organisms. These include stains of *E. coli*, salmonellae, clostridia, shigella, *Staphylococcus aureus*, protozoa and viruses.

Many of these organisms produce an enterotoxin which accelerates transport of water and salt through the bowel wall into the gut lumen causing rapid distension of the latter by fluid. Some strains of *E. coli*, particularly in Mexico, also invade the intestinal mucosa.

The main measure in the treatment of travellers' diarrhoea is to repair fluid loss. Drugs which reduce intestinal mobility are contraindicated. Antibiotics are not usually useful but should be reserved for severe salmonella or shigella (dysenteric) infections.

The ready development and transmission of r-determinants is a potent argument against the use of antibiotics for minor self-limiting attacks of travellers' diarrhoea. There is also a good chance that such infections may be resistant anyway.

Co-trimoxazole has been shown in extensive trials to be the most effective prophylactic agent for travellers' diarrhoea in Mexico and South America and may be effective for treatment. However, the microbial causes are so varied in different parts of the world that there is no universally effective preventive agent.

Enteric fever (typhoid and paratyphoid)

Where sanitation is good, enteric fever is a rare disease, but is relatively common in underdeveloped countries and occasional cases or minor epidemics from a variety of sources can break out elsewhere.

Enteric fever is one of the few important infections where chloramphenicol may need to be given. Ampicillin has less dangerous side-effects and is bactericidal but is less effective clinically than chloramphenicol. In several parts of the world co-trimoxazole has been shown to be more effective than chloramphenicol and also has the advantages of lower toxicity and a bactericidal action. More recently still trimethoprim has been reported to be more effective than co-trimoxazole in some outbreaks of enteric fever. Nevertheless, there is still a need for a safe and completely reliable antimicrobial agent to deal with typhoid fever.

Purgatives

The use of purgatives has diminished greatly over the past 200 years because of changes in ideas about the causes and consequences of constipation. At the same time the hazards of the regular use of laxatives became known. Laxatives are classified into three main groups:

1. Bulk purgatives.
2. Lubricants.
3. Irritants.

1. Bulk purgatives promote peristalsis by increasing the volume of the intestinal contents. This produces a reflex stimulation of the intestinal musculature. Bran, agar and methyl cellulose act in this way. Non-absorbed salts such as magnesium sulphate (Epsom salts) retain water in the lumen of the gut and thus act as bulk purgatives.

Guar gum is another fibrous product which produces a gel when mixed with water. This not only shortens intestinal transit time, but reduces the absorption of glucose and lipids from the intestine. It may thus prove to be an aid in the management of diabetic patients as well as acting as a purgative.

2. *Lubricant purgatives* – which mainly act in the last few feet of intestine – include liquid paraffin and dioctyl sodium sulphosuccinate. Liquid paraffin is not recommended because it can cause lipid pneumonia, paraffin granulomas in the abdominal lymph nodes and pruritus ani.

3. *Irritant purgatives* stimulate activity of the gut wall. Senna contains an anthroquinone (emodin) which acts in this way. Castor oil is itself inert, but is digested by intestinal lipase to ricinoleic acid which is irritant. Phenolphthalein has a prolonged action because the drug is absorbed by the intestine and then re-excreted via the bile back into the intestine to produce further stimulation of the gut musculature. Such recycling, known as *enterohepatic recirculation*, may prolong the action of a drug for several days. Bisacodyl is another irritant purgative which enters an enterohepatic circulation type of recycling.

SUGGESTED FURTHER READING

Anon 1987 Omeprazole. Lancet ii: 1187

Anon 1987 The influence of relapse rate on the choice of duodenal ulcer therapy. Drug and Therapeutics Bulletin 25: 77

Editorial 1982 Cimetidine and ranitidine. Lancet i: 601

Editorial 1983 Management of acute diarrhoea. Lancet i: 623

Feel J, Wormsley K G 1983 H$_2$ receptor antagonists – cimetidine and ranitidine. British Medical Journal 286: 695

Feldman M 1987 Bicarbonate, acid and duodenal ulcer. New England Journal of Medicine 316: 408

Freston J W 1982 Cimetidine: developments, pharmacology and efficacy. Annals of Internal Medicine 97: 573

Gorbach S L 1987 Bacterial diarrhoea and its treatment. Lancet ii: 1378

Gray G R, Smith I S, McWhinnie D, Gillespie G 1982 Five-year study of cimetidine or surgery for severe duodenal ulcer dyspepsia. Lancet i: 787

Harrington R A, Hamilton C W, Brogden R N, Linkewich J A, Romankiewicz J A, Heel R C 1983 Metoclopramide. An updated review of its pharmacological properties and clinical use. Drugs 25: 451

Henry D A, Johnston A, Dobson A, Duggan J 1987 Fatal peptic ulcer complications and the use of non-steroidal anti-inflammatory drugs, aspirin and corticosteroids. British Medical Journal 295: 1227

Jackson W (ed.) 1982 The clinical use of ranitidine. Medicine International Review. Medical Education Services, London

Koch-Weser J, Schulze-Delrieu K 1981 Metoclopramide. New England Journal of Medicine 305: 28

Lane M R, Lee S P 1988 Recurrence of duodenal ulcer after medical treatment. Lancet i: 1147

Laszlo J, Lucas Jr V S 1981 Emesis as a critical problem in chemotherapy. New England Journal of Medicine 305: 948

Littman A 1983 Cimetidine works for gastric ulcer, and more. New England Journal of Medicine 308: 1356

McCarthy D M 1983 Ranitidine or cimetidine. Annals of Internal Medicine 99: 551

Russell R I 1986 Protective effect of the prostaglandins on the gastric mucosa. American Journal of Medicine 81 (suppl 2A): 2

Sack R B 1986 Antimicrobial prophylaxis of travellers' diarrhoea: a selected summary. Review of Infectious Diseases 8 (suppl 2): S160

Seigel L J, Longo D L 1981 The control of chemotherapy-induced emesis. Annals of Internal Medicine 95: 352

Wade A G, Rowley-Jones D 1988 Long term management of duodenal ulcer in general practice: How best to use cimetidine? British Medical Journal 296: 971

Weir D G 1988 New drugs. Peptic ulceration. British Medical Journal 296: 195

Zell S, Carmichael J M, Reddy A N 1987 Rational approach to long term use of H$_2$-antagonists. American Journal of Medicine 82: 796

18. Toxic effects of drugs

No drug has a single action, but drugs are usually given for a single therapeutic purpose. The undesired actions of drugs are called toxic effects (or side-effects) whether or not these have a substantially harmful effect on the patient. Iatrogenic disease is a somewhat pretentious name for drug reactions or for disease resulting from any other kind of medical treatment. It is supposed to mean 'disease produced by doctors' but 'disease which produces doctors' is probably a more correct literal translation.

Toxic effects of drugs may be considered under the following headings:

1. Dose-independent actions.
2. Dose-dependent effects.
3. Drug interactions.
4. Idiosyncrasy.

1. Dose-independent toxic actions of drugs

These are mainly allergic reactions. In many cases there is no way of predicting whether a patient is going to develop an allergic reaction; the first exposure to a drug may produce no adverse reaction, but subsequent exposures are followed by allergic responses. A previous history of asthma, infantile eczema, hay fever or urticaria usually indicates an increased liability to develop allergy.

Allergy to drugs ranges from mild local itching to fatal anaphylactic shock. In general, the shorter the interval between drug administration and the onset of clinical signs of allergy, the more serious the reaction. A rough guide is that reactions which begin within half an hour may be life-threatening, while those which start on the following day are usually relatively mild.

Anaphylaxis is a dangerous early allergic response and may lead to fatal cardiovascular collapse, bronchospasm or laryngeal oedema. A serious reaction of this sort can follow an injection (or even oral administration) of penicillin in susceptible individuals. Drug treatment of this complication may be life-saving. Intramuscular adrenaline and intravenous hydrocortisone and theophylline reduce oedema of the respiratory passages and relax bronchiolar smooth muscle. In addition, respiration and circulation should be maintained.

Urticaria is a generalised acute allergic reaction affecting the skin. It consists of widespread areas of redness, itching and swelling which follow administration of a specific allergen. Local application of a cooling lotion such as calamine may relieve the irritation. Itching and swelling may also be reduced by giving an antihistamine such as chlorpheniramine (Piriton) by mouth. Antihistamines should not be applied to the skin because they themselves can cause sensitisation.

Local allergy (contact dermatitis) can be caused by a wide range of drugs. Repeated handling of procaine or streptomycin, for instance, can cause contact dermatitis. Similarly, an area of itching and swelling may appear over the site of repeated insulin injections.

Specific allergic sensitisation is frequently a result of skin medication, particularly the use of creams containimg antihistamines, antibiotics or local anaesthetics. Once an eczematous reaction has been produced it is important to avoid contact with the sensitising drug even after the lesion has healed.

It is highly questionable whether contact allergy can affect the oral mucosa.

Delayed reactions

Allergic reactions do not always follow soon after the drug has been given and toxic effects with an immunological basis can develop after a drug has been given for a long period. A delayed reaction of this sort to penicillin may take the form of arthritis and fever (serum sickness-type reaction). Similarly, reaction to the antituberculous drugs streptomycin and isoniazid can cause fever.

Immune responses to some drugs (such as the hypotensive agent hydralazine) can cause an illness similar to acute disseminated lupus erythematosus. The effects of the latter include fever, elevated erythrocyte sedimentation rate, arthritis, pleural effusion, rashes and, rarely, kidney damage.

The hypotensive drug, methyldopa, can stimulate the production of autoantibodies which attack the patients' own red cells and produce a haemolytic anaemia.

2. Dose-dependent effects of drugs

These may either be exaggerations of their therapeutic actions or side-effects unrelated to the therapeutic action.

Cytotoxic drugs such as methotrexate, cyclophosphamide and 6-mercaptopurine act as anticancer drugs or immunosuppressive agents because they inhibit cell division. However, other normal tissues of the body which undergo continuous cell division are also affected. Thus, large doses of this type of drug will inevitably lead to marrow suppression (causing anaemia, leucopenia and thrombocytopenia), inhibition of gonadal activity (producing temporary or permanent sterility), intestinal effects (with haemorrhage and diarrhoea) and suppression of hair follicle activity (producing baldness).

An example of dose-dependent toxic effects which are not part of the therapeutic action of a drug are the side-effects of the cardiac glycosides. These drugs (such as digoxin) are used because of their action on the heart in the treatment of heart failure or of rapid supraventricular arrhythmias. Large doses of such a drug also produce loss of appetite, nausea, vomiting and (in the elderly) mental changes such as confusion and excitement.

3. Drug interactions

Several types of interaction can alter the therapeutic actions of drugs.

a. Interactions outside the body. Mixing the bronchodilator drug theophylline with a wide range of other substances – including some of the antibiotics and antihistamines – produces a precipitation in vitro. Such mixtures should not be injected.

b. Interactions in the intestine can impair the absorption of drugs. An example of this is the simultaneous oral administration of tetracyclines and calcium or iron salts. The mineral binds to the tetracycline molecule and prevents absorption of both.

c. Potentiation of the actions of cerebral depressants such as the barbiturates, antihistamines or benzodiazepines is produced by ethyl alcohol. Alcohol given in addition to hypnotics can lead to dangerous respiratory depression.

d. Antagonism. An example of a drug terminating the therapeutic action of another drug is the abolition of the hypotensive effect of guanethidine by the simultaneous administration of the tricyclic antidepressives imipramine or amitriptyline. Similarly, the antihypertensive clonidine is ineffective if given with these tricyclic antidepressives.

e. Enzyme induction. Some drugs increase the ability of the body to metabolise drugs. This process of enzyme enhancement is called induction. The barbiturates phenytoin and carbamazepine are inducers of drug metabolising enzymes. One consequence of this phenomenon is that certain other substances are metabolised rapidly and their own actions are reduced in intensity and duration. Examples of drugs which are less effective if given after an inducing agent include:

Coumarin anticoagulants.
Oral contraceptive agents, androgens, oestrogens.
Hydrocortisone and synthetic glucocorticoids.
Tricyclic antidepressants.
Phenothiazine major tranquillisers.
Digitoxin.
Phenylbutazone.
Vitamin D_3 and folic acid.

Thus while a patient is continuously taking

carbamazepine or a barbiturate, oral contraceptive agents may become less effective, and pregnancy has occasionally followed. By contrast, when treatment with the enzyme-inducing drug is stopped, metabolism of many drugs slows down and an anticoagulant (for example) could cause abnormal bleeding tendencies.

Another inducing agent is the anticonvulsant drug phenytoin. Prolonged phenytoin treatment causes relative deficiency of vitamin D_3 and this in turn leads to osteomalacia. Rifampicin is also an inducing agent which can interfere with the activity of the contraceptive pill and warfarin.

f. Enzyme inhibition. The monoamine oxidase inhibitors (MAOI) block the activity of several oxidase enzymes. When a patient is being treated with a monoamine oxidase inhibitor, the administration of drugs which are normally removed by oxidation may have undesirably prolonged and intense actions. The most severe reactions are with pethidine and are usually characterised by respiratory depression, hypotension and coma. Interactions between MAOI and pethidine have occasionally been fatal.

g. Drugs binding to plasma proteins. Many drugs travel in the blood partly in a free form and partly bound to plasma proteins – particularly albumin. The active form of the drug is free and unbound. A decrease in the proportion of bound drug will therefore potentiate drug activity. Such a change may be produced when drugs compete for binding to plasma proteins. An example of this is the administration of amiodarone to a patient who is being maintained on an anticoagulant dose of a coumarin drug. The amiodarone binds preferentially to the plasma albumin and displaces the coumarin from the protein binding sites. Thus the concentration of unbound (active) coumarin rises, with a parallel increase in its anticoagulant action. The overall result is that amiodarone given to a patient maintained on a coumarin anticoagulant may lead to haemorrhage, unless the dose of the coumarin is correspondingly lowered.

Patients with a low plasma albumin bind drugs to an abnormally small extent – a larger amount remaining unbound and therefore in the active form. Thus patients with hypoalbuminaemia show increased steroid toxicity when given prednisolone.

4. Idiosyncrasy

This term, which has been argued about for generations, means no more than its common usage suggests, namely behaviour peculiar to an individual. In pharmacological terms, it means an unusual and unexplained type of adverse reaction to a drug. It is to be hoped that with increasing knowledge of factors affecting drug metabolism, disposition and excretion, the term will disappear.

Susceptibility to adverse reactions

Some patients appear to be particularly prone to toxic reactions due to certain drugs. This may be due to (a) genetic predisposition or (b) an acquired characteristic or disease.

a. Genetic factors can change the effectiveness of drugs in either direction. The antituberculous drug isoniazid is metabolised (and inactivated) by acetylation. About one-third of the population possess the capacity to metabolise isoniazid rapidly. These individuals are known as rapid acetylators, and standard doses of isoniazid will not maintain adequate antituberculous blood concentrations of the drug in these patients. On the other hand, they may be less prone to develop the toxic effects of isoniazid, even with appropriately increased dosage.

Suxamethonium is a short-acting muscle relaxant. Its effect usually lasts about 4 minutes since the action of the drug is terminated by the hydrolytic action of the plasma enzyme pseudocholinesterase. About 1 in 4000 of the population lack normal plasma pseudocholinesterase. These people appear normal in every other respect, but if they are given suxamethonium they may remain paralysed for many hours. During this time they need artificial respiration.

Patients who suffer from an inherited deficiency of the red cell enzyme glucose-6-phosphate dehydrogenase can develop acute haemolytic anaemia when given drugs such as the antimalarial pamaquine and the antibacterial nitrofurantoin. The enzyme deficiency may otherwise produce no clinical effects apart from an increased susceptibility to haemolytic jaundice.

b. Acquired factors can change drug responses in many ways and drug interactions form one type of example. For instance, previous treatment with barbiturates results in enhanced metabolism (and therefore a reduced effect) of tricyclic antidepressants and phenothiazine tranquillisers. By contrast, patients who are treated with monoamine oxidase inhibitors have excessive sensitivity to the sedative actions of pethidine and other opioids.

Diseases may alter drug responses. Two important examples are liver and kidney disorders.

i. The problems in patients with liver disease include delays in drug detoxification, abnormal brain sensitivity and coagulation defects.

Morphine and other narcotic analgesics, tricyclic antidepressants and hypnotics may produce excessive effects because their detoxification by the liver is delayed. The response to cerebral depressants (including morphine) is also exaggerated because of abnormalities in brain function which accompany liver failure.

The liver is the main site of synthesis of the plasma clotting factors. In hepatocellullar disease factors V, IX, X and prothrombin are deficient – and the administration of even small doses of anticoagulants can lead to uncontrollable haemorrhage.

ii. In renal failure, drugs which are principally excreted by the kidneys may accumulate in the body and reach toxic levels. Thus streptomycin, kanamycin, neomycin and gentamicin have to be administered less frequently (every 24 to 48 hours and not twice daily), otherwise deafness or loss of balance may develop due to VIIIth nerve damage.

Similarly digoxin and chlorpropamide which are mainly excreted by the kidneys must be used in reduced doses (or alternative drugs found) in the presence of renal failure.

Effects on fetal development (teratogenic effects)

Unlike the toxic effects described above, some drugs affect the development of the fetus and do not necessarily have any adverse action on the mother. The most striking example is, of course, the thalidomide tragedy which resulted in the birth of many hundreds of children with appalling abnormalities. Absence of limbs was the most obvious but there were very many other defects. By contrast, thalidomide appears to be a relatively safe hypnotic for adults.

A few other drugs, notably antitumour agents and the vitamin A derivative isotretinoin, have been shown clinically to be teratogenic. Isotretinoin should not be taken by pregnant women, but despite the warnings it has been estimated that in the USA several hundred babies have been born with congenital deformities, by mothers who have been taking this drug for skin disease.

In contrast to the few drugs with proven teratogenic effects on humans, virtually any drug can have this effect experimentally if given in suitable dosage at a critical stage in fetal development to some animal. Different species in fact differ widely in their vulnerability to teratogenic effects from particular drugs. This has made the testing of drugs for teratogenicity – a requirement for the acceptance of any drug by the Committee of Safety of Medicines in Britain and the Federal Drug Administration in the USA – particularly difficult.

Under the circumstances, even though few drugs have been proved to be teratogenic for man, no drugs should be given to a woman during the first 3 months of pregnancy unless it is essential to do so

Tetracycline has a limited teratogenic effect on the teeth (and skeleton) since it is incorporated in calcifying tissues. When the teeth are stained in this way, the effect is permanent and can be disfiguring. Tetracyclines should not be given during the final trimester of pregnancy or until after the sixth year of childhood (see Ch. 3).

ADVERSE REACTIONS IN DENTISTRY

These may affect the patient in ways which can be summarised as follows:

1. Adverse reactions to drugs given or prescribed for dental purposes.
2. Drugs affecting the response to dental operations.
3. Interactions between different drugs given for medical and for dental purposes.
4. Oral reactions to drugs.

Although there is natural concern about adverse reactions to drugs, it seems less widely appreciated that the disease for which the drug is given is – or could often be – a more serious source of anxiety. This is important to remember in the case of drugs used to treat heart disease, particularly ischaemic heart disease and hypertension.

1. Adverse reactions to drugs given for dental purposes

These are usually acute reactions and a cause of emergencies in the dental surgery. Examples are:

Acute anaphylactic shock following injection of a penicillin or intravenous barbiturate.

Acute porphyria (very rarely) after injection of a barbiturate such as methohexitone.

Respiratory depression or death from overdose or any other cause during anaesthesia, particularly with methohexitone.

Acute hypertension and, occasionally, death from use of high concentrations of noradrenaline (i.e. 1 : 20 000) in local anaesthetic solutions.

Adverse reactions to drugs *prescribed* for dental purposes come on after the patient has left the surgery but may occasionally be just as severe. In either case, the dental surgeon will be responsible if he has not taken an adequate history.

Examples are rashes or other reactions to an oral penicillin and gastric bleeding due to aspirin.

2. Drugs which affect the response to dental surgery

Dentistry is, for most people, a stress-provoking situation because of anxiety, pain and sometimes loss of blood. The fit patient can usually withstand such stress but drug treatment may affect his resistance in various ways as follows:

Circulatory collapse (acute hypoadrenal shock) can follow dental surgery, especially under general anaesthesia on a patient receiving systemic cortico-steroid therapy.

Prolonged bleeding may be the result of the patient being on anticoagulant therapy. This is uncommon nowadays.

3. Interactions between different drugs given for medical and dental purposes

As discussed earlier (see Chs 5 and 9) there is no evidence of clinical interactions between adrenaline or noradrenaline in dental local anaesthetics and antidepressants – either MAOI or tricyclics.

This is a myth that has arisen as a result of misinterpretation of a single series of experiments.

Severe, sometimes fatal interactions can, however, follow the administration of pethidine to a patient concurrently taking MAOI antidepressants. The latter also interact with other opioids but coma is then the usual result.

Chloral given as a sedative (very rarely nowadays) can potentiate the action of anticoagulants. Aspirin can also do so in a different way and represents a greater danger to patients taking anticoagulants, not merely by enhancing the latter's action but also because of the associated risk of gastric bleeding.

4. Oral reactions to drugs

In spite of the vast range of drugs taken by the population at large, significant oral reactions are uncommon. These reactions are nevertheless important in that the patient is unlikely to suspect that the oral symptoms are anything to do with his medical treatment, the more especially as there is often a long delay between the start of drug therapy and the onset of the reaction. The alert dental surgeon who suspects that an unusual form of stomatitis might be a drug reaction can play an important part in drawing attention to the reaction and in some cases be able to prevent the development of more severe or widespread toxic effects.

Oral reactions to drugs are varied in character and in many cases their pathogenesis is unknown, although it is probable that immunological mechanisms often play a part. It must be appreciated that the oral mucosa does not produce any counterpart to the common contact dermatitis or eczematous reactions of the skin. If a patient is sensitive to (say) nickel, a nickel-containing alloy put in the mouth will, if it provokes any reaction at all, produce the characteristic rash on the skin.

When, as is often the case, the patient is taking several drugs it is likely to be difficult or impossible to be certain which of these are the sources of trouble.

Oral reactions to drugs can be (somewhat tentatively) classified in the following way:

Local reactions

a. Chemical irritation.
b. Interference with the normal oral flora.

Systemically determined reactions

c. Depression of any aspect of marrow function, i.e. red cells, white cells or platelets.
d. Depression of the immune response.
e. Stevens–Johnson Syndrome (bullous erythema multiforme).
f. Lichen planus and lichenoid reactions.
g. Exfoliative dermatitis and stomatitis.
h. Miscellaneous.

a. Chemical irritation

The best-known example is the aspirin burn caused by a patient holding a tablet against the gum of an aching tooth. Death of the superficial epithelial cells produces a white patch.

Elderly and infirm people in hospital can get severe burns from tablets they are unable to swallow and which stick to the oral mucosa. Such patients should not be expected to swallow tablets without help; they should be given water or milk, and care must be taken to see that the tablets have in fact been swallowed, otherwise the medication may do harm and will certainly do no good.

b. Depression of the oral flora

This happens as a result of the topical use of antibiotics such as penicillin lozenges or tetracycline mouth rinses.

After a few days (in susceptible individuals within 48 hours) sufficient numbers of the normal oral bacteria are destroyed to allow the overgrowth of opportunistic organisms, particularly *Candida albicans* causing acute antibiotic stomatitis or widespread plaques of thrush. In some cases candidal infection will clear up spontaneously when the antibiotic is stopped; in other patients the balance of the oral flora seems to be permanently disturbed, and it is necessary to give a short course of an antifungal agent, such as nystatin.

Topical corticosteroids seem also capable of affecting local immune responses and promoting candidosis. The latter may occasionally be seen in patients using corticosteroid lozenges for oral ulceration or in asthmatic patients using corticosteroid inhalers. These infections do not seem to be due to systemic effects of these corticosteroids which are used, in these conditions, in minute doses and are not associated with any more widespread susceptibility to infection.

c. Depression of the bone marrow

The red cells. A few drugs can cause anaemia alone (see Ch. 12), but this is rarely severe enough to cause glossitis.

Folic acid deficiency leading to macrocytic anaemia can develop in susceptible patients on prolonged treatment with phenytoin. This can occasionally cause a severe form of aphthous stomatitis, sometimes with genital ulceration which resembles Behçet's syndrome but which responds rapidly when folic acid is given.

Folic acid deficiency can also follow prolonged treatment with co-trimoxazole but in fact rarely does so.

The white cells – agranulocytosis and aplastic anaemia. The leucocytes can be selectively depressed (leucopenia) or with all other bone marrow cells (aplastic anaemia, pancytopenia). Severe neutropenia can go on to the clinical condition of agranulocytosis characterised by necrotising bacterial infections especially of the mouth and throat. The mouth is particularly susceptible because of the persistent low-grade infection of the gingival margins and the invariable presence of chronic gingivitis or periodontitis. If resistance is much impaired, this infection becomes acute, progressive and destructive.

A wide variety of drugs can have this effect although it is uncommon. The most notorious are:

1. Antibacterials: chloramphenicol, sulphonamides and co-trimoxazole.
2. Analgesics: amidopyrine (obsolete in the UK), phenylbutazone and oxyphenbutazone.
3. Antidiabetic (hypoglycaemic) agents and antithyroid agents.
4. Cytotoxic agents.

The drug must be stopped immediately and a non-toxic bactericidal antibiotic preferably penicillin, given.

The problem has been discussed in more detail in relation to drugs affecting the blood (see Ch. 12).

Platelet depression – purpura. This may rarely be a selective effect. One of the few drugs causing this effect is apronal (Sedormid), an obsolete hypnotic, but a wide variety of other drugs have been reported as causing purpura on rare occasions.

Purpura, when drug induced, is more often the result of general marrow aplasia and is frequently the first sign, since bleeding may come from the gingival margins or be submucosal.

The drugs causing marrow aplasia are essentially those which otherwise cause leucopenia.

Purpura may also result from vascular damage and is a relatively common feature of prolonged corticosteroid therapy, particularly in older patients in whom the vessel walls are already weak.

d. Depression of immune responses

This may be the result of prolonged corticosteroid therapy for a variety of inflammatory diseases or more intensive immunosuppression for transplant surgery.

The results are usually different from those of agranulocytosis and the main effects are infective stomatitis due to viruses (usually herpes simplex) or fungi (*Candida albicans*) or both together. This is probably because the control of these types of infection is mainly dependent on cell-mediated immunity.

Persistent oral candidosis is only rarely seen in patients having moderate doses of corticosteroids. Transplant patients, on the order hand, who are given very high doses of steroids may have widespread vesiculation and ulceration due to herpes (or other viruses) or equally widespread plaques of thrush.

e. Stevens–Johnson syndrome (bullous erythema multiforme)

This is an acute mucocutaneous reaction involving mainly the mouth, eyes and skin. The drugs thought most often to be responsible are sulphonamides (particularly the long-acting types) and (rarely) phenobarbitone, but a wide variety of other drugs have been blamed on various occasions as well as herpetic and other infections. It is often impossible (as with other types of reaction) to exclude coincidence and in the majority of cases no precipitating cause can be identified.

The patients are usually young adult males. The mouth is always affected by widespread ulceration, but the most striking and characteristic feature is the swollen, cracked, bleeding and crusted lips. Other mucous membranes may be involved. The rash is variable in character and there is often conjunctivitis or more severe ocular inflammation. The disease is very rarely fatal.

The dental surgeon is likely to see mild forms of this disease where the oral changes are predominant.

f. Lichen planus and lichenoid reactions

Lichen planus is a common chronic disease involving skin and mouth in particular. It is usually 'spontaneous' but may occasionally be drug induced.

Oral lichen planus is typically characterised by fine white lines (striae) extending over a greater or lesser area of the mucosa, and often ulceration which can be extensive. Several drugs are capable of causing a clinically identical reaction or others (lichenoid reactions) which less closely resemble the idiopathic disease. Sometimes extensive ulceration (erosions) dominate the picture.

Drugs which can cause lichenoid reactions or oral ulceration include the following:

Allopurinol.
Beta blockers (rarely).
Captopril (rarely).
Chloroquine and other antimalarials.
Chlorpropamide.
Gold salts.
Methyldopa.
Non-steroidal anti-inflammatory agents, particularly phenylbutazone and indomethacin.
Penicillamine.

g. Exfoliative dermatitis and stomatitis

This is a severe reaction which because of the extensive skin damage was often fatal before effective methods of treatment became available. Exfoliative dermatitis as the name implies is characterised by widespread shedding of the skin surface. An accompanying stomatitis shows widespread erosions or ulceration. Gold, mercury and organic arsenicals are important causes but phenylbutazone, sulphonamides and barbiturates may also cause this reaction.

Occasionally the oral reaction may be more severe than the dermal reaction, at least in the early stages, so that the patient comes first to the dental surgeon. It is important to look for scaling of the skin as this reaction is so dangerous that immediate treatment is necessary.

In the case of gold and possibly of other agents, healing of the oral ulceration may leave behind a pattern of lichen planus.

h. Miscellaneous effects

Gingival hyperplasia

Phenytoin (Epanutin). Gingival fibrous hyperplasia is a well-recognised complication of the use of this drug in certain susceptible patients. The probable mechanism is that phenytoin (among many diverse properties) appears to be a collagenase inhibitor and in the gingivae where collagen turnover is high, may allow overproduction of collagen.

Provided that good oral hygiene is maintained the condition does not appear to accelerate the progress of periodontal disease and in spite of deep false pocketing the gums often remain pale and firm, and clinically are not inflamed. A high standard of oral hygiene is necessary but will not of itself cure the condition. If the patient is concerned about the appearance, gingivectomy must be carried out as necessary.

Gingival hyperplasia is *not* an indication for changing to another anticonvulsant. Phenytoin remains an effective and useful anticonvulsant and a change in treatment takes time to establish the appropriate dosage of another drug. One patient is known to have died as a result of a fit and consequent street accident during this period of restabilisation.

Yet another effect of phenytoin as mentioned earlier is to interfere with folate metabolism which, in a few susceptible subjects, can lead to folate deficiency, macrocytic anaemia and, sometimes, severe aphthous stomatitis which responds only to repair of the folate deficiency.

Cyclosporin. The immunosuppressive agent cyclosporin can cause gingival hyperplasia clinically and histologically similar to that caused by phenytoin. Moreover, cyclosporin can also cause hypertrichosis. Hypertrichosis is also a feature of the genetic form of gingival hyperplasia.

It is perhaps coincidental that phenytoin also has immunosuppressant activity, albeit much less than that of cyclosporin.

Nifedipine. The antihypertensive drug, nifedipine, can also cause gingival hyperplasia by unknown mechanisms. It does not appear to have any other effects in common with phenytoin or cyclosporin.

Gingival pigmentation

Pigmentation was a 'classic' side-effect of treatment with, or exposure to, heavy metals, particularly mercury, bismuth and lead, but is rarely seen now. Excretion of these metals in the gingival crevice or pocket leads to the deposition of black (mercury), brown (bismuth) or blue (lead) deposits. The lead line in particular is sharply defined, just short of the gingival margin and delineates the floor of the crevice or pocket.

Among currently used drugs, the anticancer agent cisplatin is probably the only one which produces a gingival line, blue or grey in colour.

Other drugs, notably the phenothiazines, can cause widespread mucosal pigmentation which may involve the gingivae.

Dry mouth

Xerostomia is a relatively common side-effect of drug treatment and is a feature of any drugs having an atropine-like action. Atropine or other anticholinergics such as propantheline (Pro-Banthine) is used to depress gastric acid secretion as an optimistic treatment of peptic ulceration. Ganglion blockers such as mecamylamine (which are obsolete for the treatment of hypertension), and amphetamines and chemically related appetite suppressants which are sympathomimetic, also (as might be expected) depress salivary secretion. Tricyclic antidepressants have a strong atropine-like action and an unpleasantly dry mouth is often one of the first things a patient notices when starting antidepressant treatment. Antihistamines and atropine-like drugs (e.g. benzhexol used in the treatment of parkinsonism) also have this effect.

The main groups of drugs likely to cause xerostomia or have other effects on the salivary glands are summarised in Table 18.1. It should be noted, however, that increased salivation is not a clinical complaint with any validity in that any excess of saliva can be swallowed unless some neuromuscular disorder interferes with this process.

Yellow cards

The Committees on Safety of Medicines and Dental and Surgical Materials provide a yellow card on which suspected adverse reactions can – and should – be reported. Dentists should appreciate that they can make a significant contribution to the recognition of adverse effects from drugs and related substances by completing and sending in these cards.

Doubt as to whether any apparent reaction is no more than coincidental should not deter anyone from sending in a card. The medical assessors are well able to evaluate such problems.

Conclusions

Serious reactions from drugs in common use are rare and a clinician may not, for instance, ever see an anaphylactic reaction to penicillin or acute hypotensive shock in a patient on withdrawal from corticosteroid treatment.

At the same time, some of these reactions are so severe that, difficult though it is, the clinician must always be prepared for the unexpected. The chances of a serious drug reaction are much reduced if these precautions are taken:

1. No drug should be given unless absolutely necessary and this is especially important during early pregnancy. Antibiotics and hypnotics in particular are grossly over-prescribed.

2. If a drug has to be given always ask if any other drugs are being taken and try to assess whether there is any danger of interaction.

3. Always ask if the patient has had any ill-effects from any drugs in the past and particularly to the drug that is to be given. This is especially important in relation to the many different penicillins, the names of which differ widely but which all share cross sensitivity.

4. It is wise to ask if there is any history of allergy as this may increase the likelihood of sensitisation or reaction to a drug.

5. Try whenever possible to use a familiar drug that has stood the test of time.

6. If an adverse reaction develops, remember to report it on a Yellow Card when the crisis has been dealt with.

Table 18.1 Drugs affecting the salivary glands

I. *Drug-induced xerostomia*
  1. Drugs with anticholinergic effects
      Atropine, ipratropium, hyoscine and analogues
      Orphenadrine, benzhexol and related anti-parkinsonian agents
      Tricyclic antidepressants
      Antihistamines
      Antiemetics (including antihistamines, hyoscine and phenothiazines)
      Major tranquillisers such as phenothiazines
      Some antihypertensives, especially ganglion blockers and clonidine
  2. Drugs with sympathomimetic actions
      'Cold cures' containing ephedrine or phenylpropanolamine
      Decongestants
      Bronchodilators
      Appetite suppressants, particularly amphetamines and diethylpropion.
II. *Drugs increasing salivation*
      Cholinesterase inhibitors (physostigmine, pyridostigmine, etc.)
III. *Drug-associated salivary swelling*
      Phenylbutazone, iodine compounds, thiouracil, catecholamines, sulphonamides, chlorhexidine and others (uncommon reaction)

SUGGESTED FURTHER READING

Anderson J A, Adkinson N F 1987 Allergic reactions to drugs and biologic agents. Journal of the American Medical Association 258: 2891
Appel G G, Neu H C 1977 Nephrotoxicity of antimicrobial agents. New England Journal of Medicine 296: 784
Bateman D N, Chaplin S 1988 Adverse reactions. I. British Medical Journal 296: 761
British Medical Journal (1977) Deaths due to drug treatment British Medical Journal 1: 1492
Brodie M J, Feely J 1988 Adverse drug interactions. British Medical Journal 296: 845
Cawson R A 1966 The problem of the newer drugs in dentistry. British Dental Journal 120: 109
Cooper J B, Newbower R S, Long C D, McPeek B 1978 Preventable anesthesia mishaps: a study of human factors. Anesthesiology 49: 399
Curtis J R 1977 Diseases of the urinary system. Drug-induced renal disorders I. British Medical Journal 2: 242
Curtis J R 1977 Diseases of the urinary system. Drug-induced renal disorders II. British Medical Journal 2: 375
D'Arcy P F, Griffin J P 1974 Drug interactions: 2. By mixing drugs before administration. Prescribing Journal 14: 38
Dundee J W 1988 Drugs and their hazards. British Medical Bulletin 44: 269

Ellis E F 1987 Adverse effects of corticosteroid therapy. Journal of Allergy and Clinical Immunology 80: 515

Geddes A M, Ball A P 1976 Interactions of antimicrobial agents. Prescribers' Journal 16: 9

Huskisson E C, Wojtulewski J A 1974 Measurement of side effects of drugs. British Medical Journal 2: 698–699

James I M 1974 Diseases affecting drug responses. British Journal of Hospital Medicine 12: 823–836

Lakshmanan M C, Hershey C O, Breslau D 1986 Hospital admissions caused by iatrogenic disease. Archives of Internal Medicine 146: 1931

Mackowiak P A, LeMaistre C F 1987 Annals of Internal Medicine 106: 728

Maxwell J D, Williams R 1973 Drug-induced jaundice. British Journal of Hospital Medicine 9: 193–200

Park B K, Kitteringham N R 1987 Adverse reactions and drug metabolism. Adverse Drug Reaction Bulletin No 122, 456

Patterson R 1988 Diagnosis and treatment of drug allergy. Journal of Allergy and Clinical Immunology 81: 380

Rawlins M D 1974 Variability of response to drugs in man. British Journal of Hospital Medicine 12: 803–811

Rawlins M D 1974 Variability in response to drugs. British Medical Journal 4: 91–94

Sherlock S 1986 The spectrum of hepatotoxicity due to drugs. Lancet ii: 440

Winstanley P A, Orme M L'E 1988 Which adverse drug interactions are really important? Adverse Drug Reaction Bulletin no 130, 488

19. Emergencies in dental practice

The dentist must have some idea of how to recognise serious emergencies and manage them, rare though they may be. His professional skill and equipment should enable the dentist to make a useful contribution and sometimes even save the patient's life. The main hazards that may have to be faced are:

1. Fainting.
2. Myocardial infarction.
3. Cardiac arrest.
4. Anaesthetic accidents.
5. Acute allergic (anaphylactic) reactions.
6. Circulatory collapse in patients on corticosteroid treatment.
7. Drug reactions and interactions.
8. Epilepsy.
9. Acute hypoglycaemia.
10. Haemorrhage.

1. Fainting

Fainting is the most common cause of sudden loss of consciousness in the dental surgery. Most patients who faint are otherwise healthy adults and the attack is precipitated by anxiety. Some patients are, however, particularly prone to fainting and frequently do so.

A fainting attack can be recognised by premonitory signs and symptoms in many cases. These include nausea, sweating and dizziness, but sometimes consciousness is lost almost instantaneously.

Fainting is caused by transient hypotension and cerebral ischaemia, so that the pulse is at first weak but soon becomes full and bounding. These attacks are not, strictly speaking, medical emergencies since they can be terminated by putting the patient flat to improve cerebral circulation. It is harmful to keep a fainting patient upright. This worsens cerebral anoxia. Traditional 'stimulants' such as spirits of sal volatile can also be given, or aromatic spirits of ammonia can be held under the nostrils. These may jerk the patient back into consciousness more quickly but are less effective than laying the patient down.

Regular fainters may be helped by sedation with diazepam (5 mg orally, on the night before and again an hour before treatment).

The most important aspect of fainting attacks is to distinguish them from more serious causes of syncope. The latter include hypoglycaemic coma and cardiovascular disturbances, notably heart block and other causes of bradycardia, atrial fibrillation and epileptic fits. In such cases the character of the pulse will indicate that there is a significant dysrhythmia.

2. Myocardial infarction

This is a common cause of death and must be recognised, as the patient's fate may be decided by the first few minutes' treatment. Several aspects of dentistry, particularly apprehension, pain or the effect of drugs could contribute to make this accident more likely in a susceptible patient.

Some patients die within a few minutes after the start of the attack and it is rash to be over-ambitious in an attempt to manage the problem. Drugs, apart from those described below, should not be used as, without continuous monitoring, they can sometimes do more harm than good.

The patient is typically a middle-aged male and may have had attacks of anginal pain or a previous infarct. The attack is characterised by the sudden onset of agonising and persistent pain in the chest, and often breathlessness due to oedema of the lungs. Pain is occasionally felt only in the left jaw. Vomiting is common and there is sometimes shock or loss of consciousness.

As soon as the emergency is recognised an assistant must immediately call an ambulance.

The essential measures to deal with the problem are:

1. Make sure the patient can breathe.
2. Relieve pain.
3. Relieve anxiety.

Respiration

A myocardial infarct frequently causes left ventricular failure and may cause pulmonary oedema. Under these circumstances the patient has great difficulty in breathing and may only be able to breathe if sitting upright. Any attempt to lay such a patient flat causes the lungs to fill with fluid and the patient, in effect, drowns. Other patients are more comfortable lying back in a supine or nearly supine position. The rule is: the patient must be placed in a position in which breathing is easiest.

Tight clothing around the neck must be loosened; 100% oxygen can be given but the patient must be reassured about what is being done, especially as there is often fear of what looks like an anaesthetic mask.

Relief of pain and anxiety

Pain and anxiety together stimulate the output of adrenaline. This in turn increases both the workload on the heart and also the excitability of the myocardium to the extent of precipitating arrhythmias. These may culminate in ventricular fibrillation and death within a few minutes. Ventricular arrhythmias are the usual cause of sudden death during a heart attack. Reducing the likelihood of arrhythmias by relieving pain and anxiety is one of the most important aspects of the initial management of this accident.

The classical treatment and still the treatment of choice is to give morphine. This effectively relieves both pain and anxiety. These benefits far outweigh theoretical dangers of depressing respiration. The difficulty is that morphine is rarely available in the dental surgery.

Pentazocine even by injection is somewhat less effective as an analgesic than morphia, but more important, fails to relieve or may even increase anxiety. Pentazocine also increases the load on the heart by raising the blood pressure and for these reasons is not recommended for myocardial infarction.

The best alternative to morphine is to give nitrous oxide with oxygen which effectively also relieves both pain and anxiety. These gases are widely used in the initial management of myocardial infarction. Up to 70% nitrous oxide may be used or premixed gases as a 50–50 mixture (Entonox) can be kept for emergency purposes. Again, the patient should be reassured about what is being done and the reasons for it.

Reassurance. This may sound a little futile but a quiet and continuous flow of encouraging talk and reassurance that everything is being done to help is of great importance. An atmosphere, or worse still, expressions of panic and despair can have a disastrous effect.

3. Cardiac arrest

The most important aspects of management are as follows:

1. Prevention. It is of the utmost importance to do everything possible to prevent the likelihood of cardiac arrest. This means that patients with cardiovascular disease must be appropriately managed and that anaesthetics must be given skilfully with full oxygenation.

2. The dentist should be aware of and alert to the possibility of cardiac arrest and be able to recognise it when it happens.

3. The dentist and his team should know what to do in such an emergency and also the extent of their limitations.

4. Speed of response is most important and, once the emergency is recognised, the dental team should be able to institute cardiopulmonary resuscitation immediately.

It is hardly possible to be alert to the onset of

cardiac arrest without knowing under what circumstances it is likely to develop.

Causes of cardiac arrest

There are many recognised causes of cardiac arrest, but only a few are relevant to dentistry or are at all likely to happen in the dental surgery.

1. Coronary artery disease and myocardial infarction. These are probably the commonest precipitating causes. Ventricular fibrillation or cardiac arrest are the usual causes of sudden death shortly after a myocardial infarct. Clinically, ventricular fibrillation is indistinguishable from arrest.

2. Hypoxia and hypercapnia. Hypoxia is thought to be the most common cause of cardiac arrest during anaesthesia. Both hypoxia and accumulation of carbon dioxide act together to depress the myocardium and can also interact with anaesthetic agents, notably halothane.

3. Anaesthetic agents. The halogenated hydrocarbons, most notoriously chloroform but even to some extent halothane, sensitise the myocardium to catecholamines, particularly in the presence of hypoxia and hypercapnia.

4. Drugs. Cardiac arrest can be caused by overdose of a wide variety of drugs other than anaesthetics but of these probably only adrenaline is important in dentistry. Nevertheless, the latter, when used in a concentration of not more than 1 : 80 000, remarkably rarely causes any ill-effects. Dysrhythmias culminating in cardiac arrest might develop if the patient has unstable cardiac rhythm due to coronary artery disease (especially after a myocardial infarct), if the solution is injected intravenously by accident or if excessive amounts are given. As mentioned earlier, halothane and related halogenated hydrocarbons sensitise the myocardium to the effects of adrenaline.

5. Anaphylactic reactions to drugs, such as penicillin, can also lead to cardiac arrest as a consequence of severe hypotension and hypoxia.

6. Severe hypotension. This, whatever the cause, predisposes to cardiac arrest. Apart from anaphylactic reactions to drugs or myocardial infarction, acute hypotension can also develop in a dental patient who has been on systemic corticosteroids and who has had dental surgery, particularly under general anaesthesia without adequate prophylactic administration of corticosteroids.

Management

The most important features can be summarised again as follows:

1. Awareness of and alertness to the possibility of cardiac arrest.
2. Clinical diagnosis.
3. Immediate establishment of cardiopulmonary resuscitation.

Clinical diagnosis

Diagnosis depends on the recognition of only two signs, namely:

1. Unconsciousness.
2. Absence of arterial pulses.

The patient is often also of an ashen-grey colour and there may still be weak gasping respiration if arrest is very recent.

Although there are other signs, such as increasing dilatation of the pupils, with loss of reaction to light, and loss of measurable blood pressure, it is dangerous to waste time looking for them.

If doubt still remains about an unconscious patient with absent pulses, the only other useful measure is to listen for heart sounds. If no stethoscope is available, the dentist has to put his ear to the patient's chest.

As with any other condition involving acute cerebral hypoxia and loss of consciousness, there can be convulsions with or without incontinence.

It is not possible to distinguish clinically between ventricular fibrillation and cardiac arrest, and in any case they have the same effect on the patient.

Cardiopulmonary resuscitation

Once cardiac arrest has been recognised, resuscitation must be started immediately. It is very difficult for a single operator to do this unaided. The main measures are as follows:

1. If collapse is sudden and arrest very recent, one or two sharp blows on the mid-sternum should

be given. These should be really vigorous thumps with the side of the closed fist. They may be sufficient to restart the heart or may stop ventricular fibrillation. Although a thump on the chest may be beneficial in this way, some regard it as dangerous in that it may precipitate ventricular fibrillation.

2. Shout for help.

3. Put the patient on a firm flat surface such as the floor. However, it is by no means easy to lift a heavy patient out of a dental chair. If, therefore, the chair allows the patient to be laid supine, then it may be more satisfactory to carry out resuscitation in this way with the operator and his assistant standing beside the chair.

4. Clear the airway and keep it clear by extending the neck and holding the jaw forward.

5. Start external cardiac compression immediately. The operator kneels beside the patient and places one hand over the other on the patient's lower sternum. The sternum is depressed about 1.5–2 inches (4–5 cm) at the normal heart rate, i.e. about 60 times a minute. Compression must be forceful and the danger of cracking a rib must be disregarded. The optimal pressure is about 40 or 50 kg and this is provided by allowing the weight of the upper part of the operator's body to be applied through stiffly extended arms.

6. Give artificial ventilation during external cardiac massage. This must be done either as a mouth-to-mouth procedure or using a face mask and oxygen. The lungs must be inflated, preferably with oxygen, between each six or eight compressions of the sternum.

7. Get an assistant to telephone for help as soon as these measures have been started.

Unless the operator is skilled in its use, he should not waste time in trying to pass an endotracheal tube. The dentist should, however, have available as emergency equipment, a self-inflating bag respirator with an oxygen supply. A plastic airway should be put in the patient's mouth and the mask applied firmly with the resuscitation bag attached. The aim is to inflate the patient's lungs with oxygen pressure and the chest should be visibly expanded at each respiration. Passive recoil of the chest wall causes spontaneous expiration as soon as the pressure is removed.

If a self-inflating bag respirator is not available, mouth-to-mouth respiration can be used, preferably with an intervening Brook airway.

During artificial respiration the patient's nose must be closed. Deep inflations are given by the operator and time allowed for passive recoil of the chest. If there is not even an airway available, direct mouth-to-mouth resuscitation, with an intervening gauze pad and the nose occluded, must be given.

Cardiac massage and artificial ventilation should be alternated; six compressions to one ventilation is probably about right. Wherever possible, one operator should carry out cardiac compression and the other should manage ventilation. External cardiac massage is tiring, and if another person is available he should take over as soon as the first operator shows signs of fatigue.

Resuscitation should be continued until there are signs of restoration of blood pressure and a good spontaneous pulse. Other signs of success are contraction of the pupils, return of reflex activity such as the blink reflex and reaction of the pupils to light, lightening of unconsciousness and purposeful spontaneous movements – not, that is to say, the jerking movements of convulsions.

If these signs fail to appear the attempt at resuscitation should still go on until expert help arrives, but if no signs of recovery appear within 15 minutes recovery is unlikely.

After recovery the patient should be admitted to hospital for correction of the systemic effects of circulatory arrest and measures taken to prevent recurrences.

Causes of failure

The most common mistakes are:

1. Giving external cardiac compression without artificial ventilation.

2. Giving artificial ventilation without external cardiac compression.

3. Failing to clear the airway or to make sure that it remains open by hyperextending the head adequately.

4. Failing to close the nose during mouth-to-mouth respiration.

5. Failing to get a close fit with the mask when using a bag respirator.

6. Failing to make sure that ventilation is adequate, as indicated by the movement of the chest.

7. Timidity in applying external cardiac compression, and as a result using insufficient force to compress the heart.

8. Failing to release pressure on the chest completely between compressions and preventing cardiac filling as a consequence.

9. Compressing the chest too rapidly to allow enough time for the heart to fill between compressions.

10. Putting the hands in the incorrect position.

11. Failing to act sufficiently quickly and fretting about details rather than getting on with the essentials of external cardiac compression and artificial ventilation.

4. Anaesthetic accidents

These have caused deaths of dental patients and have produced a good deal of adverse publicity. Probably the chief danger associated with general anaesthesia is that of failing to maintain adequate oxygenation. Most anaesthetic agents also lower the blood pressure and these two factors contribute to even more severe reactions such as, occasionally, cardiac arrest. The main dangers are:

1. Respiratory obstruction.
2. Respiratory failure.
3. Overdose of the anaesthetic agent.
4. Cardiac arrest.
5. Anaphylactic reactions, particularly to intravenous agents.
6. Acute hypotension in corticosteroid-treated patients or in patients sitting upright.

Respiratory obstruction. The airway must be cleared using a finger, swabs or, preferably, suction. If this fails, tracheostomy may have to be performed.

Respiratory failure is usually caused by overdose of the anaesthetic agent, particularly one of the intravenous barbiturates, or by hypoxia or a combination of both.
The treatment is:

1. To stop the anaesthetic.
2. To make sure the airway is clear.

3. To give intermittent positive pressure artificial ventilation immediately. This should preferably be by means of a face mask and oxygen.

Overdose. The treatment is the same as for respiratory failure. If the patient has been given a narcotic analgesic as premedication or to enhance the anaesthetic effect, naloxone should be given. Naloxone is of no help for overdose of barbiturates or other non-narcotic anaesthetic agents.

Cardiac arrest. Recognition is difficult if the patient is already unconscious and there is thus a good argument for continuously monitoring the pulse.

Features suggestive of cardiac arrest in an anaesthetised patient are sudden pallor, weakening or cessation of respiration and, later, wide dilatation of the pupils.

In addition to the factors contributing to cardiac arrest discussed earlier, it is also suggested that an excessively anxious patient may be more likely to develop severe dysrhythmias culminating in ventricular fibrillation or arrest.

Anaphylactic and related reactions. Intravenous anaesthetic agents, such as methohexitone, can occasionally cause anaphylactic reactions. As discussed earlier, anaphylactic reactions to penicillin can also happen during a general anaesthetic.

Acute hypotension in corticosteroid-treated patients. This is discussed later.

5. Acute anaphylactic reactions

Penicillin is the most common cause of acute anaphylactic reactions. Similar reactions due to histamine release by intravenous anaesthetics can also develop.

A severe reaction to penicillin may start within 30 seconds of an injection, but may develop half an hour or more after oral penicillin because of its slower absorption. In general, the quicker the onset the more severe the reaction. A reaction starting 30 minutes after an injection is unlikely to be very severe.

The clinical picture is variable as described in Chapter 3. The main features in severe cases are bronchospasm with wheezing, but more important, circulatory collapse with a deep fall in blood pressure due to widespread vasodilatation and increased capillary permeability. Consciousness is lost and the patient may become cyanotic; death can quickly follow if treatment is delayed or inappropriate. Although this is a rare reaction to penicillin, the drug has been given on so vast a scale that over the years it has caused many deaths.

Management of anaphylactic reactions

As soon as the diagnosis is made the patient should be laid flat, with the legs raised, to maintain cerebral blood flow. Adrenaline (1 ml of 1 : 1000) should be given by intramuscular injection, but before the drug is given the plunger of the syringe should be withdrawn to make sure the needle is not in a vein. The adrenaline should be followed immediately by 200 mg of hydrocortisone sodium succinate (Efcortelan) into a vein. There should be no delay in giving hydrocortisone in the hope that adrenaline alone may be effective.

The adrenaline has the advantage of acting rapidly. It increases cardiac output and also decreases capillary permeability in the skin and splanchnic regions. Adrenaline also combats some of the effects of histamine. The action of adrenaline is relatively shortlived and administration can be repeated every 15 minutes, if necessary, until the patient responds.

Hydrocortisone takes an hour or so to take effect but maintains the blood pressure for some hours and combats the continued effect of the antigen–antibody reaction.

Another measure, ancillary to giving adrenaline, is to give an antihistamine, such as chlorpheniramine by slow intravenous injection.

After recovery the patient should be sent to hospital for a period of observation and must be given a card warning against the use of penicillin in the future.

6. Circulatory collapse in patients on corticosteroid treatment

The response of patients on long-term corticosteroid treatment to surgery is unpredictable, but near fatal circulatory collapse has been seen in patients taking as little as 5 mg of prednisone a day after dental extractions under intravenous methohexitone. Since large doses of corticosteroids given for a short period are safe – and for these patients may be life-saving – the policy should lean towards being over-protective. All patients, therefore, who are having systemic corticosteroids, and even those who have had these drugs in the past, are at risk. It has been suggested that cortical function may take up to 2 years to recover, but this may be an overestimate. Corticosteroid skin preparations used lavishly, particularly for widespread eczema, also have systemic effects and have been known to cause severe reactions.

Types of dental treatment hazardous for these patients are surgical treatment of any type including extractions, especially under anaesthesia, or so-called sedation with methohexitone. Local anaesthesia is much safer.

The following principles are a general guide for the management of patients under systemic corticosteroid treatment:

a. Major oral surgery must be carried out in hospital.

b. Minor operations including extractions should preferably be carried out under local anaesthesia, but an intravenous corticosteroid should be given prophylactically.

c. If even a brief general anaesthetic is unavoidable, then a corticosteroid must be given prophylactically. At least 100 mg of hydrocortisone succinate should be given intravenously just before the operation and the patient's condition carefully watched throughout. At the first sign of a falling blood pressure or pallor with a rapid but weak pulse, immediate corticosteroid supplementation (100–500 mg intravenously) must be given.

d. For extractions under local anaesthesia 100 mg of hydrocortisone should be given intravenously and repeated if there is the least doubt as to the patient's condition.

e. These patients should be kept under observation for at least an hour after operation.

f. If inadequate amounts of corticosteroids have been given or if for any other reason the patient shows signs of circulatory collapse, 500 mg of hydrocortisone should be given immediately, the patient laid flat, but with the legs raised, and an ambulance called. Artificial ventilation with oxygen may be necessary in the interim.

g. Restorative dentistry under local anaesthesia is probably not dangerous. There is probably no need for corticosteroid supplementation but, on the other hand, there should be no hesitation in giving large amounts intravenously if circulatory collapse seems imminent.

The suggestion of doubling the patient's normal dose of corticosteroid the day before and on the day of treatment is probably quite ineffective, as relatively enormous doses (that is hundreds of milligrams) are needed to prevent or manage circulatory collapse.

7. Drug reactions and interactions

Although these can be disastrous or even fatal, drug reactions and interactions have probably received more publicity than they deserve. Apart from anaphylactic reactions discussed earlier, very few endanger life, but these include the following:

a. Noradrenaline when used as a vasoconstrictor in high concentration, i.e. 1 : 20 000 has been known to cause acute hypertension resulting in cerebral haemorrhage or death. Quite apart from its dangers, noradrenaline has no advantages and should not be used in local anaesthetic solutions. The treatment is, if possible, to give an α blocker such as phentolamine.

There is no clinical evidence of such reactions to adrenaline used in normal concentration and quantity.

b. Monoamine oxidase inhibitors can cause severe reactions with opioids, particularly pethidine. The reaction can be very sudden in onset. Monoamine oxidase inhibitors also interact with indirectly acting sympathomimetic agents, that is, drugs such as ephedrine (used as a nasal decongestant) to cause acute severe hypertension. The treatment is to give an α blocker such as phentolamine. Adrenaline or noradrenaline do not cause these reactions.

c. General anaesthetic agents are one of the chief causes of fatal accidents in the dental surgery although this is not necessarily a direct effect of the drug but, as described earlier, a cumulative effect of several factors associated with general anaesthesia. Nevertheless, apart from the dangers of overdose, particularly of intravenous agents, there are the dangers of anaphylactic reactions. Intravenous barbiturates in particular potentiate the effect of antihypertensive agents and may produce a dangerous fall in blood pressure.

d. As already described, patients on *long-term corticosteroid treatment* when exposed to stress can suffer circulatory collapse as a result of adrenal suppression.

8. Epilepsy

Epilepsy is usually well controlled with modern drugs but very occasionally an epileptic can have an attack in the dental surgery. A major fit is characterised by the sequence of sudden loss of consciousness, stiffening of the body due to generalised muscular contraction (tonic stage), a convulsion in which there are jerking movements of the body (clonic stage) and finally recovery.

The tongue may be bitten between the clenched teeth and there may be incontinence. The attack is usually quickly over but the patient is sometimes drowsy or confused for several hours afterwards. Many epileptic patients are reluctant to admit to their disability, although they may mention that they have 'blackouts'. As a consequence an attack will usually catch the dental surgeon by surprise.

Some epileptic patients have swollen gums, a complication of prolonged treatment with phenytoin, and this may be a useful sign. There is, however, no effective treatment for the attack itself but, if it can be done quickly enough, a pad of gauze should be put between the teeth to prevent the tongue from being bitten. The patient should also be prevented from injuring himself on surrounding objects during the convulsion. After an attack an epileptic patient should be accompanied home to prevent accidents due to postepileptic confusion.

When attack follows attack in quick succession, the condition is called *status epilepticus*. This can be fatal. The standard and most effective treatment is to give intravenous diazepam. After the initial period of response to a single dose of diazepam, the fits may recur and further injections will be needed. It is therefore important that this dangerous medical emergency be treated in hospital as soon as possible.

9. Acute hypoglycaemia

Hypoglycaemia affects diabetic patients who have had an overdose of insulin or who have been prevented from eating at the proper time. This in turn may be because of dental treatment.

The early features of a hypoglycaemia attack are very similar to those of fainting, but instead of quick recovery there is deepening coma. The patient is often aware of what is happening and may be able to warn the dentist in the early stages. The treatment is to give sugar (at least four lumps in a sweetened drink) and this may be repeated if symptoms are not completely relieved.

If consciousness is completely lost, sterile intravenous glucose (20–40 ml of a 50% solution) should be given. During the brief recovery that the latter should provide, sugar should be given by mouth. Subcutaneous *glucagon* is another satisfactory treatment.

If there is any doubt about the cause of loss of consciousness in a diabetic, insulin must *never* be given. Insulin can be lethal to a patient in hypoglycaemic coma.

10. Haemorrhage

Although haemorrhage may be occasionally alarming for dentist and patient alike, a major vessel is unlikely to be opened during dental surgery and hence the patient is unlikely to lose any dangerous quantity of blood if promptly dealt with.

The most prolonged bleeding is likely to come from an unsuspected haemophiliac. This can be controlled by giving antihaemophilic factor. It is necessary, therefore, to control the bleeding as well as possible (by means of a pressure pad and supporting the patient's jaw with a firm barrel bandage) and to get the patient admitted to hospital as quickly as possible where antihaemophilic factor can be given.

Continued bleeding due to local causes is much more common and is only an emergency in the sense that the dentist may be woken up at 3 o'clock in the morning to deal with it. The simplest and most effective treatment is to give a local anaesthetic, to tidy up the socket and to suture it.

Once the bleeding has been controlled, the patient (or relatives) can be asked about any bleeding tendencies and particularly if there is any such family history. If the patient has haemophilia, suturing will not stop the bleeding and the patient will have to be admitted to hospital. This is occasionally the way by which previously unsuspected haemophilia is discovered.

When there is persistent bleeding without systemic cause a fibrinolytic inhibitor such as tranexamic acid may be effective. This may be at least partially effective even in the presence of a haemorrhagic defect until definitive treatment becomes available.

SUGGESTED FURTHER READING

Anon 1986 Immediate primary care of a suspected heart attack. Drug and Therapeutics Bulletin 24: 89
Ellis C, Fidler J 1982 Drugs in pregnancy: adverse reactions British Journal of Hospital Medicine 28: 575
Hanashiro P K, Wilson J R 1986 Cardiopulmonary resuscitation: a current perspective. Medical Clinics of North America 70: 729
L'Estrange Orme M 1983 Major drug interactions. Hospital Update 7: 1013
Lipkin D P, Reid C J 1988 Myocardial infarction: the first 24 hours. British Medical Journal 296: 947
McEwan H P 1982 Drugs in pregnancy: prescribing. British Journal of Hospital Medicine 28: 559
Patterson R, Anderson J 1982 Allergic reactions to drugs and biologic agents. Journal of the American Medical Association 248: 2637
Prescott L F 1983 New approaches in managing drug overdosage and poisoning. British Medical Journal 287: 274
VanArsdel P P 1981 Drug allergy, an update. Medical Clinics of North America 65: 1089
Venning G R 1983 Identification of adverse reactions to new drugs. II. How were 18 important adverse reactions discovered and with what delays? British Medical Journal 286: 289

Appendix I:
The antibiotic prophylaxis of infective endocarditis

A Working Party of the British Society for Anti-microbial Chemotherapy made the following recommendations for patients at risk requiring extractions, scaling or periodontal surgery:

A. Patients not requiring a general anaesthetic and no special risks

(i) Patients who are not allergic to the penicillins. Adults – 3 g amoxycillin orally 1 hour before the operation, taken in the presence of the dentist or DSA. For children under 10, half the adult dose; for children under 5, a quarter of the adult dose.

(ii) Patients allergic to penicillin. Adults – 1.5 g erythromycin stearate given orally under supervision 1–2 hours before the dental procedure followed by a second dose of 0.5 g 6 hours later. For children under 10, half the adult dose; for children under 5, a quarter of the adult dose.

Note: High dose (3 g) amoxycillin is now considered to be suitable for patients who have received a penicillin within the previous month.

B. Patients requiring a general anaesthetic but who are not allergic to the penicillins

Amoxycillin 1 g intramuscularly in 2.5 ml of 1% lignocaine before induction plus 0.5 g of amoxycillin orally 6 hours later.
OR oral amoxycillin 3 g, 4 hours before induction and repeated as soon as possible after recovery,
OR oral amoxycillin 3 g plus oral probenecid 1 g, 4 hours before induction.

C. Patients who should be referred to hospital

Special risk patients, who should be referred to hospital, are:

(a) those who have had a previous attack of infective endocarditis (thus indicating susceptibility to the disease), and

(b) patients who are to have a general anaesthetic, but who have a prosthetic heart valve.

It is suggested that special risk patients who are not allergic to the penicillins, should receive: amoxycillin 1 g intramuscularly in 2.5 ml of 1% lignocaine plus gentamicin 120 mg intramuscularly immediately before induction. A further 0.5 mg of amoxycillin should be given orally 6 hours later.

Patients (in any of these subgroups) who are allergic to the penicillins should be given: vancomycin 1 g by slow intravenous infusion over 60 min followed by 120 mg of gentamicin intravenously before induction.

The doses given above are for adults. Half the adult dose should be given to children under 10 and a quarter of the adult dose for children under 5. In the case of vancomycin the dose for children is 20 mg per kg.

Additional measures

1. It was suggested that application of an antiseptic such as 0.5% chlorhexidine to the gingival margins before the dental procedure could reduce the severity of any resulting bacteraemia and may usefully supplement antibiotic prophylaxis in those at risk.

2. The Working Party emphasised the need for regular dental care for the maintenance of optimal dental health in those at risk. Good dental health should reduce the frequency and severity of any bacteraemias and also reduce the need for extractions.

3. More important still is that, even when antibiotic cover has been given, *patients at risk should be instructed to report any unexplained illness*. Infective endocarditis is often exceedingly insidious in origin and can develop 2 or more months after the operation which might have precipitated it. Late diagnosis considerably increases both the mortality or disability among survivors.

4. Patients at risk should carry a warning card to be shown to their dentist at each visit to indicate the danger of infective endocarditis and the need for antibiotic prophylaxis.

Appendix II:
Viral hepatitis B – high-risk groups

1. Sexually promiscuous individuals (especially male homosexuals).*

2. Intravenous drug abusers.*

3. Patients receiving untreated blood products, plasma or blood transfusions repeatedly, such as haemophiliacs.*

4. Patients on haemodialysis.

5. Immunosuppressed or immunodeficient patients, especially transplant patients.

6. Residents and staff of long-stay institutions, especially for the mentally handicapped.

7. Medical and paramedical staff of renal dialysis units.

8. Tattooing, acupuncture or blood transfusion, especially in the Far East.

9. Patients from the Third World, especially Africa and Asia.

10. Certain other disorders, especially Down's syndrome, polyarteritis nodosa.

11. Sexual partners of patients with hepatitis or any of the above groups.

12. Some chronic liver diseases.

---

* These are also high-risk groups for Acquired Immune Deficiency Syndrome (AIDS).

Index